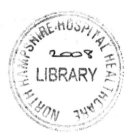
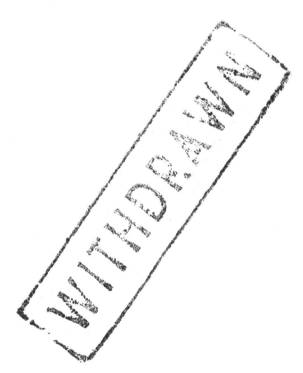

OXFORD MEDICAL PUBLICATIONS

Emergencies in Clinical Surgery

Emergencies in Clinical Surgery

Edited by

Chris Callaghan

Clinical Lecturer in Surgery
University of Cambridge
and Honorary Specialist Registrar
Addenbrooke's Hospital
Cambridge, UK

J. Andrew Bradley

Professor of Surgery
University of Cambridge
and Honorary Consultant Surgeon
Addenbrooke's Hospital
Cambridge, UK
and

Christopher J. E. Watson

Reader in Surgery
University of Cambridge
and Honorary Consultant Surgeon
Addenbrooke's Hospital
Cambridge, UK

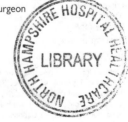

OXFORD
UNIVERSITY PRESS

OXFORD
UNIVERSITY PRESS

Great Clarendon Street, Oxford OX2 6DP

Oxford University Press is a department of the University of Oxford.
It furthers the University's objective of excellence in research, scholarship,
and education by publishing worldwide in

Oxford New York

Auckland Cape Town Dar es Salaam Hong Kong Karachi
Kuala Lumpur Madrid Melbourne Mexico City Nairobi
New Delhi Shanghai Taipei Toronto

With offices in

Argentina Austria Brazil Chile Czech Republic France Greece
Guatemala Hungary Italy Japan Poland Portugal Singapore
South Korea Switzerland Thailand Turkey Ukraine Vietnam

Oxford is a registered trade mark of Oxford University Press
in the UK and in certain other countries

Published in the United States
by Oxford University Press Inc., New York

© Oxford University Press, 2008

British Library Cataloguing in Publication Data
Data available

Library of Congress Cataloging in Publication Data
Oxford handbook of emergencies in clinical surgery / Chris Callaghan ... [et al.].

Typeset by Cepha Imaging Private Ltd., Bangalore, India
Printed in Italy
on acid-free paper by
LegoPrint SpA

ISBN 978–0–19–921901–8

10 9 8 7 6 5 4 3 2 1

Preface

The image of a senior surgeon performing a life-saving operation is often seen on TV or in the movies. But the operation is just one piece in the jigsaw that is emergency surgery. The less glamorous, but equally important jobs of making the diagnosis and optimizing the patient preoperatively are usually left to the juniors. Once the senior surgeon is tucked up in bed, it is the task of the junior staff to recognize the postoperative complication, and to wake the boss with the bad news. But in this era of reduced working hours, junior surgeons are finding that their exposure to surgical emergencies is limited. Changes to night-time working practices also mean that relatively inexperienced doctors may be covering more than one specialty.

We believe that a quick-reference, practical guide to common emergencies in general surgery and related specialties is therefore needed more than ever. *Emergencies in Clinical Surgery* aims to make the life of junior surgeons easier. We have tried to write in an easily accessible, concise style, and the book is in a pocket-sized format that means that readers should be able to refer to it on the ward, or on the way down to the emergency department. Extensive cross-references are used throughout.

The first section deals with approaches to the sick surgical patient, communication, and how to prepare the patient for emergency surgery, endoscopy, and interventional radiology. The 'Problem-based emergency surgery' section is concerned with the assessment and management of trauma emergencies, the acute abdomen, and ward emergencies. Generic postoperative complications are discussed in the ward emergencies chapter. Conditions are cross-referenced to more detailed topics in the 'Disease-based emergency surgery' section. This contains a fuller description of individual diseases with comments on initial and further investigations and management. Specific early complications after surgery, endoscopy, and interventional radiology are also dealt with. As neurosurgery, cardiothoracic surgery, and neonatal paediatric surgery are performed in specialist centres, early postoperative complications for these subspecialties are not covered. The final section describes how to perform common procedures, along with their indications, contraindications, and post-procedure care.

Emergency surgery is constantly evolving and some of the issues covered are controversial. With an eye on future editions, we welcome feedback, both positive and negative. Please send comments via http://www.oup.co.uk.

We believe that emergency surgery is an exciting and challenging branch of medicine. We hope that this book makes it a less stressful one.

Chris Callaghan
J. Andrew Bradley
Christopher J. E. Watson

Contents

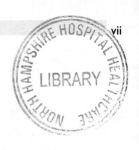

Detailed contents

Part 3 **Disease-based emergency surgery**

16 Orthopaedic surgery   **405**

17 Neurosurgery   **427**

Acknowledgements

We would like to thank the following for their advice and assistance.
- Katherine Brown, Consultant Colorectal Surgeon, Luton and Dunstable Hospital, Luton
- Sarah Cheslyn-Curtis, Consultant HPB and Paediatric Surgeon, Luton and Dunstable Hospital, Luton
- Simon Dwerryhouse, Consultant Upper GI Surgeon, Addenbrooke's Hospital, Cambridge
- Richard Moxon, Consultant Radiologist, Bedford Hospital, Bedford
- Duraisamy Ravichandran, Consultant Breast and Endocrine Surgeon, Luton and Dunstable Hospital, Luton
- David Waine, Specialist Registrar in General and Respiratory Medicine, Heartlands Hospital, Birmingham

Our special thanks go to Raaj Praseedom, Consultant HPB and Transplant Surgeon, Addenbrooke's Hospital, Cambridge.

Contributors

J. Andrew Bradley

Professor of Surgery, University of Cambridge, and Honorary Consultant Surgeon, Addenbrooke's Hospital, Cambridge, UK
Chapters 6, 10, and 11

Chris Callaghan

Clinical Lecturer in Surgery, University of Cambridge, and Honorary Specialist Registrar, Addenbrooke's Hospital, Cambridge, UK
Chapters 1, 2, 3, 5, 8, 12, 14, 19, and 20

Adel Helmy

Academic Clinical Fellow, Department of Neurosurgery, University of Cambridge and Addenbrooke's Hospital, Cambridge, UK
Chapters 3 and 17

Peter J. Hutchinson

Senior Academy Fellow, University of Cambridge and Honorary Consultant Neurosurgeon, Addenbrooke's Hospital, Cambridge, UK
Chapters 3 and 17

Eric Lim

Consultant Thoracic Surgeon, Royal Brompton Hospital, London, UK
Chapters 3, 18, and 20

Nikhil Misra

Specialist Registrar in General Surgery, Peterborough District Hospital, Peterborough, UK
Chapter 7

Shafi Mussa

Specialist Registrar in Cardiothoracic Surgery, Papworth Hospital, Cambridge, UK
Chapters 3, 18, and 20

Dermot O'Riordan

Consultant General Surgeon, West Suffolk Hospital, Bury St Edmunds, UK
Chapter 7

Lee van Rensburg

Consultant Orthopaedic Surgeon, Addenbrooke's Hospital, Cambridge, UK
Chapters 3, 16, and 19

Harbinder Sharma

Consultant Urological Surgeon, Bedford Hospital, Bedford, UK
Chapters 15 and 20

Matthew Wallard

Specialist Registrar in Urology, Ipswich Hospital, Ipswich, UK
Chapters 15 and 20

Christopher Watson

Reader in Surgery, University of Cambridge, and Honorary Consultant Surgeon, Addenbrooke's Hospital, Cambridge, UK
Chapters 4, 9, and 13

Symbols and abbreviations

&#x1F4D5;	cross-reference
&#x2757;	important
▶▶	very important
↑	increased
↓	decreased
↔	normal
>	greater than
<	less than
≥	greater than or equal to
≤	less than or equal to
±	with or without
&#x1F4A3;	controversial
ΔΔ	differential diagnosis
AAA	abdominal aortic aneurysm
AAST	American Association for the Surgery of Trauma
ABG	arterial blood gas
ABPI	ankle-brachial pressure index
ACE	angiotensin converting enzyme
ACS	acute coronary syndrome **or** abdominal compartment syndrome
AF	atrial fibrillation
AICD	automatic internal cardiac defibrillator
ALI	acute lung injury
ALP	alkaline phosphatase
ALT	alanine aminotransferase
AMPLE	allergies, medications, pregnancy/past medical history, last meal/drink, events/environment
AP	anteroposterior **or** acute pancreatitis
APTT	activated partial thromboplastin time
ARDS	acute respiratory distress syndrome
AST	aspartate aminotransferase
ATLS®	Advanced Trauma Life Support
AVN	avascular necrosis
AVPU	alert, responds to voice, responds to pain, unresponsive

AXR	abdominal X-ray
bd	twice a day
BMI	body mass index
BNF	British National Formulary
BP	blood pressure
bpm	beats per minute
Ca	calcium
CABG	coronary artery bypass grafts
CBD	common bile duct
CBG	capillary blood glucose
CCF	congestive cardiac failure
CCK	cholecystokinin
CCrISP™	Care of the Critically Ill Surgical Patient
CCU	coronary care unit
CHD	common hepatic duct
CHF	congestive heart failure
CK	creatine kinase
CLO	Campylobacter-like organism
CO_2	carbon dioxide
COPD	chronic obstructive pulmonary disease
CPAP	continuous positive airways pressure
CPP	cerebral perfusion pressure
CPR	cardiopulmonary resuscitation
CRP	C-reactive protein
CSF	cerebrospinal fluid
CSU	catheter specimen of urine
CT	computed tomography
CTPA	CT pulmonary angiogram
CTU	CT urogram
CVP	central venous pressure
CXR	chest X-ray
DDAVP®	1-desamino-8-D-arginine vasopressin
DIC	disseminated intravascular coagulation
DKA	diabetic ketoacidosis
DPL	diagnostic peritoneal lavage
DRE	digital rectal examination
DVT	deep venous thrombosis
ECG	electrocardiogram
EDH	extradural haemorrhage
ERCP	endoscopic retrograde cholangiopancreatography

EUA	examination under anaesthesia
FAST	focused abdominal sonography for trauma
FBC	full blood count
FDPs	fibrinogen degradation products
FES	fat embolism syndrome
FFP	fresh frozen plasma
FiO_2	inspired oxygen fraction
FV	femoral vein
G&S	group and save
GA	general anaesthesia
GB	gall bladder
GCS	Glasgow Coma Scale or Score
GFR	glomerular filtration rate
GGT	gamma-glutamyltranspeptidase
GI	gastrointestinal
GOO	gastric outlet obstruction
GORD	gastro-oesophageal reflux disease
GTN	glyceryl trinitrate
h	hour(s)
Hb	haemoglobin
hCG	human chorionic gonadotropin
H_2O	water
HCO_3^-	bicarbonate
HDU	high dependency unit
HELLP	haemolysis, elevated liver enzymes, low platelet count
HIV	human immunodeficiency virus
HR	heart rate
HRT	hormone replacement therapy
IAH	intraabdominal hypertension
IAP	intraabdominal pressure
IBD	inflammatory bowel disease
ICP	intracranial pressure
ICS	intercostal space
IDDM	insulin-dependent diabetes mellitus
IHD	ischaemic heart disease
IJV	internal jugular vein
IM	intramuscular
IMA	inferior mesenteric artery
INR	international normalized ratio
ITU	intensive therapy unit

IV	intravenous
IVC	inferior vena cava
IVU	intravenous urogram
JVP	jugular venous pressure
K	potassium
KUB	kidneys, ureters, bladder
LA	local anaesthesia
LBBB	left bundle branch block
LDH	lactate dehydrogenase
LFTs	liver function tests
LIF	left iliac fossa
LMP	last menstrual period
LMWH	low molecular weight heparin
LSV	long saphenous vein
LUQ	left upper quadrant
LV	left ventricle
LVF	left ventricular failure
LVH	left ventricular hypertrophy
M, C, & S	microscopy, culture, and sensitivities
MABP	mean arterial blood pressure
Mg	magnesium
MI	myocardial infarction
min	minute
MRC	Medical Research Council
MRCP	magnetic resonance cholangiopancreatography
MRI	magnetic resonance imaging
MRSA	methicillin-resistant *Staphylococcus aureus*
MSU	midstream urine
Na	sodium
NAI	non-accidental injury
NBM	nil by mouth
NG	nasogastric
NJ	nasojejunal
NSAID	nonsteroidal anti-inflammatory drug
NSTEMI	non-ST elevation myocardial infarction
NSTI	necrotizing soft tissue infection
O_2	oxygen
od	once a day
OGD	oesophagogastroduodenoscopy
OPSI	overwhelming post-splenectomy infection

$PaCO_2$	arterial partial pressure of CO_2
PaO_2	arterial partial pressure of O_2
PCA	patient-controlled analgesia
PCD	phlegmasia caerulea dolens
PCNL	percutaneous nephrolithotomy
PE	pulmonary embolism
PEA	pulseless electrical activity
PEFR	peak expiratory flow rate
PO	orally, by mouth
PPI	proton pump inhibitor
PPM	permanent pacemaker
PR	per rectum
prn	as required
PSA	prostate-specific antigen
PT	prothrombin time
PTC	percutaneous transhepatic cholangiography
PU	peptic ulcer
PUD	peptic ulcer disease
PVD	peripheral vascular disease
qds	four times a day
RBCs	red blood cells
RIF	right iliac fossa
RR	respiratory rate
RUQ	right upper quadrant
s	second(s)
SAH	subarachnoid haemorrhage
SaO_2	arterial oxygen saturation
SC	subcutaneous
SDH	subdural haemorrhage
SIRS	systemic inflammatory response syndrome
SMA	superior mesenteric artery
SMV	superior mesenteric vein
SOAP	subjective, objective, assessment, plan
SOB	shortness of breath
SPC	suprapubic catheter
STEMI	ST-elevation myocardial infarction
SV	subclavian vein
TB	tuberculosis
tds	three times a day
TIPSS	transjugular intrahepatic portosystemic shunt

TPN	total parenteral nutrition
TURP	transurethral resection of the prostate
U&Es	urea and electrolytes (and creatinine)
UC	ulcerative colitis
UK	United Kingdom
USS	ultrasound scan
UTI	urinary tract infection
VF	ventricular fibrillation
V/Q	ventilation/perfusion
VT	ventricular tachycardia
VTE	venous thromboembolism
WBC	white blood cell
WCC	white cell count

Part 1

Emergency surgery—the basics

Introduction

Approaches to the emergency surgical patient

The 'three speeds'

Ask a medical student what they would do in almost any clinical situation, and most of them will reply 'I would take a full history, and then perform a thorough examination'. This mantra is drummed into all of us at medical school, and for most patients it is entirely suitable. Unfortunately, this approach is, at best, inefficient and, at worst, dangerous when dealing with the sickest surgical patients.

❶ Acutely unwell surgical patients have life- or limb-threatening diseases, the immediate management of which can often be initiated without the requirement for detailed history-taking.

The spinal reflex of 'history and then examination' must therefore be modified, and the approach to the surgical patient tailored appropriately. Emergency surgical patients can be approached in one of three ways (Fig. 1.1).

The emergency trauma patient in resus (ATLS® approach, 📖 p.42)

This approach is best used for patients suffering from trauma with life- or limb-threatening injuries. The priority is to identify these injuries by examining the systems likely to cause death most rapidly. Airway problems kill before breathing problems, which kill before circulatory problems, etc. Once a life-threatening injury is identified **it must be treated successfully** before moving on to the next step in the algorithm.

In clinical practice, these patients are usually assessed by the trauma team, and each member of the team can be assigned a role (e.g. breathing or circulation), allowing assessment and treatment to occur in parallel, rather than in series. Note that a limited history is only taken in the secondary survey.

The sick HDU/ward patient (CCrISP™ approach, 📖 p.132)

Patients who have had, or who are about to have, major surgery are at risk of developing significant complications, including shock, sepsis, and hypoxia. These problems require immediate management, as above, but clues to the underlying diagnosis often reside in the patient's notes and bedside charts. After identification and treatment of life-threatening airway, breathing, and circulatory problems, sit down and review their charts, notes, and lab results before returning to take a focused history and examination. Decide if the patient is stable or unstable: stable patients require a thorough daily management plan while unstable patients require definitive investigations and management, including the consideration of returning to theatre. This approach is taught in the Royal College of Surgeons of England CCrISP™ course.

The well HDU/ward patient (SOAP approach)

Most patients you see on the ward or in HDU can be assessed in this way. A focused **subjective** history leads on to an **objective** examination of the operation site and related systems, with concurrent review of the observation charts, fluid balance sheet, drug chart, and relevant lab results. Make it a habit to make an **assessment** (diagnosis) with each patient—an entry in the notes stating 'Day 2 post-anterior resection, clinically improving' gives more information to night staff who have never seen your patient before than just 'Plan: continue'. Stand back and look at the patient—for each tube going into or coming out of your patient, there should be a **plan**, e.g.

- epidural, remove tomorrow;
- catheter, leave until epidural out, and mobile;
- pelvic drain, out today;
- intravenous fluids, continue until oral intake improves;
- nasal cannula, continue until O_2 sats > 94% on air.

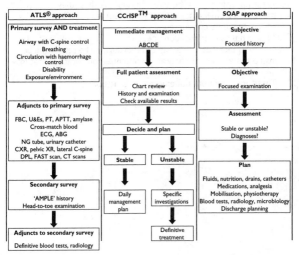

Fig. 1.1 Emergency surgical patients can be approached in one of three ways, depending on the clinical circumstances. (The CCrISP™ flow chart is adapted with permission, from Anderson, I.D. (ed.) (1999). *Care of the critically ill surgical patient*, p. 8. Arnold, London.)

Assessing the patient

Of course, with all of these algorithms, you must first be able to recognize which patients are sick. The unconscious, hypotensive, multiply injured patient brought to the emergency department after a high-speed road traffic accident should be recognizable as 'sick' by all. What is more difficult to spot is the slowly deteriorating postoperative patient who doesn't seem 'quite right'. Physiological scoring systems such as the Modified Early Warning Score (MEWS) may be used to prompt nurses to call the surgical and/or ITU teams, but these systems shouldn't replace clinical judgement and common sense.

Assess the patient, initiate basic treatment, and review them in no more than a few hours' time. If they're not better, call your senior for help.

- ❶ An abnormal respiratory rate is the single best clinical predictor of physiological deterioration.
- ❶ When in doubt over which approach is appropriate, use an algorithm 'higher' up the hierarchy than you suspect might be necessary.

In order to help the reader to distinguish between true emergencies that require immediate assessment and management, and those that are less urgent, this book uses four icons.

- ☺ A true emergency. These need to be dealt with in the first 1–2min and then a consultant should be called. These emergencies should be memorized.
- ☺ These patients need to be assessed very quickly as they can rapidly shift into the emergency category if not sorted soon. Senior help/ advice should be considered.
- ① Although these patients don't need to be seen straight away, they must be assessed quickly and thoroughly. The reader will be instructed to think carefully about potential complications that may develop.
- ② These are urgent but not emergency conditions.

Communication

As a junior doctor on-call you are the centre of the communication web. Managing emergency patients requires you to communicate **clearly** and **effectively** with patients, their relatives, colleagues, ward, theatre and technical staff, and, finally, your boss. With experience you will become a better communicator, but some common-sense basics are given below.

- Patients who are in pain, anxious, intoxicated, or sedated are difficult to communicate with. Despite this, you should tell them what is happening and why, even if you're unsure if they can hear or understand you. Reducing their anxiety will decrease their pain, sympathetic response, and cardiorespiratory stress.
- Patients' relatives should be kept informed. Make sure a quiet, clean, well-lit room is available and bring a nurse with you. Make sure that they are sitting comfortably and that you introduce yourself. Be honest, and don't be afraid to admit that you don't know the answer. Document these discussions in the notes and record who is present.
- Communication with ancillary, theatre, and laboratory staff can be stressful as they may not appear to appreciate the urgency of the situation. This is usually because no-one has told them. Let them know the clinical scenario, and within what timescale you would like their assistance.
- Hand over personally to the nurse responsible for your patient and give them clear information on what has happened, the management plan, and any target physiological values. Don't expect them to have read your notes—do you read theirs?

❶ Above all keep calm, treat everyone with respect and courtesy, and think how you would feel if you were in their shoes.

When to call the boss (and what to say)

Seniors need to be kept informed and should not be left to discover sick, poorly managed patients on the morning ward round. The essential question you must ask yourself is 'Can I confidently and competently manage this patient safely until my boss reviews them routinely?'. If you have doubts, call them. The phone is your friend.

If you do need to call your boss you **must** be appropriately prepared. Stop and think.

- What do you want from your boss—advice, urgent assessment, or their presence in theatre? Tell them clearly what you are asking of them at the beginning of the phone call. If it's early in the morning, give them time to wake up.
- Do you have **all** the information you need: patient details, history and examination findings, blood results, X-rays? Are drug charts, fluid balance charts, and case-notes nearby in case you need to refer to them?
- What are your working diagnosis and differential diagnoses? What is your plan? Seniors appreciate being called by juniors who have clearly thought about the options.
- Are you in an appropriate frame of mind or environment to make an important phone call? Calm down, sit down, and close the door.

If you're working with a senior with whom you're not familiar, contact them early during your on-call to introduce yourself. Ask them if they would prefer to be called at a certain time to discuss all new patients, or if they are happy to be called as you see fit. Ask colleagues who have worked with them previously what their management preferences are.

There are a few situations where the on-call consultant should be called immediately. These include if a patient:
• dies unexpectedly;
• requires emergency ITU/HDU admission or assessment;
• has a postoperative complication that requires a return to theatre;
• requires emergency assessment/treatment from another consultant;
• may require major emergency surgery.

Documentation
Once the emergency patient has been assessed and stabilized, make a legible, concise, but fully informative entry in the case-notes as a priority. This is especially important in patients requiring transfer to another hospital or team. Your documentation must include:
• your signature, name (in capitals), grade, bleep number, and specialty;
• the time (use the 24h clock) and date;
• the name of your on-call consultant;
• where you are assessing the patient, e.g. HDU, emergency department.

❶ Don't forget that emergency patients are often the focus of subsequent morbidity and mortality audits or medicolegal actions. Accurate documentation is essential.

Teamwork
As you become more senior you will be expected to co-ordinate your juniors. This can be your most challenging task.
• Find out at the start of your on-call period whom you will be working with and what their fixed commitments are during the day. If you haven't worked with them before, let them know when you want to be called and what you expect of them.
• Get to know your juniors, and enjoy their company. Understand that they will know more than you about some things. Find out what.
• Offer to help them out if you're quiet. They'll appreciate it, and you'll feel less guilty about asking them to do the boring jobs.
• With modern shifts, handovers are becoming more frequent. Smooth handover is a priority—meet with the rest of your team 20–30min before you start handover to prepare appropriately.
• Foster a feeling of teamwork and mutual respect. You won't enjoy your job without it. This is hard to do. For tips, watch a consultant you admire on their ward round. What do they do to make the team productive and happy? Emulate them.

Preparing the patient for surgery

Preoperative assessment

Before a patient requiring emergency surgery arrives in theatre, they have travelled along a complex assessment and management pathway. Steps along this pathway include:
- formulation of a working diagnosis;
- assessment of co-morbidity and pre-morbid functioning;
- confirmation that emergency surgery is appropriate;
- consideration of the timing of emergency surgery;
- preoperative optimization;
- arrangement of theatre;
- consent and marking;
- anaesthetic assessment.

The correct performance of each of these steps is crucial if the surgery is to be successful and if morbidity and mortality are to be minimized. Senior surgical, anaesthetic, and medical colleagues are often involved. Anaesthetic assessment is performed by the on-call anaesthetist.

Formulation of a working diagnosis

History-taking, examination, and investigations lead to a working diagnosis. In emergency situations this stepwise process is altered (📖 p.4). Understanding that emergency surgery is needed is usually more important than making an exact diagnosis (📖 p.102).

Assessment of co-morbidities and pre-morbid functioning

Many emergency surgical patients are fit and well and do not require extensive assessment before surgery. However, it is essential that a past medical history is taken, focusing on cardiorespiratory disease, as well as past surgical and anaesthetic history and history of allergies. In elderly patients it is particularly important to assess pre-morbid functioning. This process may uncover issues that raise questions about:
- whether it is appropriate to offer emergency surgery;
- whether discussion with on-call physicians is required;
- the grade of surgeon and anaesthetist required;
- the need for preoperative admission to ITU/HDU for optimization;
- the anaesthetic technique used, e.g. spinal versus GA;
- the type of surgery performed;
- the requirement for postoperative ITU/HDU care.

On history-taking include the following.
- Check for a history or symptoms consistent with MI, dysrhythmias, angina, heart failure, diabetes, peripheral vascular disease, stroke, smoking, alcoholism, COPD.
- Ask about mobility and exercise tolerance.
  - Can they walk outside and do they need a frame or stick to do so?
  - How far can they walk and what stops them?
  - Can they walk up a flight of stairs unaided?

On examination:
- look specifically for signs of heart failure and COPD.

Old notes are invaluable. Check for:
- recent outpatient letters;
- results of recent investigations, especially echocardiograms, lung function tests, and serum creatinine;
- old operation notes.

Although most investigations are ordered to assist in diagnosing the current surgical problem, other investigations may be necessary to help assess fitness for emergency surgery (Box 2.1).

> **Box 2.1. General indications for emergency preoperative investigations to assess fitness***
>
> - FBC: males > 50 years; all females of child-bearing age; symptoms or signs of anaemia; sepsis; major surgery expected.
> - U&Es: age > 50 years; history of diuretic use; symptoms or signs of dehydration; sepsis; major surgery expected.
> - LFTs: history of chronic liver disease or alcoholism.
> - PT/INR, APTT: sepsis; warfarin use; active bleeding; history of chronic liver disease.
> - Venous blood glucose: if CBG > 10mmol/L; diabetics.
> - ABG: sepsis; SaO_2 < 95% on pulse oximetry; history of significant respiratory disease; tachypnoea.
> - CXR: possibility of malignancy or TB; history of cardiorespiratory disease; symptoms or signs of cardiorespiratory disease.
> - ECG: males > 50 years; females > 60 years; history of cardiorespiratory disease; tachycardia or bradycardia on examination.
> - Urine pregnancy test: all females of child-bearing age.
> - Sickle cell test: Afro-Caribbean patients with unknown sickle status. Request Hb electrophoresis if positive.
>
> * See also local guidelines.

These assessments enable an estimate of the morbidity and mortality of emergency surgery and anaesthesia to be made.

Is emergency surgery appropriate?
In the majority of patients with conditions requiring emergency surgery it is obvious that surgery is appropriate, i.e. the benefits outweigh the risks. However, some groups of patients are unlikely to survive major emergency surgery. Those who do survive may require months in hospital and are unlikely to be able to regain their previous level of functioning. In the following patient groups, the utility of surgery should be considered carefully:
- those with multiple significant co-morbidities associated with poor pre-morbid functioning;
- those with pre-existing malignancy with a poor prognosis;
- those with advanced disease that is unlikely to be helped by surgery.

❶ These decisions can be difficult and must be made by experienced surgeons on a case-by-case basis after discussion with the patient and their family. Assessment by senior anaesthetists and/or physicians to assist in estimating prognosis is often invaluable.

❶ Even though surgery may be deemed appropriate by the anaesthetic and surgical teams, the patient may decline consent when the expected mortality and morbidity are communicated.

Timing of surgery

In situations where life or limbs are not threatened, surgery under GA or regional anaesthesia (e.g. spinal) takes place once the patient has been NBM for a suitable period of time (see Box 2.2) and a space on the emergency theatre list is available. When the clinical urgency of the situation precludes a delay, anaesthesia can take place regardless of the fasting period, but with a significantly higher risk of aspiration. In some situations (e.g. bowel obstruction, peritonitis), the stomach is unable to empty.

Reasons for delaying emergency surgery beyond the required starvation time and the wait for theatre availability include:
* preoperative resuscitation and optimization (📖 p.16);
* availability of anaesthetic and/or surgical expertise;
* availability of beds on HDU/ITU.

❶ A decision to delay emergency surgery is usually made after discussion between senior surgeons and anaesthetists. Reasons should be carefully documented in the notes and the patient and family kept informed.

Box 2.2 Approximate NBM times before surgery

* After food or opaque fluids (e.g. tea/coffee with milk): 6–8h
* After clear fluids: 2–4h

❶ These times are approximate, as emergency surgical patients have delayed gastric emptying due to pain and opioid use. If in doubt, discuss with the on-call anaesthetist.

Preoperative optimization: introduction

Abnormalities in fluid balance, electrolytes, metabolism, and coagulation are common in patients requiring emergency surgery. General (or regional) anaesthesia and subsequent surgery under these circumstances carry significant risk. As part of the surgical on-call team one of your tasks is to return the patient's physiological state to as near normal as possible before surgery. Patients with multiple co-morbidities, especially cardiorespiratory disease, may benefit from admission to HDU or ITU preoperatively. Intensive monitoring and insertion of a central venous line, arterial line, and urinary catheter enables optimization of oxygenation and fluid and electrolyte abnormalities. Discuss with senior surgical and anaesthetic colleagues.

❶ Close liaison between the on-call surgical, anaesthetic, and medical teams is necessary.

Preoperative fluid management

- The majority of preoperative surgical patients are dehydrated to some degree and require fluid resuscitation with crystalloids (e.g. normal saline or Hartmann's).
  - ❶ Dextrose 5% is not an adequate resuscitation fluid due to the rapid movement of H_2O into the intracellular space, as opposed to confining itself to the extracellular space.
- Patients with haemorrhagic shock can be temporarily resuscitated with either crystalloids or colloids, but will eventually need blood products and intervention (surgical, endoscopic, or radiological) to stop the bleeding.
- Patients with presumed good LV function (e.g. patients < 60 years old with good exercise tolerance and no history or signs of cardiorespiratory disease, and those with good LV function on recent echocardiogram) can be aggressively resuscitated with a 20mL/kg fluid bolus if hypotensive (or 10mL/kg bolus if not).
  - If shock, sepsis, or significant dehydration are present, insert a urinary catheter to guide resuscitation and aim for > 0.5mL/kg/h urine output.
  - Further 10–20mL/kg fluid boluses may be needed.
- Patients with cardiac failure or significant cardiorespiratory disease require regular monitoring during fluid resuscitation with a 5mL/kg bolus.
  - Insert a urinary catheter to guide resuscitation (0.5mL/kg/h may be acceptable urine output).
  - Review clinically every 1–2h looking for fluid overload.
  - Central venous line ± arterial line insertion may be necessary to monitor CVP and BP. Central line insertion is often easier when some fluids have already been given peripherally.
- Fluid overload may sometimes be apparent at presentation, usually due to cardiac failure. Fluid restrict, treat with IV diuretics (e.g. furosemide 40mg), and discuss with the on-call physicians. Exclude liver or renal disease as a cause for fluid retention. These patients have high perioperative mortality.

Preoperative electrolyte correction

Before starting treatment for abnormal electrolytes, always check that the sample was not haemolysed or taken from a drip arm.

Potassium

❶ Correction of hypo- or hyperkalaemia is essential before anaesthesia to avoid intraoperative dysrhythmias.

Hypokalaemia

- Mild hypokalaemia (2.5–3.5mmol/L) can be corrected by adding 20–40mmol of potassium chloride to each litre of IV fluids at a maximum rate of 10mmol/h. KCl irritates peripheral veins. Don't replace K^+ aggressively if the urine output is poor.
- Severe hypokalaemia (< 2.5mmol/L) or those with fluid overload may require concentrated potassium chloride (40mmol in 100mL of NS) to be given via a central venous line over 2h.
  - ❶ This requires cardiac monitoring in CCU/HDU/ITU as excessive K^+ causes cardiac arrest.

Hyperkalaemia

- ❶ Early identification and rapid treatment of hyperkalaemia is essential, as severe hyperkalaemia can lead to cardiac dysrhythmias and eventually cardiac arrest. Hyperkalaemia usually indicates severe physiological dysfunction and is associated with high perioperative mortality. Inform the on-call anaesthetist. Pre- or postoperative ITU is often required.
- ❶ Always request an emergency ECG. If ECG changes consistent with hyperkalaemia are present (i.e. first-degree heart block, flattened P waves, tall T waves, ST segment depression, widened QRS > 0.12s, dysrhythmias), then give 10mL of 10% calcium gluconate slowly IV to stabilize the myocardial cell membrane. Calcium gluconate does **not** lower serum potassium.
- Mild hyperkalaemia (5.5–6mmol/L): rehydrate with IV fluids to promote urinary K^+ excretion and give nebulized salbutamol 5mg qds.
- Moderate hyperkalaemia (6.1–6.5mmol/L): treat as above + give 5–10 units of short-acting insulin (e.g. Actrapid®) in 50mL of 50% dextrose IV over 30min. CBG must be monitored at least hourly.
- Severe hyperkalaemia (> 6.5mmol/L): treat as above + urgent discussion with an intensivist to consider haemodialysis or haemofiltration.
- Treatment of the underlying cause is essential for all severities of hyperkalaemia, i.e. stop K^+ infusions, oral K^+ supplements, and drugs that cause ↑ K^+ (e.g. ACE inhibitors, angiotensin II receptor blockers, K^+-sparing diuretics, NSAIDs). Treat renal dysfunction, metabolic acidosis, rhabdomyolysis, and haemolysis.
- ❶ Monitor response to treatment with at least twice-daily U&Es, more regularly in those with moderate or severe hyperkalaemia.
- ❶ If significant renal dysfunction is present with any degree of hyperkalaemia, or if hyperkalaemia is refractory to treatment, discussion with a nephrologist or intensivist is recommended to consider haemodialysis or haemofiltration
- ❶ IV furosemide lowers serum K+ but should be used sparingly in emergency surgery patients who are not fluid overloaded, due to

the risks of dehydration. Polystyrene sulphonate resins (e.g. calcium Resonium®) bind potassium in the gut, but need to be given orally or as an enema, and should therefore be avoided in preoperative patients.

Sodium

There is rarely enough time to fully correct significant sodium abnormalities preoperatively.

Hyponatraemia

- Hyponatraemia is often due to GI losses in preoperative surgical patients. Replace losses with normal saline. Avoid hypertonic saline.
- Postoperative hyponatraemia is usually due to excess water (dextrose)—usually best managed by fluid restriction to 1L/24h.
- ❶ Serum Na^+ should not rise by > 20mmol/L/day in acute hyponatraemia due to the risk of central pontine myelinosis.

Hypernatraemia

- Significant hypernatraemia (> 150mmol/L) is rare in surgical patients. Seek advice.
- Check serum Na^+ at least daily.

Preoperative oxygenation

- Correct hypoxia ($SaO_2 < 95\%$) with supplemental O_2. First perform ABG analysis while the patient is breathing room air.
- Use nasal cannulae if < 3L/min required, or a face-mask if more is necessary to maintain O_2 sats > 94%.
- In those with COPD, re-check ABGs regularly to ensure that CO_2 retention does not occur. If $PaCO_2$ is rising, reduce the O_2 flow and re-check. Discuss with the on-call anaesthetists and physicians if PaO_2 remains poor.

Preoperative correction of haematological abnormalities

Anaemia

- In patients with chronic anaemia and Hb < 8g/dL, first send blood for serum B_{12}, folate, and iron studies before transfusing to Hb of 10g/dL with packed RBCs.
  - One unit of packed RBCs increases Hb by ~ 1g/dL. Give each unit over 2–3h.
  - IV furosemide is not needed unless a history of cardiac failure is present.
- In actively bleeding patients with Hb < 10g/dL, give packed RBCs stat.

❶ In unstable patients do not delay theatre while waiting to correct Hb. Surgery stops bleeding.

Thrombocytopenia

Patients with platelets < 100 x 10^9/L and those with known platelet disorders should be discussed with the on-call haematologist to discuss platelet transfusion and other treatments. Aim for platelets > 50 x 10^9/L in those undergoing surgery.

Coagulopathy

- Coagulopathy is commonly due to warfarin or liver disease. Both prolong PT/INR. Stop warfarin.
- Patients with INR > 1.4 may require FFP for surgery.
  - FFP is given at 10–15mL/kg, and each bag contains 300–350mL.
  - FFP has a duration of action of 6–12h.
  - Give each bag stat if the patient is actively bleeding, or over 1–2h each if not (and time is available).
  - Re-check INR before surgery to ensure INR < 1.5.
  - Also give vitamin K 1mg by slow IV injection if INR > 2.5. Give 10mg if subsequent warfarinization is not needed. Vitamin K takes 12–24h to have an effect.
  - In patients on warfarin with life- or limb-threatening haemorrhage, other concentrated clotting factors may be indicated. Discuss with the on-call haematologist.
- Patients requiring surgery who are on IV infusions of unfractionated heparin should have the infusion stopped at least 6h before surgery. Check that the APTT ratio is < 1.3 before theatre.
  - If patients are actively bleeding, stop the infusion and discuss with the on-call haematologist about giving protamine IV.
- Patients on high-dose LMWH therapy should have their treatment stopped or reduced to prophylactic doses if surgery is expected within 24h.
  - Those who are actively bleeding or require surgery within 24h need to be discussed with the on-call haematologist. The action of LMWH can only be partially reversed by protamine.
- If DIC is suspected (↓ platelets, ↑ PT/INR, ↑ APTT, ↓ fibrinogen, ↑ FDPs), identify and treat the underlying cause and discuss with the on-call haematologist.

- Likewise, those with congenital coagulation disorders (e.g. haemophilia A and B, von Willebrand's disease), should be discussed with the on-call haematologist.
- Uraemic patients (those on dialysis) have platelets that function poorly. Discuss the use of desmopressin (e.g. DDAVP®) with the on-call haematologist. Desmopressin raises plasma von Willebrand factor levels.
- Hypothermia impairs platelet function and the coagulation cascade, and causes fibrinolysis. These abnormalities are not detected in the laboratory, where tests are run at 37°C. Actively warm patients who are hypothermic (≤ 35°C) with hot air blankets (e.g. Bair Hugger™).

Preoperative optimization of chronic medical conditions

Chronic medical conditions are unlikely to improve significantly in the short time available before major emergency surgery. In general, the priorities are to liaise closely with anaesthetic colleagues and to recognize medical emergencies.

Diabetes

- Maintenance of tight glycaemic control perioperatively reduces postoperative morbidity. These benefits must be balanced against the risk of unrecognized hypoglycaemia in the sedated postoperative patient.
- Before major emergency surgery, start an insulin IV infusion ('sliding scale') on patients with IDDM or tablet-controlled diabetes 6–8h preoperatively (see Box 2.3). Stop long-acting insulin and long-acting oral hypoglycaemics the night before, if possible.
- Patients with diet-controlled diabetes do not require an insulin sliding scale unless CBG > 15mmol/L.
- ❶ Diabetic ketoacidosis (CBG > 20mmol/L with pH < 7.2 or HCO_3^- < 15mmol/L) is a medical emergency. Discuss with the on-call physician immediately.

❶ Most hospitals have their own protocols and insulin sliding scale proformas.

Box 2.3 An IV insulin infusion regimen

- Give 1000mL 5% dextrose + 20mmol KCl 10-hourly. Reduce rate if risk of fluid overload.
- Add 50U of short-acting soluble insulin (e.g. Actrapid®) to 50mL of normal saline and run according to the blood glucose via a syringe driver. Measure CBG 2–4-hourly.
  - CBG < 5mmol/L: 0mL/h
  - CBG 5.1–10mmol/L: 1mL/h
  - CBG 10.1–15mmol/L: 2mL/h
  - CBG 15.1–22mmol/L: 4mL/h
  - CBG > 22mmol/L: 5mL/h

❶ The regimen may need to be altered if CBG is consistently > 10mmol/L or < 5mmol/L.

Atrial fibrillation Ventricular rates > 100/min may require IV digoxin or amiodarone. Discuss with the on-call anaesthetist or physician.

▶▶ If rate > 200/min, systolic BP < 90mmHg, chest pain, or presence of pulmonary oedema, give high-flow O_2, get IV access, and seek emergency medical help. Cardioversion may be needed (📖 p.158).

Ischaemic heart disease

- Patients with stable angina require careful analgesia, fluid balance, and electrolyte management.

- Those with recent worsening angina or angina at rest are at high risk of perioperative myocardial ischaemia and death. Discuss with the on-call anaesthetist and physician regarding admission to ITU/HDU for optimization.

Hypertension

Systolic BP > 200mmHg or diastolic > 100mmHg may require emergency preoperative treatment, especially if associated with symptoms, e.g. headache, LVF. Exclude urinary retention, pain, and fluid overload first, and then discuss with the on-call anaesthetist.

Congestive heart failure/left ventricular failure

- If aggressive IV fluid resuscitation is needed, invasive monitoring (urinary catheter, central venous line, arterial line) is required. Consider admission to ITU/HDU for optimization.
- Emergency echocardiography may be useful to determine LV function and guide fluid resuscitation.

Chronic obstructive pulmonary disease

- Prescribe qds nebulized bronchodilators (e.g. salbutamol 2.5mg and ipratropium 250mcg).
- For those with a productive cough, emergency chest physiotherapy may be beneficial.
- Check ABGs regularly to exclude CO_2 retention and alter FiO_2 accordingly.

Preoperative thromboembolism prophylaxis

- Prevention of postoperative venous thromboembolic disease requires a risk assessment to be performed (see Box 2.4). Check local protocols.
- Contraindications to LMWH include active bleeding, suspected haemorrhagic stroke, abnormal baseline PT/INR and APTT, and previous adverse reaction to heparin. Prescribe graduated compression stockings instead.
- Contraindications to compression stockings include peripheral vascular disease and diabetic neuropathy.
- Intermittent pneumatic compression devices may be used in theatre and, increasingly, on the wards.
- LMWH should not be given less than 12h before surgery as this may preclude epidural/spinal anaesthesia. Check with the on-call anaesthetist about the planned route of anaesthesia.

Thromboembolism prophylaxis in patients on warfarin

- Mechanical aortic valve replacement, DVT/PE more than 3 months ago, AF and no history of stroke (or AF and stroke more than 3 months ago):
  - Reverse warfarin and give 1mg vitamin K IV if needed (📖 p.22).
  - Start high-dose prophylactic LMWH (e.g. 40mg enoxaparin SC od) with compression stockings, calf pump, and early mobilization.
  - Re-start warfarin after surgery when safe to do so, and stop LMWH when INR > 2.
- DVT/PE within 3 months, recurrent DVT/PE while on warfarin, AF with arterial embolism, AF with stroke within 3 months, AF with recurrent stroke on warfarin, mechanical mitral valve replacement:
  - Reverse warfarin and give 1mg vitamin K IV if needed (📖 p.22).
  - Start an IV unfractionated heparin infusion (📖 p.334), aiming for APTT ratio 1.5–2.5, with compression stockings, calf pump, and early mobilization.
  - Re-start warfarin after surgery when safe to do so, and stop the heparin infusion when INR > 2.

Box 2.4 Thrombosis risk assessment and prophylaxis

Strong risk factors (score 3)
- Major orthopaedic surgery or trauma
- Major pelvic or abdominal surgery
- Expected confinement to bed > 72h
- Past history of DVT/PE
- Major active medical illness
- MI within 3 months
- Known thrombophilia

Moderate risk factors (score 2)
- Post-thrombotic syndrome, phlebitis, venous ulcers
- Malignancy

Weak risk factors (score 1)
- Pregnant or within 6 weeks of delivery
- HRT or combined oral contraceptive pill within 4 weeks of surgery
- Age > 60 years
- BMI > 30kg/m^2
- Lower limb paralysis
- Family history of DVT/PE
- Major surgery within previous 6 months

Prophylaxis
- Total score 0: early mobilization and thigh-length graduated compression stockings only.
- Total score 1–3: standard prophylaxis dose LMWH* (e.g. enoxaparin 20mg od SC) with thigh-length graduated compression stockings. Mobilize early.
- Total score > 3: high prophylaxis dose LMWH (e.g. enoxaparin 40mg od SC) with thigh-length graduated compression stockings. Mobilize early.

* Patients with significant renal impairment accumulate LMWH and are at risk of bleeding complications postoperatively. Consider dose reduction or check factor Xa levels.

Other preoperative optimization considerations

Group and save and cross-matching

- All patients undergoing major emergency surgery should have at least a valid G&S. A full cross-match can be performed within 30min in an emergency. After transfusion, the original G&S remains valid for 72h. After this time another G&S needs to be sent.
- Packed RBCs need to be available for emergency vascular surgery, surgery for trauma, surgery on those actively bleeding, surgery on those with Hb < 10g/dL. If unused, the units are available for 24h before being re-allocated.
- See individual chapters for recommendations and follow local maximum blood ordering schedules.

❶ Inform the anaesthetist and operating surgeon whether packed RBCs have been cross-matched.

Bowel preparation

Oral bowel preparation is contraindicated for emergency abdominal surgery.

Gastric distension

Patients with frequent vomiting, those with suspected bowel obstruction, and patients with gastric distension on X-ray or CT require NG tube placement (📖 p.498).

Nutrition

Patients with pre-existing malnutrition are at high risk of postoperative complications and intraoperative placement of an NG/NJ feeding tube, feeding jejunostomy, or a central venous line for TPN should be considered.

Current medications

- With few exceptions (e.g. warfarin), continue all medications, including on the morning of surgery. This applies particularly to cardiac medications. Give with a sip of water more than 2h preoperatively.
- Patients on long-term therapy of ≥ 5mg of prednisolone (or equivalent) per day require replacement with IV hydrocortisone.
  - Prescribe 25–50mg hydrocortisone IV to be given at induction.
  - In major surgery, give 25–50mg hydrocortisone IV tds for 2–3 days.
  - In moderate surgery, give 25–50mg hydrocortisone IV tds for 1 day.
  - Return to the usual oral corticosteroid dose after this.
- Patients with known Addison's disease or hypopituitarism should be discussed with the on-call physician.

Arranging theatre

Each hospital has its own way of booking and arranging emergency surgery. In general, the case must be booked with the emergency theatre coordinator (usually a senior theatre nurse or operating department practitioner) and then discussed with the on-call anaesthetist. Cases proceed in booking order unless there is a clinical imperative. 'Out of hours' emergency surgery may occasionally be necessary (Box 2.5).

❶ These processes can take a significant amount of time and be a source of considerable stress and frustration. Good communication skills are **essential** (📖 p.8).

Booking the case

- Phone the theatre coordinator and ask to book a case. Some hospitals require a booking sheet to be filled in. You'll need the following information:
  - patient name, sex, date of birth, hospital number, and ward;
  - working diagnosis;
  - operation to be performed;
  - surgeon's name and bleep number;
  - name of the admitting consultant;
  - infection risk, e.g. MRSA, hepatitis B/C, HIV, TB;
  - position of the patient on the table.
- Inform the theatre coordinator if any specialized instruments are needed, e.g. disposable laparoscopic instruments, deep retractors for obese patients.
- It is always a good idea to find out how the emergency list is progressing and to ask when your patient may be going to theatre. This will help you plan your time more effectively.
- Call the on-call radiographer if portable X-ray is required (e.g. on-table cholangiography, angiography). Give them as much notice as possible, and then call again just before surgery starts.

Anaesthetic issues

- It is good practice to discuss all patients placed on the emergency list with the on-call anaesthetist. You'll need the following information:
  - patient name, sex, date of birth, hospital number, and ward;
  - working diagnosis, operation to be performed, and surgeon;
  - significant co-morbidities and allergies;
  - recent blood, CXR, and ECG results;
  - G&S or cross-match availability;
  - time of last oral intake and what was ingested;
  - previous anaesthetic problems.
- Patients with multiple co-morbidities, sepsis, or shock, and those requiring major surgery may require urgent anaesthetic review and discussion with the on-call senior anaesthetist. Involve the anaesthetic and/or ITU team **early**.

Discussion with other on-call surgical teams

- If you believe that your patient takes **clear** clinical priority, you must discuss this with the theatre coordinator and the on-call team looking after the other patient to get permission to 'jump the queue'.
- Clinical priority may be difficult to decide. Other factors to consider include:
  - the age of the patient (emergency paediatric cases take priority);
  - the time already spent waiting on the emergency list;
  - the expected duration of surgery and the impact on hospital resources (a 10min incision and drainage of an abscess may enable a patient to be sent home the same day).

❶ Discussions between specialties can be difficult. Be courteous and honest at all times. If you are unable to agree on an acceptable strategy with your colleagues, then inform your consultant. They may need to discuss the issue with their counterpart.

Box 2.5 'Out of hours' emergency surgery

In the UK, many emergency theatres in smaller hospitals close between 23.00 and 08.00, except for life- or limb-threatening conditions. If you feel that opening theatre is necessary, discuss with the on-call consultant and get their backing before approaching the list coordinator and on-call anaesthetist. 'Out of hours' surgery may have a significant cost implication as a theatre team may need to be called in. Discussion between the on-call surgical consultant and anaesthetic consultant may be necessary.

Consent and marking

Consent and marking policies vary between countries, and occasionally, between hospitals. The information on consent in the next section is in accordance with English law (see *www.dh.gov.uk/consent*). These issues may be complex and have significant medicolegal consequences—if in doubt, discuss with your senior.

Consent

- The basic principles for seeking consent are the same for elective and emergency surgery, although the quantity of information given in an emergency may be limited.
- Check that you are qualified to seek consent.
  - Are you able to perform the procedure?
  - If not, have you been adequately trained in seeking consent for that procedure?

❶ The ultimate responsibility for the consent process is borne by the person carrying out the procedure.

Adult consent (≥ 18 years old)

Check that the patient is competent to give consent. An interpreter may be required. The following need to be addressed.

- Are they able to comprehend and retain information relating to the decision?
- Are they able to weigh and use the information in coming to a decision?
- Is there an absence of duress, i.e. is the consent voluntary?

❶ If an adult patient is not competent to give consent, no-one else can give it on their behalf, including family members. You may still treat the patient if you believe that the treatment would be in their best interests. Discuss with your seniors.

❶ If an adult patient is competent to give consent but is unable to sign the form, an independent witness can confirm oral or nonverbal consent.

Paediatric consent (< 18 years old)

- Children 16–17 years old are assumed to have competence to give or withhold consent. Check for competence as above. Parents may wish to countersign consent forms, although they cannot overrule the decision of a competent 16–17 year old. If a child aged 16 or 17 is not competent to give consent, the parents can make the decision on their behalf.
- Children < 16 years old may be competent to give consent, but are not assumed to be so. Ideally, their parents should be involved in the consent process. If the child is competent and gives consent to a procedure, a parent cannot overrule their decision. However, if a competent child < 16 refuses consent a parent can overrule this decision.

❶ 'Parents' as used above indicates a person with legal parental responsibility. Unmarried fathers, stepparents, grandparents, and foster parents do not automatically have legal parental responsibility.

Issues to be covered in seeking consent

Ideally, these should include:

- the working diagnosis;
- the aims of the surgery;
- the alternatives to surgery, and their risks and benefits;
- the type of anaesthetic expected (although the final decision rests with the on-call anaesthetic team);
- the expected incision and what the operation entails;
- other procedures that may be required during surgery (especially the possibility that a stoma may be needed);
- possible complications and risks;
- likelihood of requiring a blood transfusion (Box 2.6);
- any drains, catheters expected to be placed;
- need for HDU/ITU postoperatively;
- expected inpatient stay and recovery time;
- the approximate duration of the surgery.

❶ You should mention 'significant risks that would affect the judgement of a reasonable patient'. 'Significant' has not been defined in English law.

❶ Occasionally, patients refuse detailed information on the basis that they do not wish to know. You must ensure that at least basic information is given and that their reluctance to discuss details is documented in the notes.

Box 2.6 Jehovah's Witnesses

Jehovah's Witnesses regard the transfusion of packed RBCs, WBCs, platelets, whole blood, or FFP as unacceptable on religious grounds. Some Jehovah's Witnesses also refuse albumin, immunoglobulin, factor VIII, recombinant factor VIIa, and cell-saver devices, although this is an individual decision. Most Jehovah's Witnesses carry advance directives detailing their beliefs regarding blood products. Where advanced directives exist, the patient's wishes must be adhered to, even in life-threatening emergencies. This is not the case in children < 16 years old.*

❶ Discuss the patient's wishes regarding blood and blood product transfusion preoperatively and document this discussion in the notes. Specific consent forms are available.

❶ It is essential to inform the on-call surgical and anaesthetic consultants if emergency surgery on a Jehovah's Witness is required.

* Association of Anaesthetists of Great Britain and Ireland. *Management of anaesthesia for Jehovah's Witnesses*, 2nd edn, 2005. www.aagbi.org

---

Emergency theatre list delays

Delays with the emergency list are a common source of complaints from patients and their relatives. The consent-seeking process is a good time to remind patients that it is very difficult to predict when they may be going to theatre due to the nature of emergency surgery. Make sure that you inform the patient as soon as possible if theatre has been delayed and record this in the notes.

Preoperative marking
This should take place whenever surgery involving one side occurs.

Principles of safe preoperative marking
- Verify the side against documentation and imaging.
- Involve the patient in the process to check that the correct side is being marked. Marking should take place before pre-medication.
- Marking should be performed by the operating surgeon (or deputy).
- Use an indelible marker to draw an arrow that extends near to the intended incision. The arrow should be visible after skin preparation and draping. Some surgeons initial the arrow, others write an abbreviation of the operation on the abdomen (e.g. Lap Appx, Lap Chole).
- ❶ Some hospitals use marking verification checklists that need to be filled in even if marking is not required. Transfer of the patient to theatre may be delayed if these have not been filled in.
- Any emergency bowel surgery (especially on the large bowel) may result in stoma formation. During working hours, contact the stoma nurse specialist to mark potential stoma sites (Box 2.7).
  - ❶ The possibility that a stoma may be needed must be discussed with the patient fully before siting a stoma. This should be documented on the consent form.

Box 2.7 Siting a stoma
- Mark the waistband line with the patient standing, if possible.
- The stoma is best brought out through the rectus sheath, inferior to the waistband line, on a flat area not crossed by creases that appear on sitting, standing, or bending. Creases will cause a stoma to leak.
- The stoma should be away from the ribs, bony landmarks, old scars, and the anticipated incision.
- The patient should be able to see the stoma when in a sitting position.
- Mark stoma sites on the right (ileostomy) and left (colostomy).
- When the optimum site is identified, mark with a permanent marker pen.

Preparation for endoscopy

Consent for endoscopy is usually obtained by the endoscopist or endoscopy nurse. Check local policies.

Oesophagogastroduodenoscopy (OGD)

The timing of OGD is determined by clinical urgency.
- Emergency OGD is performed on patients with significant upper GI bleeds who are unstable.
  - Place 2 x large-bore peripheral IV cannulae.
  - Have recent FBC, PT/INR, and APTT results available, and correct INR if > 1.4 (📖 p.22).
  - Have cross-matched packed RBCs available.
- Urgent OGD is usually performed for patients with upper GI bleeds who are haemodynamically stable.
  - Keep NBM for 6h before.
  - Place an IV cannula and adequately resuscitate if bleeding.
- Ensure that antibiotic prophylaxis is given for those with a prosthetic heart valve or previous endocarditis.

Flexible sigmoidoscopy/colonoscopy

Lower GI endoscopy is less commonly performed on an urgent or emergency basis. Most patients with PR bleeding do not require inpatient lower GI endoscopy as bleeding usually stops spontaneously (📖 p.280).
- Preparation for inpatient flexible sigmoidoscopy:
  - low residue diet for 24h before;
  - NBM for 2h before;
  - phosphate enema 1h before.
- Preparation for semi-urgent in-patient colonoscopy:
  - low residue diet starting 3 days before;
  - clear fluids for 24h before;
  - bowel cleansing solutions (e.g. Fleet, Picolax) the day before.
- ❶ Follow local protocols for bowel preparation.
- For patients with active GI bleeding requiring urgent flexible sigmoidoscopy or colonoscopy, prepare as for an emergency OGD. Bowel preparation is not required as blood is a laxative.
- Ensure that IV antibiotic prophylaxis is given for those with a prosthetic heart valve or previous endocarditis.

Endoscopic retrograde cholangiopancreatography (ERCP)

It is rare for an ERCP to be performed out-of-hours. Most cases can wait until the next planned list. Indications include severe obstructive jaundice, acute cholangitis not responding to IV antibiotics, and severe acute gallstone pancreatitis.
- Recent FBC, U&Es, LFTs, amylase, PT/INR, and APTT results should be available. Correct if INR > 1.4 (📖 p.22). Request G&S.
- The patient should be NBM for 6h beforehand.
- Place an 18G IV cannula in the right arm as the patient will be lying on their left-hand side for the procedure.
- Most units give routine antibiotic prophylaxis, e.g. oral ciprofloxacin 500mg PO 2h before ERCP. Check local policies.
- Ensure that IV antibiotic prophylaxis is given for those with a prosthetic heart valve or previous endocarditis.

Preparation for interventional radiology

Emergency interventional radiology is commonly performed for bleeding patients not amenable to surgical intervention, those with thromboembolic vascular disease, or patients with renal outflow obstruction requiring a nephrostomy. Consent for emergency radiological intervention is usually obtained by the radiologist. Food and fluid restrictions are not required, but many patients are NBM in case emergency surgery is needed.

- ❶ Have recent FBC, U&Es, PT/INR, and APTT results available, and correct if INR > 1.4 (📖 p.22).
- ❶ When contrast is used, ensure that IV hydration is optimal to reduce the risks of contrast-induced nephrotoxicity.
- ❶ Contrast can induce lactic acidosis in diabetics on metformin. Discontinue metformin on the day of the procedure and re-start 2 days later.
- In patients with renal outflow obstruction:
  - antibiotic prophylaxis is required if signs of infection are present. Check with the urologist.
- If the patient is actively bleeding:
  - place 2 x large-bore peripheral IV cannulae;
  - have cross-matched packed RBCs available.
- In patients undergoing revascularization procedures:
  - mark the affected limb beforehand;
  - palpate peripheral pulses beforehand and document your findings.

Part 2

Problem-based emergency surgery

Trauma emergencies

Trauma principles

This chapter describes an approach to major, life-threatening trauma that seeks to reduce morbidity and mortality within the 'golden hour' after injury, when simple interventions can save life and limb. Despite the wide range of injuries that may occur, there is a small number of basic principles that underpin trauma management, as described here.

The ATLS® approach

The Advanced Trauma Life Support (ATLS®) course was developed by the American College of Surgeons in the late 1970s. The ATLS® philosophy is to assess and stabilize each organ system according to priority, i.e. treat the greatest threat to life first. This initial phase is known as the **primary survey** and consists of immediate assessment and management of the following (ABCDE).
- Airway with cervical spine protection.
- Breathing.
- Circulation with haemorrhage control.
- Disability (neurological assessment).
- Exposure/environment.

❶ Once a life-threatening injury is identified it must be successfully treated before the next system is assessed. A definitive diagnosis does not need to be reached before treatment is begun.

❶ If at any point the patient deteriorates, the primary survey must be repeated from 'A'.

Once the patient is stabilized and the primary survey is completed, additional investigations and procedures can be performed ('adjuncts to the primary survey'). When stability is achieved, and the observations are improving, the **secondary survey** can be started. This involves a thorough head-to-toe examination ('tubes or fingers in every orifice') and a brief history. This may need to be delayed for hours or days after admission, e.g. after recovery from trauma laparotomy. Note that, although a description of the scene and information from the ambulance crew are vital, history from the patient is sometimes less important, and can wait until the secondary survey.

Transfer to another hospital may be required, especially for those patients with significant head injuries, major burns, or penetrating chest trauma.

A summary of an emergency trauma pathway is shown in Fig. 3.1. This algorithm applies to both blunt and penetrating trauma, and to children, pregnant women, and the elderly.

❶ Standard protective clothing should be worn, i.e. face mask, eye protection, water-proof apron, gloves, and leggings, shoe covers, and cap/gown as required. Practice safe sharps handling.

❶ ATLS® was developed in order to train often inexperienced doctors to approach major trauma in a logical, safe manner. Occasionally, experienced senior clinicians and trauma teams may approach trauma in a more focused way, bypassing steps in the pathway. However, doctors involved in the management of patients with trauma emergencies should undergo ATLS® training.

Mechanism of injury

Knowing the mechanism of injury assists in determining which injuries are likely to be present. Injuries are broadly classified into blunt and penetrating.

- Blunt injuries tend to involve multiple organ systems and body compartments as the energy delivered to the patient is spread over a wide area.
- Penetrating injuries (e.g. stab wounds, firearm injuries) generally involve organs lying in the line of penetration. The injuries caused by high energy firearms (e.g. military or hunting rifles) are an exception, as bullets traveling at high velocity cause extensive tissue cavitation.

Injuries may occur via a number of different mechanisms. For example, blast injuries cause tissue damage in at least three ways:

- barotrauma due to the expanding pressure wave, leading to ruptured tympanic membranes, lung contusions, pneumothoraces, air emboli, intestinal rupture, etc.;
- penetrating injuries from shrapnel and flying objects;
- blunt injuries when the patient is thrown against a solid object or the ground.

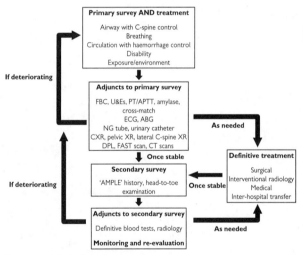

Fig. 3.1 An algorithm for emergency trauma management.

Certain mechanisms of injury are associated with specific injury patterns, e.g.:

- fall from a height on to feet: calcaneal fractures, vertical shear pelvic fractures, thoracolumbar vertebral wedge fractures;
- frontal impact in a vehicle (unrestrained): head injury, cervical spine fracture, myocardial contusion, traumatic aortic rupture, liver/spleen laceration, femoral fractures, hip fracture–dislocations.

Despite these patterns, in high energy trauma, patients can injure almost any organ or structure. Patients with high cervical spine injuries, severe open head injuries, and complete aortic transection are very unlikely to survive to hospital.

Triage

When more than one trauma victim is present, an assessment must be made to decide prioritization. This process is triage, meaning 'to sort'. In the majority of instances in the developed world the capabilities of the receiving hospital are not exceeded, and triage is therefore based on the 'ABCs', i.e. those with airway problems are treated before those with breathing difficulties, etc. When there are mass casualties and the hospital's capabilities are exceeded, e.g. natural disasters, terrorist incidents, triage should be based on the patient's chance of survival with the least resources expended.

❶ These decisions are difficult and need to be made by senior clinicians.

Airway with cervical spine protection

The primary survey begins with assessment of the patient's airway. Protection of the cervical spine is essential (Box 3.1). Early recognition of those at risk of airway obstruction is important, e.g. patients with head, neck, or facial trauma, facial burns, or reduced level of consciousness from any cause. In the heat of the moment it is easy to forget the simple things.

▶▶ All patients with significant trauma should have high-flow O_2 at 10–12L/min via a non-rebreathing mask. This includes those with COPD; hypoxia will kill faster than CO_2 narcosis.

▶▶ Ask for a pulse oximeter, ECG electrodes, and non-invasive BP cuff to be connected. These will give you basic observations throughout the resuscitation.

The on-call anaesthetist is usually a member of the trauma team, and often takes over airway control on arrival. You must ensure that the patient survives until then.

Box 3.1 Cervical spine protection

Assume that **all** patients with significant blunt trauma have a C-spine injury. Those with an altered level of consciousness or blunt trauma above the level of the clavicle are at especially high risk. C-spine protection is most commonly provided using an appropriately sized and fitted semi-rigid collar + sandbags/fluid bags next to head + tape across the forehead and chin stuck to the bed.

❶ All components are necessary to protect the C-spine.

If the collar/sandbags/tape need to be removed (e.g. for examination or intubation) C-spine protection must be maintained using in-line immobilization, i.e. a trained colleague standing at the patient's head with the flat of each hand firmly placed on each side of the patient's head. C-spine protection should not be removed until the C-spine has been cleared (📖 p.80).

❶ In the combative, restless patient, it may be preferable to release the restraints rather than have the patient strain and fight against them. This decision should only be made by a senior clinician appropriately trained in the assessment of spinal injuries. Consider sedation and intubation to allow CT to exclude a head or spine injury.

Examination

Examine for signs of airway obstruction, or those disorders likely to lead to obstruction.

❶ Patients able to speak or shout clearly are unlikely to have immediately life-threatening airway problems.

Look
- At the patient: agitation, cyanosis.
- At the patient's face and neck: facial trauma or burns, neck wounds.
- In the mouth: blood, vomit, broken teeth, foreign bodies, airway burns.

❶ Suck out any oropharyngeal liquid immediately. If gastric contents are present, rotate the entire patient laterally (using the spinal board) and then suction. Remove any foreign bodies with forceps, if easily accessible.

Listen
- To breath sounds at the mouth: air movement, added noises (e.g. snoring, gurgling, stridor).
- To the voice: hoarseness (laryngeal oedema or fracture).

Feel
- The face: facial fractures.
- The larynx and neck: palpable laryngeal fractures (may also have subcutaneous emphysema).

Immediate management
❶ Patients with facial or airway burns or laryngeal fractures are likely to develop airway obstruction. Senior anaesthetic review is required **immediately**.

A stepwise approach to airway management is taken. Start with the simplest manoeuvres; ascend the 'ladder' as needed to maintain the airway. The C-spine must remain protected at all times.

Simple manoeuvres
- Suction the oropharynx and remove foreign bodies.
- Chin lift and jaw thrust.

❶ Do not tilt the head due to the risk of C-spine injury.

Simple airway devices
Patients with severe head injuries or intoxication may lose oropharyngeal muscular tone, causing the tongue to fall backwards, and obstructing the airway. Chin lift/jaw thrust opens the airway, and this can be maintained by insertion of a simple airway device.
- Nasopharyngeal airway.
  - The diameter should be equal to that of the patient's little finger.
  - Often better tolerated than the oropharyngeal airway.
  - Do not insert in those with a significant head injury due to the risk of intubating a skull base fracture.
- Oropharyngeal airway.
  - The length should be equal to the distance from the corner of the patient's mouth to their earlobe.
  - Insert upside-down, and rotate 180° to lie over the tongue. Do not use this insertion technique in children.
  - Poorly tolerated in the conscious patient.

In patients where a definitive airway will eventually be required (e.g. severe head injury), but you do not have the expertise to insert an endotracheal tube, maintain the airway with a simple airway device until an appropriately trained colleague arrives. If ventilation is poor, use a bag-valve-mask attached to high-flow O_2.

❶ The use of laryngeal mask airways is not encouraged in trauma patients as they do not provide a definitive airway.

Definitive airway

This is defined as a tube in the trachea with the cuff inflated, O_2 attached, and secured with tape. Indications for a definitive airway include the following.

- Need for airway protection:
  - facial fracture, airway burns, laryngeal fracture;
  - risk of aspiration due to airway contamination with blood, vomit, etc.;
  - reduced level of consciousness, e.g. severe head injury (GCS < 9) or intoxication.
- Need for ventilation:
  - apnoea, poor inspiratory effort, or inability to maintain oxygenation using face mask and high-flow O_2;
  - severe head injury requiring therapeutic hyperventilation.

Examples of a definitive airway include an endotracheal tube (orotracheal or nasotracheal) and surgical cricothyroidotomy.

- Endotracheal intubation.
  - Intubation should only be undertaken by those trained and experienced in the technique and the use of sedating and paralysing drugs.
  - Details on how to intubate are beyond the scope of this book.
  - ❶ A patent airway maintained using a simple technique is better than multiple failed attempts at intubation.
- Repeated failure at orotracheal intubation when a definitive airway is essential mandates surgical cricothyroidotomy (🕮 p.536).

❶ Emergency open tracheostomy is difficult, bloody, and slow. Percutaneous tracheostomy is not used in the trauma setting due to the need for neck hyperextension.

Jet insufflation

When a definitive airway is unable to be placed due to lack of equipment or expertise, a large cannula can be inserted through the cricothyroid membrane to enable temporary oxygenation (Fig. 3.2).

- Insert a 12–14G IV cannula attached to a 5mL syringe, aspirating as you pass through the cricothyroid membrane in the midline.
- Stop once air is aspirated and advance the plastic cannula while removing needle.
- Attach the cannula to a three-way tap and wall O_2 at 15L/min.
- Oxygenate for 1s, allow exhalation for 4s, and continue.
- This can be used for 30–45min. Barotrauma and CO_2 accumulation may occur before then.

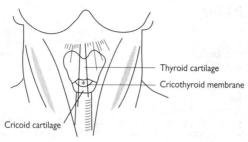

Fig. 3.2 Anatomy of the cricothyroid membrane. (Adapted, with permission, from Wyatt, J.P. et al. (1999). *Oxford handbook of accident and emergency medicine*, 1st edn, p. 345. Oxford University Press, Oxford.)

Breathing

The following immediately life-threatening thoracic injuries should be identified and treated in 'B': tension pneumothorax (📖 p.463), open pneumothorax (📖 p.462), massive haemothorax (📖 p.464), and flail chest (📖 p.456).

Examination

Inspection

- Of the patient: cyanosis, pallor.
- Of the chest: tachypnoea, shallow respirations, asymmetrical chest movement, paradoxical chest wall motion, chest wall bruising, open chest wounds.

Palpation

- Of the trachea in the sternal notch: tracheal deviation.
- Of the chest: tenderness, bony crepitus, flail segments, subcutaneous emphysema.

Chest percussion (apices and bases)

- Hyperresonance, dullness.

Chest auscultation (apices and bases)

- Normal air entry, decreased air entry.

❶ Percussion and auscultation can be difficult in a noisy resuscitation room.

Immediate management

Tension pneumothorax:

- Needle thoracic decompression with a large-bore cannula in the 2nd intercostal space, mid-clavicular line (📖 p.516).
- Insert an intercostal chest drain (📖 p.522).

❶ This is a clinical diagnosis; do **not** wait for a CXR.

Open pneumothorax

- Apply a square sterile non-adherent occlusive dressing large enough to cover the entire defect, taped securely on three sides to act as a flap valve.
- Insert an intercostal chest drain (📖 p.522) remote from the wound site.
- Discuss surgical closure with a cardiothoracic surgeon.

Massive haemothorax

- Before inserting a chest drain, IV fluid resuscitation is essential. Insert two peripheral large-bore IV cannulae. Take bloods and cross-match 4–6 units of packed RBCs. Give 1000mL of warmed Hartmann's solution as a bolus through each cannula.
- Insert an intercostal chest drain (📖 p.522).
- If initial chest drain output is > 1500mL of blood, transfuse with packed RBCs and **immediately** refer to a cardiothoracic surgeon for emergency thoracotomy.

❶ This is a clinical diagnosis; do **not** wait for a CXR.

Flail chest

- Ensure adequate oxygenation and analgesia. Have a low threshold for intubation and mechanical ventilation. Check ABGs regularly.
- Avoid overhydration as this will exacerbate the effects of the underlying pulmonary contusion.
- Patients with large flail segments causing difficulty with ventilation should be referred to a cardiothoracic surgeon for consideration of operative fixation.

Further investigations

An ABG and a supine AP CXR should be performed as adjuncts to the primary survey.

Circulation with haemorrhage control

The recognition and correction of shock are the prime aims here. Shock can be defined as inadequate tissue perfusion and oxygenation.

Shock

In trauma patients, the cause of shock can be haemorrhagic or non-haemorrhagic. Haemorrhagic shock is much more common.

Haemorrhagic shock

- Clinical features depend on the volume of blood lost (Table 3.1).
- Blood loss can be from one or more of five compartments (Box 3.2).
- Normal adult blood volume is 70mL/kg.

Non-haemorrhagic shock

- Cardiogenic, e.g. cardiac tamponade (📖 p.474), myocardial infarction, myocardial contusion.
- Tension pneumothorax (📖 p.463). This is usually detected in 'B'.
- Neurogenic, i.e. spinal cord injury causing loss of sympathetic tone, peripheral vasodilatation, and hypotension in the absence of a tachy-cardia.
- Septic shock (📖 p.482): rare unless presentation is delayed or pen-etrating abdominal injuries are present.
- Anaphylactic shock (rare in trauma patients).

Table 3.1 Clinical features of haemorrhagic shock in adults and blood loss

Variable	Class I	Class II	Class III	Class IV
% blood volume lost	< 15	15–30	30–40	> 40
Heart rate	< 100	> 100	> 120	> 140
Systolic BP	↔	↔	↓	↓↓
Pulse pressure	↔ or ↑	↓	↓	↓↓
Respiratory rate	14–20	20–30	30–40	> 35
Mental state	↔	Anxious	Confused	Lethargic
Urine output (mL/h)	↔	20–30	< 20	Negligible

Adapted from the ATLS® Course Manual, 7th Edition, Table 1, p74, with the permission of the American College of Surgeons.

❶ This is a rough guide only. The patient's age and medication history (e.g. β-blockers) will alter the physiological response to blood loss. Young, fit patients may mask signs of haemorrhage before decompensating dramatically.

Box 3.2 Sources of haemorrhagic shock

- Thorax
- Abdomen
- Pelvis (e.g. pelvic fracture)
- Thigh (a femoral fracture can cause blood loss of up to 1500mL)
- Peripheral wounds

This is nicely summarized as 'One on the floor and four more'.

❶ In adults, intracranial bleeding cannot cause haemorrhagic shock due to the relatively small intracranial volume. Coning will occur before shock.

Examination

- General inspection: pallor, mental state, blood on the floor.
- Limbs.
  - Peripheries: cool to touch.
  - Pulse: tachycardia, ↓ pulse volume.
  - Recent BP reading.
- Neck.
  - Inspection: tracheal deviation, distended neck veins, bruises.
  - **❶** Distended neck veins are a feature of both cardiac tamponade and tension pneumothorax. Differentiate between the two by chest examination. Cardiac tamponade and tension pneumothorax can occur without distended neck veins due to blood loss.
- Heart/chest.
  - Inspection: penetrating injuries, bruises.
  - Auscultation: muffled heart sounds (cardiac tamponade), murmurs.
- Abdomen.
  - Inspection: penetrating injuries, bruises (especially seatbelt), distension, evisceration of omentum or small bowel.
  - Palpation: tenderness, guarding, rigidity.
  - Percussion: tenderness, epigastric tympanism indicating acute gastric dilatation (📖 p.205).
  - Auscultation: quiet or absent bowel sounds.
  - **❶** Intraperitoneal blood can be present without overt signs of peritonitis.
  - **❶** Accurate examination of the abdomen can be made difficult by distracting injuries, intoxication, head or spinal cord injuries.
- Pelvis.
  - Look: bruises, deformities.
  - Feel: mobility of the pelvis on compression.
  - **❶** Test for pelvic fractures only once (📖 p.72).
- Thighs.
  - Look: swelling, deformity.
  - Feel: tenderness.

❶ If this examination fails to identify the cause of the hypotension, check for signs of a spinal cord injury (neurogenic shock).

Immediate management

Treatment is initiated as if haemorrhage is the cause of shock, unless there is clear clinical evidence otherwise.

Obtain adequate intravenous access
- Insert **at least** 2 x large-bore (14–18G) peripheral cannulae in the arms. Do not place a cannula distal to a limb injury, as extravasation of fluid may result.
- If this is not possible, gain IV access elsewhere:
  - long saphenous vein (just anterior to the medial malleolus) via cutdown (📖 p.526);
  - insertion of a central venous line into the femoral, subclavian, or internal jugular veins (📖 p.528). Avoid femoral lines in a patient with a fractured pelvis due to the risk of fluid extravasation.
- ❶ Poiseuille's law states that flow through a tube is proportional to the 4th power of the radius, and inversely proportional to the length. A short, fat cannula is **far superior** to a long, thin central venous line for rapid fluid resuscitation.
- Take blood for FBC, U&Es, LFTs, amylase, PT, and APTT. Consider toxicology studies, and blood βhCG in females of child-bearing age. If class II–IV haemorrhagic shock is present, cross-match 4–6 units of packed RBCs.
  - The type of packed RBCs requested should vary with clinical urgency.
  - Fully cross-matched packed RBCs may take an hour to prepare; type-specific blood should be available within 15min.
  - Patients with exsanguinating haemorrhage require type O packed RBCs. Females of child-bearing age should have type O Rhesus negative blood. At least 2 units should be immediately available.

Begin aggressive IV fluid resuscitation
- Start 1000mL of warmed Hartmann's solution through each cannula, given as rapidly as possible (☀ Box 3.3).
- ❶ Massive fluid resuscitation can cause hypothermia, causing coagulopathy, and increasing mortality. Keep the patient warm (📖 p.60).
- Patients with class III or IV haemorrhagic shock will also require packed RBCs given as a bolus. Discuss the use of blood products early with the on-call haematologist.

Haemorrhage control

Replacing lost fluid is a temporizing measure. Ongoing blood loss must be halted and early haemorrhage control is **essential**.
- Stop peripheral bleeding with firm pressure directly over the bleeding site. Padded tourniquets can be used in exsanguinating haemorrhage.
- ❶ Do not attempt to clamp bleeding vessels as further damage to neurovascular structures may ensue.
- Reduce and splint long bone fractures, especially femoral fractures (e.g. with a Thomas splint).
- Splint suspected pelvic fractures (📖 p.73).
- Laparotomy (📖 p.71) and/or thoracotomy (📖 p.67) are often required.

- Surgical exploration of penetrating vascular injuries may be necessary (📖 p.337).
- Interventional radiology may be used (e.g. to control bleeding associated with pelvic fractures), but availability is limited.
- ❶ Regular clinical assessment is vital to determine the patient's response to fluid resuscitation. In blunt trauma, the response to fluid boluses gives an indication of the likely need for surgery (📖 p.64).

Box 3.3 Evolving strategies in the management of haemorrhagic shock

Although ATLS® guidelines recommend 2L of Hartmann's given as a bolus for adults with haemorrhagic shock, other resuscitation strategies may be superior.

- Some surgeons advocate fluid resuscitation with hypertonic saline (with or without dextran) given as a 250mL bolus. The results of randomized controlled trials are awaited.
- Patients with penetrating torso trauma appear to benefit from 'permissive hypotension', i.e. limited fluid resuscitation to maintain a palpable pulse, consciousness, and systolic BP of approximately 90mmHg, before rapid transfer to theatre for control of haemorrhage. This strategy may prevent re-bleeding from damaged blood vessels that may occur with large volume fluid resuscitation. Patients with blunt trauma often have head injuries and permissive hypotension in this setting is detrimental.
- Patients with severe injuries who are likely to need massive blood transfusions (≥ 10 units packed RBCs in 24h) may benefit from early blood component therapy using FFP, packed RBCs, and platelets in a ratio of 1:1:1. Recombinant factor VIIa should also be considered. This has been called 'damage control resuscitation'.

Treatment for non-haemorrhagic shock
Cardiac tamponade (📖 p.474)
- Perform immediate pericardiocentesis (📖 p.534).
- Discuss transfer to a cardiothoracic centre.

Tension pneumothorax (📖 p.463)
- Needle thoracic decompression with a large-bore cannula in the 2nd intercostal space, in the mid-clavicular line (📖 p.516).
- Insert an intercostal chest drain (📖 p.522).

Neurogenic shock
- Give further crystalloid fluid resuscitation.
- Fluid overload can occur, and central venous lines are useful to measure CVP.
- Atropine boluses (300mcg IV) may be required if bradycardia is present.
- Consider inotropes if hypotension persists despite adequate filling.

Septic shock (📖 p.482)
- Give further crystalloid fluid resuscitation.

- Start broad-spectrum IV antibiotics (e.g. cefuroxime 1.5g tds with metronidazole 500mg tds) after taking blood, urine, wound, and sputum samples for culture.
- Fluid overload can occur, and central venous lines are useful to measure CVP—consider inotropes if hypotension persists despite adequate filling.
- Drain the source of sepsis using surgical or radiological techniques.

Further investigations

- ECG to exclude myocardial ischaemia and myocardial trauma.
- Pelvic XR as part of the trauma series to identify a pelvic fracture.
- CXR to identify haemothoraces.
- Patients with multiple possible sites of haemorrhage who are haemo-dynamically unstable may benefit from either DPL or a FAST scan to identify an intraabdominal source of bleeding. Patients who are rela-tively haemodynamically stable can undergo abdominal and pelvic CT scanning to achieve the same goal (🕮 p.70).

Disability (neurological assessment)

A rapid neurological examination is required. The level of consciousness should be established and the pupils examined. Also check for gross peripheral neurological signs.

Examination

Level of consciousness

Use either the AVPU scale or the Glasgow Coma Scale (GCS). If AVPU is performed, document GCS during the secondary survey.

- AVPU.
  - **A**lert spontaneously.
  - Responds to **V**oice.
  - Responds to **P**ain.
  - **U**nresponsive.
- GCS (Box 3.4).

Pupils Check size and reactivity.

Peripheral neurological examination Check gross strength and sensation in all four limbs.

Immediate management

Moderate or severe head injury (📖 p.78)

- Prevent secondary brain injury: ensure adequate oxygenation and airway protection, avoid hypotension, and treat seizures.

❶ Discuss with neurosurgical colleagues before giving mannitol, sedatives, or inducing hyperventilation (📖 p.430).

Suspected spinal cord injury (📖 p.80)

- Maintain C-spine protection.
- Treat neurogenic shock (📖 p.55), if present.

☛ The use of high-dose IV methylprednisolone in spinal cord trauma is controversial. Discuss with neurosurgical or orthopaedic colleagues first.

Further investigations

- CBG: exclude hypoglycaemia as a cause of decreased level of consciousness.
- Spinal X-rays. A lateral C-spine X-ray may be performed as part of trauma series. If a vertebral fracture or spinal cord injury is suspected clinically, X-rays of the entire spinal column are required.
- Once the patient is haemodynamically stable, perform CT head or spinal CT, as indicated. Spinal MRI may be required later.

Box 3.4 The Glasgow Coma Scale (GCS)

An accurate and reproducible method of assessing level of consciousness is essential. The GCS is a global assessment of consciousness; as it is not intended to pick out focal deficits the best response must always be used (see Table 3.2). A detailed neurological exam is needed to pick up focal deficits. The three components of the GCS have different prognostic significance so the GCS must always be broken down. The verbal scale varies with age (📖 p.91).

- ❶ The component of most relevance to the neurosurgeon is the motor response and particular attention must be paid to this assessment as it is often done badly (see Table 3.3).
- Coma can be defined as the inability to obey commands, speak, or open eyes to pain. 90% of patients with a GCS < 9 will fulfil these criteria and therefore GCS < 9 is regarded as an empirical definition of coma.
- ▶▶ Patients with GCS < 9 have an impaired ability to maintain patency of their upper airway and thus require a definitive airway.

Table 3.2 The Glasgow Coma Scale

Score	Eye opening	Verbal response	Motor response
1	None	None	None
2	To pain	Incomprehensible	Extensor response
3	To speech	Inappropriate	Abnormal flexion
4	Spontaneous	Confused	Normal flexion
5		Oriented	Localizes to pain
6			Obeys commands

Table 3.3 Assessing the motor score of the GCS*

Score	Response
1	No response despite sustained, severe stimulus
2	Elbows extended, forearm pronated, wrist flexed, fingers flexed
3	Elbows flexed, forearm pronated, wrist flexed, fingers flexed
4	Elbows flexed, forearm supinated, hand stays below level of clavicle
5	Hand reaches above level of clavicle
6	Patient can stick out tongue or squeeze fingers to verbal command

* A reliable way to assess motor score is to exert sustained pressure over the supraorbital nerve and assess the best response from the upper limbs.

Exposure/environment

Examination
- Undress the patient completely.
  - Clothes should be cut off using heavy scissors to ensure that spinal immobilization is maintained.
  - Removal of clothes covering the back may have to wait until a log-roll is performed.
- Take the patient's temperature, if necessary with a low-reading thermometer.

Immediate management
- Keep the patient warm.
  - The room temperature in the resus area should be kept warm.
  - Cover with pre-warmed blankets or use an external warming device (e.g. Bair Hugger™).
  - All IV fluids should be warm, or put through a warming device.
  - Uncover the patient only when necessary.
  - Remove spilt bodily fluids rapidly to prevent cooling through evaporation.

Adjuncts to the primary survey

As part of the primary survey, a number of procedures and investigations should be performed. Monitoring must also be connected. As polytrauma patients require the attention of a trauma team, members not involved in the assessment/management of 'A' through to 'E' should ensure that the adjuncts are completed.

Procedures

Urinary catheterization (📖 p.504)

• Look for signs of a urethral injury (📖 p.390) first, i.e. blood at the meatus, scrotal or perineal bruising, signs of a pelvic fracture, high-riding or impalpable prostate on DRE.
• Catheterization is essential before performing a DPL to prevent bladder injury.
• Perform dipstick urinalysis, and urine βhCG in all females of child-bearing age.

NG (Ryle's) tube insertion (📖 p.498)

• This can be difficult in awake, supine patients. Vomiting or aspiration can occur during insertion, so make sure that suctioning equipment is available. Turn the patient on their side maintaining spinal protection with log roll, or using a spinal board.
• If basal skull fracture is suspected, or significant facial trauma is present, use the orogastric route to prevent intracranial insertion.

Fracture immobilization

• Any obvious long bone fractures not reduced as part of 'C' should be reduced to an approximate anatomical position and immobilized in a splint or with in-line traction.
• Check distal pulses before and after moving any limb.

Investigations

• Bloods: these are usually taken with IV access insertion during 'C'.
• ABG: repeat regularly in those with chest trauma and chronic lung disease.
• ECG.
  • Especially in those with pre-existing cardiorespiratory disease, chest trauma, and where MI is suspected.
  • If dysrhythmias are present, consider myocardial contusion, hypoxia, hypovolaemia, or electrolyte abnormalities.
• X-rays.
  • Patients with significant blunt trauma should have an AP supine CXR and an AP pelvic X-ray during the primary survey, as these may influence management.
  • A cross-table lateral C-spine film should also be performed, but this can often wait until the secondary survey, as long as adequate spinal protection is maintained.
  • These three films are collectively referred to as a 'trauma series'.
• DPL or FAST scanning (📖 p.70) may be useful in the detection of occult intraabdominal bleeding.

- CT scanning.
  - Previously, CT scanning was only used on trauma patients who were haemodynamically normal, due to the risks of moving critically ill patients away from the resuscitation area for prolonged periods.
  - With multidetector helical CT scanners, rapid image acquisition means that the time spent aware from resus is decreasing. Some hospitals have CT scanners adjacent to resus, reducing this time further. This has meant that CT scans are increasingly used at the end of the primary survey in those with polytrauma and some haemodynamic instability (transient responders (🕮 p.64)).

❶ The decision to transfer relatively unstable patients to CT **should be made by senior colleagues only**. The radiology department is poorly equipped to deal with a deteriorating polytrauma patient—avoid the 'doughnut of death'!

Monitoring

- ECG.
- Non-invasive BP measurement.
  - Ensure that the correct cuff size is used and that frequent measurement does not significantly slow IV fluid infusions.
- Pulse oximetry.
  - This is a valuable method of determining the heart rate and SaO_2, but will **not** detect $PaCO_2$ and therefore will not measure adequacy of ventilation.
  - Poor peripheral perfusion, shivering/movement, dysrhythmias, intense ambient light, and carboxyhaemoglobinaemia can cause false readings.
  - ❶ Do not place the sensor distal to a BP cuff or a limb injury.
- Intubated patients require expired CO_2 monitoring.

After the primary survey

The end of the primary survey is an ideal point to re-assess the patient's progress and decide further treatment or interhospital transfer. The patient's airway should be unobstructed. Immediately life-threatening cardiothoracic injuries should have been identified and treated. Patients with haemorrhagic shock should be regularly re-assessed to determine their response to initial fluid resuscitation.

- Rapid responders. May not require immediate surgery but will need imaging (usually CT) to locate the source of bleeding once they are haemodynamically stable enough to leave resus.
- Transient responders. The re-appearance of signs of shock despite adequate fluid resuscitation with crystalloids and blood indicates that ongoing bleeding is present and surgery is likely. Exclude causes of non-haemorrhagic shock (e.g. myocardial contusion).
- Non-responders. Require immediate surgery once non-haemorrhagic causes of shock are excluded. Mortality is high.

Definitive treatment

In trauma patients this usually means surgery. Interventional radiology may also be important, e.g. to stop bleeding associated with pelvic fractures.

Patient transfer

The majority of hospitals in the UK have acute general surgery and orthopaedic specialties on-site with 24h imaging and theatre facilities. Transfer for definitive treatment is most commonly needed for neurosurgical or cardiothoracic expertise. Transfer outside of the emergency department is hazardous. Check the following.

- The receiving team are fully aware of the mechanism of injury, patient co-morbidities, injuries sustained, interventions, and response to treatment.
- You know where to send the patient, and which team will be responsible for their care when they arrive. This must be clearly communicated to the transport personnel and the medical staff accompanying the patient.
- An ATLS®-trained colleague with appropriate experience accompanies the patient with the necessary equipment and drugs should deterioration occur en route.
- Send all relevant documentation including blood results, observation charts, and images (hard copy or on CD/DVD). Send any cross-matched blood as well.

❶ Decisions regarding the requirement for transfer and its timing are often complex and require the involvement of seniors. Established transfer protocols should be adhered to.

❶ Transfer by air has its own problems, e.g. reduced atmospheric pressure leading to expansion of pneumothoraces. Accompanying staff should be specifically trained in air transfer procedures.

The secondary survey

This consists of a head-to-toe examination and a brief, focused history (AMPLE). It should only begin when the primary survey and adjuncts are completed, immediately life-threatening injuries have been treated, and physiological parameters are improving. Further investigations may be required after the secondary survey is completed (e.g. limb X-rays).

History
- **A**llergies.
- **M**edications.
- **P**regnancy/**P**ast medical history.
- **L**ast meal/drink.
- **E**vents/**E**nvironment surrounding trauma.

Head-to-toe examination
This is an in-depth examination looking and/or feeling in every orifice, and palpating every joint. Start at the head and work down. Here are some points to remember.
- A log roll requires at least 4 adequately trained staff to perform the roll, and one doctor to remove the spinal board and examine the back.
- A full neurological, musculoskeletal, and vascular examination is performed. Check specifically for compartment syndrome (📖 p.412) and limb ischaemia (📖 p.337).
- Re-assess the GCS and pupils.
- Check visual acuity and remove contact lenses. Look in the ears and nose.
- Perform a vaginal examination. A DRE should have been performed before urinary catheterization as part of the primary survey adjuncts.
- Examine closely the fluid draining from any catheters inserted, including intercostal chest drains. In this way, iatrogenic and previously occult traumatic injuries may be revealed.

❶ Any deterioration in vital signs during the secondary survey requires a repeat primary survey (📖 p.42).

❶ The secondary survey may have to wait until after theatre/transfer. Prior to transfer from resus, clearly document if a secondary survey is still required.

Cardiothoracic trauma

Trauma to the thorax varies in its presentation, from relatively minor conditions requiring expectant management to the immediately life-threatening requiring emergency surgery.

Cardiothoracic injuries requiring detection and immediate management during the primary survey can be remembered by the mnemonic 'ATOM FC', i.e. **a**irway obstruction (🕮 p.46), **t**ension pneumothorax (🕮 p.463), **o**pen pneumothorax (🕮 p.462), **m**assive haemothorax (🕮 p.464), **f**lail chest (🕮 p.456), and **c**ardiac tamponade (🕮 p.474). These injuries should be detected in 'B' or 'C'. Other cardiothoracic injuries may become apparent after investigations performed as adjuncts to the primary survey, especially the CXR (Box 3.5), or during the secondary survey. These injuries include:

- simple pneumothorax (🕮 p.460);
- haemothorax (🕮 p.464);
- pulmonary contusion (see below);
- blunt cardiac injury (see below);
- tracheobronchial injury (🕮 p.466);
- traumatic aortic rupture (🕮 p.472);
- traumatic diaphragmatic rupture (see below);
- oesophageal perforation (🕮 p.200).

History
- Significant blunt trauma to the chest, or penetrating trauma to the chest or upper abdomen.
- Shock, SOB, and chest pain are common.

Examination
The examination of the chest is covered elsewhere (🕮 p.50).

❶ A full chest examination requires a log roll to examine the back.

Investigations
- FBC: to detect ↓ Hb, although Hb is often ↔ in acute haemorrhage.
- ABG: to detect and quantify ↓ PaO_2 and ↑ $PaCO_2$.
- ECG: to determine heart rate, rhythm and conduction abnormalities, and identify myocardial ischaemia and/or contusion.
- Cardiac biomarkers (e.g. troponin I/T): useful in suspected myocardial contusion.
- CXR: An AP supine CXR must be taken as an adjunct to the primary survey in significant blunt trauma, and in penetrating injuries of the neck, chest, and abdomen (Box 3.5).
  - If a patient is stable, and spinal injuries have been excluded, an erect CXR should also be performed to exclude small haemo/pneumothoraces.
- CT chest: the gold standard investigation for the detection of haemo/pneumothorax and pulmonary contusion.
  - Widely used for the investigation of suspected traumatic aortic or diaphragmatic rupture and oesophageal perforation.
  - Should only be performed in haemodynamically stable patients due to the risks of transfer.
- In haemodynamically stable patients a wide variety of other investigations may be of use, e.g. bronchoscopy, thoracoscopy, contrast studies.

Box 3.5 Interpretation of the trauma CXR

A systematic approach is essential to ensure that pathology is not missed. Examine each anatomical structure in turn, beginning centrally and working to the periphery

• Mediastinum: look for widening (traumatic aortic rupture), mediastinal air (tracheobronchial injury, oesophageal rupture, pneumoperitoneum), displacement of main bronchi (traumatic aortic rupture), and a globular heart (haemopericardium).
• Diaphragm: look very carefully for evidence of a diaphragmatic rupture (see 'Traumatic diaphragmatic rupture', this section).
• Lung fields: look for haemothorax, pneumothorax, and patchy parenchymal changes (pulmonary contusion or aspiration).
• Bones: look for fractures of the ribs, scapulae, or clavicles. Fracture patterns may suggest other injuries (e.g. aortic rupture).
• Soft tissues: look for subcutaneous emphysema (may highlight an otherwise occult pneumothorax).
• Tubes/lines/foreign bodies: check the placement of endotracheal tubes, central venous lines, NG tubes, and intercostal chest drains. Displacement of an NG tube to the right may indicate traumatic aortic rupture. Look for radio-opaque foreign bodies.

❶ Check the technical details of the film carefully. Supine films make detection of haemothoraces and pneumothoraces more difficult. AP films magnify the heart and mediastinum.

Management

• The majority of patients with cardiothoracic injuries can be managed by relatively simple measures such as intercostal chest drain insertion, IV fluid resuscitation, analgesia, and supplemental O_2.
• Only a minority of patients require emergency surgery, ideally performed in the operating room by an experienced cardiothoracic surgeon. Temporizing measures such as multiple chest drains or pericardiocentesis may be necessary.
• Rarely, emergency thoracotomy in resus may be indicated (Box 3.6).

Box 3.6 Emergency room thoracotomy

Emergency room thoracotomy is indicated in **penetrating** chest trauma where the patient is pulseless but with myocardial electrical activity.
• Access to the intrathoracic organs is most commonly gained via an anterior thoracotomy or median sternotomy, depending on which organ is most likely to be injured.
• Occasionally, bilateral anterior thoracotomies may be joined across the midline to form a 'clamshell' incision.
• Control of haemorrhage, removal of pericardial blood, cross-clamping of the descending thoracic aorta, and open cardiac massage can be achieved.

❶ Patients in **asystole** after penetrating chest trauma and those with pulseless electrical activity after **blunt** chest trauma are not candidates for emergency room thoracotomy, as the prognosis is universally dismal.

Pulmonary contusion

This is common, and potentially life-threatening, especially in those with pre-existing lung disease. It is usually seen in association with other injuries, e.g. rib fractures, pneumo/haemothorax. The accumulation of blood within the pulmonary parenchyma impairs oxygenation and causes hypoxia (shunting).

Clinical features

- Symptoms may be due to hypoxia, or associated injuries.
- Signs are non-specific and include tachypnoea and decreased air entry. Hypoxia may cause confusion and agitation.

Investigations

- CXR: shows patchy parenchymal infiltrates with ΔΔ aspiration pneumonia. These radiographic signs may take time to develop.
- CT chest: highly sensitive.
- ABG: quantifies the severity of hypoxia.

Management

Management is supportive.

- Give supplemental O_2 to maintain PaO_2 > 8kPa. Consider CPAP or mechanical ventilation, as required.
- Avoid excessive IV fluid resuscitation—central venous line placement may be useful.
- Chest physiotherapy to encourage coughing and adequate analgesia (e.g. PCA, intercostal nerve blocks, epidural) are essential.
- The development of pneumonia (i.e. pyrexia, worsening hypoxia, purulent sputum, ↑ WCC) should trigger aggressive treatment with broad-spectrum IV antibiotics.
- ❶ Manage on HDU/ITU, depending on the level of respiratory support required.

Blunt cardiac injury and myocardial contusion

Blunt cardiac injury can lead to myocardial contusion, rupture of cardiac chambers, or valvular disruption. Myocardial contusion is the most common of these injuries. Rupture of a cardiac chamber presents as cardiac tamponade (📖 p.474), whilst heart valve disruption (usually mitral or aortic valves) presents as acute LVF secondary to valvular regurgitation.

- ❶ Clinical evidence of acute valvular regurgitation in the setting of trauma should prompt immediate senior cardiology and cardiac surgical involvement to stabilize the patient prior to valve repair or replacement.
- Myocardial contusion may be asymptomatic or have significant haemodynamic consequences with compromised cardiac output. In addition, damage to the cardiac conduction system may cause dysrhythmias.

Clinical features

- Overlying sternal and rib fractures are common; consider myocardial contusion in all patients with sternal tenderness and sternal fractures on lateral sternal X-rays.
- Chest pain is common, and ↓ cardiac output may cause dyspnoea.
- Signs include shock and ↑ JVP in the absence of cardiac tamponade or tension pneumothorax.

Investigations

- The diagnosis is suggested by ECG changes, e.g. multiple ventricular ectopics, sinus tachycardia, AF, new bundle branch block, and ST segment changes.
- Echocardiography may show wall motion abnormalities.
- The diagnosis is confirmed with elevated cardiac biomarkers (e.g. cardiac troponin I/T).

Management

- Continuous ECG monitoring for at least 24h post-injury due to the risk of dysrhythmias. Discontinue after 24h free of cardiac dysrhythmias.
- For recurrent ventricular ectopics, consider an IV lidocaine bolus of 1mg/kg, then an IV infusion at 2–4mg/min.
- Hypotension may require the use of inotropes or an intra-aortic balloon pump if severe.
- ❶ Monitor on HDU/ITU and involve senior cardiology and cardiac surgical colleagues.

Traumatic diaphragmatic rupture

This may occur after blunt or penetrating trauma. Penetrating trauma tends to lead to small tears that can present many months or years later with diaphragmatic hernias. Blunt thoracic and abdominal trauma can lead to large radial diaphragmatic tears with subsequent herniation of abdominal contents into the chest. When the right hemidiaphragm is injured, the liver commonly obliterates the defect and prevents acute herniation.

Clinical features

- Often clinically occult. Large hernias can cause severe dyspnoea with decreased air entry on auscultation.
- ❶ Consider this as a ΔΔ for haemothorax. This emphasizes the importance of the finger-sweep during intercostal chest drain insertion (📖 p.522).

Investigations

- The diagnosis is usually first suspected on CXR findings:
  - irregular or unclear diaphragmatic outline;
  - elevated hemidiaphragm;
  - mass-like density above the diaphragm. This may have air within it (a 'loculated haemo/pneumothorax');
  - NG tube lying above the diaphragm.
- The diagnosis may also become apparent after insertion of an intercostal chest drain, when a finger-sweep reveals abdominal contents.
- Diagnosis can be confirmed with a CT chest/abdomen, upper GI contrast study, video-assisted thoracoscopy, or at laparotomy or thoracotomy.

Management

- If not already present, pass an NG tube to decompress the stomach.
- Repair surgically via the abdomen or the chest (open or thoracoscopic). Laparotomy is usually preferred to enable reduction and assessment of the abdominal contents.

Abdominal and pelvic trauma

The abdomen and pelvis should be assessed during the primary survey as part of 'C', as both may be the source of considerable blood loss. Because the pelvic cavity is protected by the bony pelvis, significant trauma to intrapelvic organs is usually associated with pelvic fractures.

Abdominal trauma

Blunt abdominal trauma most commonly damages the spleen (50%), liver (40%), and small bowel (5%), while penetrating trauma commonly involves the liver (40%), small bowel (30%), and diaphragm (20%).

Clinical features
- Significant blunt or penetrating trauma to the abdomen, pelvis, or lower chest.
- Shock and/or abdominal pain are common.
- Examination of the abdomen is covered elsewhere (📖 p.53, p.102).
- ❶ A DRE and vaginal examination should be performed to look for blood.
- ❶ A full abdominal examination requires a log roll to examine the back and gluteal regions.

Investigations
- FBC, U&Es, LFTs, amylase: to detect ↓ Hb, renal impairment, liver dysfunction, and pancreatic injury, respectively.
- CXR: supine films can detect diaphragmatic injury. An erect CXR is more sensitive than a supine film for detecting free subdiaphragmatic gas.
- Supine AXR: rarely useful in blunt trauma. Loss of a psoas shadow may indicate a retroperitoneal haematoma. Free gas is easy to miss.
- FAST scan.
  - A USS performed in the resus room looking for intraperitoneal or intrapericardial fluid (blood) in 4 locations (RUQ, LUQ, pelvis, pericardium).
  - Especially useful in hypotensive patients with multiple injuries due to blunt trauma, in order to detect intraperitoneal bleeding.
  - Is non-invasive and repeatable, but sensitivity is highly operator-dependent. Cannot reliably detect retroperitoneal bleeding.
- CT abdomen and pelvis.
  - Can detect intraperitoneal blood and is the investigation of choice for suspected retroperitoneal bleeding. Can identify and grade specific organ injury.
  - Non-invasive, but risk of reactions to contrast.
  - Should only be performed in haemodynamically stable patients due to the risks of transfer.
- DPL.
  - Detects intraperitoneal bleeding or perforation.
  - Periumbilical insertion of a peritoneal dialysis catheter can be performed in resus under LA. Lavage is performed with 1000mL of warmed Hartmann's and the effluent is sent for laboratory analysis.
  - A positive test is defined as: gross blood (> 10mL) or GI contents aspirated, or > 100,000 RBC/mm^3, ≥ 500 WBC/mm^3, or a Gram stain with bacteria present in the effluent fluid.

- Highly sensitive, but invasive, and has largely been replaced by FAST scans and CT. Relative contraindications include advanced pregnancy, cirrhosis, obesity, and coagulopathy. A urinary catheter and an NG tube must be inserted first.
- Laparotomy: indications are listed in Box 3.7.
  - ❶ Where a clear indication for laparotomy exists, further imaging is contraindicated.
- In haemodynamically stable patients, a wide variety of other investigations may be of use, e.g. upper or lower GI endoscopy, contrast studies.

Box 3.7 Indications for trauma laparotomy

- Blunt abdominal trauma with hypotension despite attempted fluid resuscitation and signs of intraperitoneal bleeding, including a positive FAST scan or DPL.
- Blunt abdominal trauma with a ruptured hemidiaphragm.
- Blunt or penetrating abdominal trauma with free gas seen on imaging.
- Penetrating abdominal trauma and hypotension despite attempted fluid resuscitation.
- Penetrating abdominal trauma with protruding viscera (usually small bowel or omentum).
- Penetrating abdominal trauma with upper GI, lower GI, or genitourinary bleeding.
- Signs of peritonitis after either blunt or penetrating trauma.
- Gunshot wounds to the abdomen.

Management

- Blunt injuries to the liver (📖 p.236), spleen (📖 p.252), pancreas (📖 p.250), and kidney (📖 p.386) detected on CT can often be managed non-operatively. Intraperitoneal bladder ruptures require laparotomy (📖 p.388).
- Stab wounds to the anterior abdominal wall: Up to 30% do not penetrate the peritoneal cavity. If there are no indications for trauma laparotomy, one of the following options can be followed.
  - Admission for observation and repeated examinations every 2–4h. If the patient remains well after 24h, consider discharge.
  - Wound exploration under LA. If the parietal peritoneum has been breached, laparotomy is indicated. Often difficult to perform due to inadequate instruments or lighting, patient obesity, or small wound size.
  - Diagnostic laparoscopy. Can accurately identify a peritoneal breach, requiring conversion to laparotomy.
  - DPL. A positive test mandates laparotomy.
- Stab wounds to the back or flanks. If there are no indications for trauma laparotomy, one of the following options can be followed.
  - Admission for observation and repeated examinations every 2–4h. If the patient remains well after 24h, consider discharge.
  - CT abdomen and pelvis with IV, oral, and rectal contrast to identify retroperitoneal injuries.
  - Thick musculature prevents wound exploration.

- Laparotomy (Box 3.7).
  - Usually through a full-length midline incision.
  - Ensure that 4–8 units of packed RBCs are cross-matched.
  - In patients with significant co-morbidities, multiple or complex intraabdominal injuries, a 'damage control' laparotomy is the best policy, i.e. to do the minimum needed to control bleeding and contamination with packing of potential spaces. Definitive repair and anastomoses can be performed 24–48h later once the patient has been stabilized on ITU.

Fractures of the pelvis and trauma to pelvic organs

Fractures of the pelvic ring occur only after significant blunt trauma. Therefore, other major injuries are often present. Pelvic fractures themselves can cause life-threatening haemorrhage and can damage intra-pelvic organs (e.g. rectum, bladder, urethra, vagina).

The bony pelvic ring usually breaks in two places: look at the rami and pubic symphysis for the anterior injury and look at the sacrum, sacroiliac joints, and posterior ilium for the posterior injury. Posterior injuries are often best appreciated on CT. There are 3 mechanisms by which major pelvic fractures can occur (Fig. 3.3).

- Anteroposterior compression ('open book' fracture). Compression is in the AP plane, leading to opening of the sacroiliac joint. These injuries are associated with significant blood loss due to tearing of the pelvic venous plexus and increased pelvic volume.
- Vertical shear. The affected hemipelvis shears proximally through the sacroiliac joint, e.g. after falling from a height on to one leg. This is also associated with significant blood loss.
- Lateral compression. Follows a blow from the side, pushing in the lateral wall of the pelvis. This is generally a stable injury, and is not associated with as much blood loss as the other injury patterns. Injury to pelvic organs is common.

❶ Combined injuries are also possible.

Clinical features

- History of a significant mechanism of blunt injury.
- Shock and/or lower abdominal pain are common.
- Inspect the scrotum and perineum looking for evidence of coexistent pelvic organ trauma:
  - blood at the urethral meatus or anus;
  - perineal/scrotal bruising or swelling.
- Bony pelvic deformity, leg rotation, or leg length discrepancy.
- Pain and/or instability on manipulation of the pelvic ring.
  - **❶** This must only be performed **once**, due to the risk of worsening any pelvic haemorrhage.
- Perform a DRE looking for a high-riding prostate, blood, or palpable bone fragments. Check perianal sensation and tone, as fractures through the sacrum may damage sacral nerve roots.
- Perform a vaginal examination looking for blood or palpable bone fragments.
- **❶** Blood in the rectum or vagina suggests a mucosal injury, most commonly by bone fragments (open fracture) or other penetrating objects.

Investigations
- AP pelvic X-ray as part of the trauma series.
- Before inserting a urinary catheter, perform a retrograde urethrogram if a urethral injury is suspected (📖 p.390). Once catheterized a cystogram may be required if bladder injury is suspected (📖 p.388).
- Pelvic CT: once stabilized, fracture configuration is better appreciated on CT, and can allow planning for definitive repair.

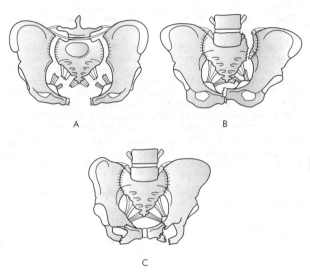

A   B

C

Fig. 3.3 (a) AP compression injury. (b) Vertical shear injury. (c) Lateral compression injury.

Management
- ❶ Aggressive IV fluid resuscitation ± blood products is required.
- The management of bladder (📖 p.388) and urethral (📖 p.390) trauma is discussed elsewhere.
- Penetrating injuries to the rectum require laparotomy for repair ± defunctioning colostomy.

The emergency treatment of pelvic fractures depends upon the facilities and expertise available.
- AP compression fractures require **immediate** closing of the book. Manoeuvres include:
  - applying a pelvic binder (e.g. a sheet wrapped around the pelvis and tied tightly anteriorly to reduce an 'open book' fracture);
  - internally rotating the legs;

- inserting an anterior pelvic external fixator. This is usually placed in the operating theatre, but occasionally can be done in resus.
- Vertical shear fractures: the aim is to reduce and stabilize the pelvis, e.g.:
  - ipsilateral leg traction and a pelvic binder or sheet;
  - placement of an anterior external fixator to hold the anterior component of the pelvic injury.
- Lateral compression fractures require very little emergency active treatment. If the pelvis feels unstable a pelvic binder may be placed. Beware of overtightening the binder as this will lead to further displacement.

If a patient with AP compression or vertical shear fractures remains haemodynamically compromised despite a pelvic binder/anterior external fixator and aggressive fluid resuscitation, emergency application of a C-clamp may be needed to stabilize the posterior injury. Where the expertise exists, emergency angiography and embolization of bleeding vessels will help reduce blood loss. If angiography is not available and an anterior external fixator and C-clamp do not restore haemodynamic stability, laparotomy and packing of the pelvis could be considered.

❶ Haemodynamic instability may also be due to ongoing blood loss from other sources, especially intraabdominal. Consideration should be given to early laparotomy. Senior input and close liaison between orthopaedic and general surgeons is mandatory.

❶ Definitive treatment of pelvic fractures is often complex and is best performed in specialist units.

Head trauma

Although head injuries can be classified by their mechanism (penetrating or blunt), or anatomy (scalp laceration, skull vault/base fracture, or intracranial haemorrhage), perhaps the most useful classification in the emergency setting is by severity. This is based on the GCS (📖 p.59) to give a score from 3 to 15:

- mild head injuries (GCS 14–15);
- moderate head injuries (GCS 9–13);
- severe head injuries (GCS 3–8).

The GCS is usually taken during the primary survey. The GCS, combined with an examination of the pupils, guides initial emergency head injury management (see rest of this section). During the secondary survey, an accurate history (where available) and detailed examination are essential.

❶ Patients with significant head injuries often have cervical spine injuries as well (📖 p.80).

History
- Mechanism of injury.
- Changes to the level of consciousness since injury.
- Presence and duration of amnesia (retrograde, antegrade).
- Episodes of vomiting or convulsions.
- Presence of headache and severity.
- Other neurological symptoms, e.g. weakness, altered sensation.
- Symptoms of a basal skull fracture (📖 p.446).
- Medication history, especially sedatives and anticoagulants.
- Recent ingestion of alcohol and illicit drugs.
- Social situation (presence of a telephone and responsible adults at home, transport).

Examination
- Scalp (lacerations, signs of skull fractures (📖 p.446)).
- Ears (bruising, CSF otorrhoea, haemotympanum, deafness).
- Nose (CSF rhinorrhoea, anosmia).
- Eyes (periorbital bruising, subconjunctival haemorrhage, pupil size and reflexes, movement, visual acuity).
  - ▶▶ A unilateral fixed, dilated pupil ('blown pupil') indicates an expanding intracranial haematoma causing transtentorial herniation. This is a neurosurgical emergency (📖 p.431).
- Cranial nerve I–XII examination.
- Peripheral neurological examination (tone, power, reflexes, co-ordination, sensation).

Investigations
The principal investigation for head injuries is the head CT. Indications for an urgent head CT include:
- GCS < 13 at any point since the injury;
- GCS < 15 at 2h post-injury;
- focal neurological deficit;

- suspected open or depressed skull fracture (📖 p.446);
- suspicion of basal skull fracture (📖 p.446);
- post-traumatic seizure;
- more than one vomit since the injury (use clinical judgement with children ≤ 12 years old);
- retrograde amnesia of > 30min duration;
- history of loss of consciousness or amnesia post-head injury plus:
  - age ≥ 65, *or*
  - coagulopathy, *or*
  - significant mechanism of injury (e.g. pedestrian hit by car, fall from > 1m height, fall down > 5 stairs).

❶ GCS < 15 should not be assumed to be due to intoxication until a significant head injury has been excluded.

❶ Skull X-rays should not be used as a surrogate for head CT as skull fractures are difficult to see and X-rays do not detect intracranial haemorrhage.

Management

Emergency management varies, depending on the severity of the head injury. The principles of management include the following.
- Prevention of secondary brain injury:
  - good oxygenation and airway protection;
  - maintenance of euvolaemia.
- Control of raised intracranial pressure (📖 p.430):
  - seizure control (📖 p.430);
  - prevention of infection.
- Frequent reassessment to detect complications, e.g. further intracranial haemorrhage.
- Close co-operation with the regional neurosurgical service. Indications for discussing a patient with a neurosurgeon include:
  - a new, potentially surgically significant abnormality on imaging;
  - persisting neurological abnormality despite normal imaging.

Mild head injuries (GCS 14–15)

The overwhelming majority of patients with a mild head injury have no underlying pathology and recover spontaneously. The aim of management is to detect the small subgroup with intracranial bleeds that may deteriorate unexpectedly.

Management

- CT head, if indicated.
- Admission for observation is required if any of the following apply:
  - abnormal head CT (requires discussion with a neurosurgeon);
  - GCS < 15, ongoing vomiting, or severe headache, even if head CT is normal;
  - CT head is required but cannot be performed, e.g. due to unavailability or lack of co-operation of the patient;
  - other issues, e.g. intoxication with alcohol/illicit drugs, other injuries, suspicion of non-accidental injury, lack of adequate adult supervision at home, significant mechanism of injury.

- If admission is required:
  - if GCS < 15, neurological observations are needed every 30min until GCS is 15;
  - if GCS = 15, neurological observations are needed every 30min for 2h, then hourly for 4h, then every 2h;
  - any new focal neurological abnormality, seizures, pupillary changes, or ↓ GCS should prompt immediate review and consideration of emergency CT head;
  - anti-emetics and IV fluids may be required if vomiting is present, especially in children;
  - give simple analgesia (paracetamol, ibuprofen) for headache.
- After observation for 12h (usually overnight), the patient can be discharged if:
  - headache and vomiting have resolved;
  - eating and drinking normally;
  - GCS 15 and neurologically normal;
  - a responsible adult can observe the patient for the next 48h.
- Before discharge, give the patient a head injury information sheet and emphasize that they must return to hospital immediately if they develop further vomiting, worsening headaches, or neurological signs.

Moderate head injuries (GCS 9–13)

The majority of these patients have abnormal CT scans, but may not require neurosurgery. A patient with a moderate head injury may deteriorate rapidly, and close observation is essential.

Management

- ❶ Treat life-threatening thoracic and abdomino-pelvic injuries first to achieve good oxygenation and haemodynamic stability.
- Request emergency CT head in all cases once haemodynamically stable. Discuss the results with the local neurosurgeon on-call, and transfer as required.
- If transfer is not required, admit to HDU/ITU and request half-hourly neurological observations.
- Maintain SaO_2 > 95% with supplemental O_2, as required.
- Give IV fluids, insert a urinary catheter, and keep urine output > 0.5mL/ kg/h.
- Difficulty in maintaining an airway mandates intubation and mechanical ventilation.
- ❶ If deterioration occurs, contact the neurosurgeons immediately.

Severe head injuries (GCS 3–8)

The patient is likely to have sustained a life-threatening head injury requiring emergency neurosurgery. Early discussion with a neurosurgeon is essential and transfer is likely.

Management

- ❶ Treat life-threatening thoracic and abdomino-pelvic injuries first to achieve good oxygenation and haemodynamic stability. This may require laparotomy/thoracotomy before a head CT.

- Intubation is required as they are unlikely to be able to protect their own airway. Give 100% O_2, and avoid hyperventilation unless requested by a neurosurgeon.
- ❶ Obtain an accurate GCS and examine the pupils before the patient is sedated or paralysed.
- Request emergency CT head in all cases once haemodynamically stable. Patient transfer should not be delayed while waiting for a CT head.
- Begin therapies to decrease intracranial pressure (e.g. mannitol, anti-convulsants) only after discussion with a neurosurgeon.

Spinal trauma

In all blunt trauma patients, spinal column injury should be assumed and actively excluded, although the priority is spinal protection and immobilization while life-threatening injuries are dealt with. Once this has been achieved, spinal imaging can occur, although this should not interfere with interhospital transfer.

The spinal column consists of 7 cervical (C), 12 thoracic (T), and 5 lumbar (L) vertebrae, as well as the sacrum and coccyx. C1 is also known as the atlas, while C2 is known as the axis. The spinal cord ends at the L1 vertebra in adults and, below this, the cauda equina continues on within the spinal canal.

Although ~ 50% of spinal injuries occur in the cervical region, remember to exclude bony and ligamentous injury to the whole spine. If spinal injury is identified, look hard for a second injury. Interpretation of spinal X-rays can be difficult, especially in children < 10 years old. A detailed description of the interpretation of spinal X-rays is beyond the scope of this book. Spinal cord injury without a radiographic abnormality (SCIWORA) can occur, and is more common in children.

Patients with spinal trauma are managed by orthopaedic or neurosurgical specialists, depending on local practice.

History of significant blunt trauma ± neck/back pain or peripheral neurological symptoms.

❶ All patients with significant blunt injuries above the level of the clavicle are at high risk of C-spine trauma.

Examination
- Neurogenic shock may be present (📖 p.52).
- Examination of the spinal column requires a log roll.
  - The spinal column should be inspected and palpated along its length, noting the location of any wounds, swellings, tenderness, crepitus, or palpable defects.
  - Where spinal column injury is suspected, a full peripheral neurological examination is necessary, including an assessment of proprioception and vibration sense. Look for a motor and sensory level. Dermatomes are shown in Fig. 3.4.
  - Perform a DRE to assess external anal sphincter tone and check perianal sensation.

❶ It is possible to clinically exclude spinal injury in an alert, orientated patient as long as all 5 exclusion criteria are met: no head injury, no drugs or alcohol, no spinal pain or tenderness, no abnormal neurology, no significant other 'distracting' injury (i.e. may 'distract' the patient from complaining about a possible spinal injury).

Investigations

C-spine X-rays (Box 3.8)
- The 3 standard X-ray views of the C-spine in trauma are the lateral, AP, and open mouth (peg) views. If the C7–T1 junction is not clearly seen on the lateral, further views can be performed, e.g. the swimmer's or oblique views. These are often difficult to interpret.

- Indications include midline neck pain, bruising, swelling, tenderness, deformity, or neurology attributable to the C-spine.
- A lateral C-spine view is obtained as part of the trauma series in patients with multiple blunt trauma. This detects 75–90% of C-spine injuries. If CT is not indicated, and the patient is haemodynamically stable, lateral and open mouth views are also required.
- ❶ In the polytrauma patient, CT of the C-spine is often performed.

Box 3.8 Interpretation of C-spine X-rays (Fig. 3.5)

A systematic approach is **essential** in order not to miss injuries.

❶ The interpretation of paediatric C-spine X-rays requires considerable expertise.

Lateral view
Use the 'ABC' system:
- Adequacy: occiput to T1 upper border seen, appropriate penetration with minimal rotation or projection.
- Alignment: the anterior vertebral bodies, posterior vertebral bodies, posterior spinal canal, and tips of the spinous processes must all be aligned. The spinous processes must all point to the same place. Anterior subluxation of C2 on C3 may be physiological in children (pseudosubluxation).
- Bones: individually outline the components of every vertebra, looking for fractures.
- Connective tissues: pre-vertebral soft tissue thickness should be < 5mm at the inferior border of C3. The atlanto–dens interval should be < 3mm in adults and < 4–5mm in children. Intervertebral disc spaces should be equal throughout the C-spine.

AP view The tips of the spinous processes and transverse processes make straight lines. Malalignment indicates malrotation (e.g. unifacet dislocation).

Open mouth (peg) view
- The joint spaces between C2 and the lateral masses of C1 should be symmetrical, as should the distance from the C1 lateral masses to the peg.
- Look for fractures through the peg, especially its base.

T- and L-spine X-rays
- The standard views are AP and lateral.
- Indications include midline back pain, bruising, swelling, tenderness, deformity, or neurology attributable to the T- or L-spine.
- If a fracture of the C-spine is identified plain X-rays of the T- and L-spine are also required.

CT C-spine (skull base to T1–4)
Indications include:
- GCS < 13 on initial assessment;
- intubated patients (open mouth view is unreliable);
- a C-spine fracture is seen or suspected on plain X-rays;

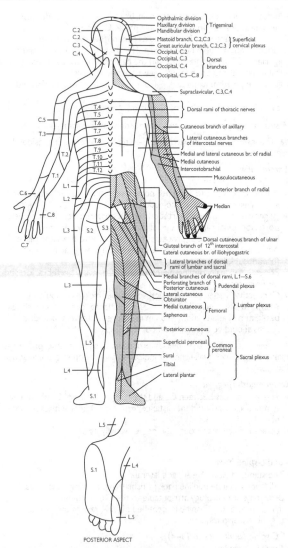

Fig. 3.4 (a) Dermatomes and cutaneous nerves. (Reproduced, with permission, from Wyatt, J.P., *et al.* (1999). *Oxford handbook of accident and emergency medicine*, 1st edn, pp. 402–3. Oxford University Press, Oxford.)

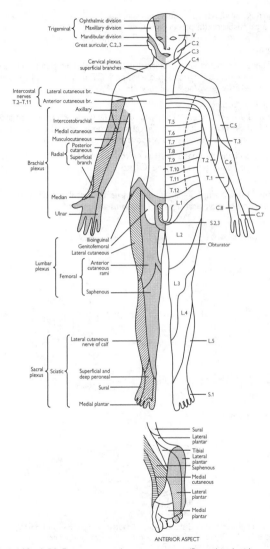

ANTERIOR ASPECT

Fig. 3.4 (*Cont.*) **(b)** Dermatomes and cutaneous nerves. (Reproduced, with permission, from Wyatt, J.P., *et al.* (1999). *Oxford handbook of accident and emergency medicine*, 1st edn, pp. 402–3. Oxford University Press, Oxford.)

- plain X-ray views are inadequate;
- clinical suspicion despite normal C-spine X-rays;
- in the polytrauma patient, where CT of other regions is being performed.

❶ There is an increased risk of irradiation to the thyroid gland in children < 10 years old. In this age group, discuss neck CT with the radiologists and orthopaedic surgeons/neurosurgeons first.

CT of T- or L-spine

Indicated if there are any abnormal, suspicious or poorly visualized areas identified on plain X-ray, or if clinical suspicion is high. The scan should include the entire vertebral body above and below the level of injury.

❶ It is difficult to image the upper thoracic spine on plain X-rays— consider extending the C-spine CT to T4 in high-energy polytrauma patients.

Spinal MRI Obtain if significant soft tissue or vascular injuries are suspected, or if neurological signs or symptoms are present.

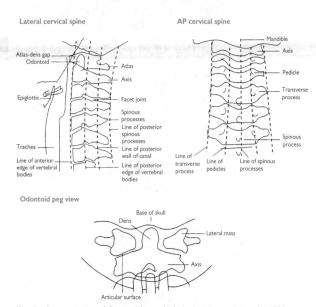

Fig. 3.5 Interpretation of C-spine X-rays. (Adapted, with permission, from Wyatt, J.P., et al. (1999). *Oxford handbook of accident and emergency medicine*, 1st edn, p. 401. Oxford University Press, Oxford.)

Management

- If the C-spine X-rays are normal, CT is not indicated, and neck pain/ tenderness and abnormal neurology are not present, the C-spine can be cleared.
  - ❶ Only clinicians with appropriate training and experience should decide whether or not to clear the spine and remove spinal protection.
- The C-spine can be declared 'stable' for nursing care after normal C-spine X-rays and C-spine CT. These should be reported on by an experienced trauma radiologist or orthopaedic or neurosurgical specialist.
- If spinal injury is suspected or identified:
  - maintain strict C-spine protection and spinal immobilization;
  - treat neurogenic shock (📖 p.55), if present;
  - insert a urinary catheter and NG tube.

❶ Discuss with neurosurgical or orthopaedic colleagues **immediately**. Only specialists should decide if an injury is stable or unstable.

❶ Transverse fractures through the thoracolumbar vertebrae (Chance fractures) are associated with retroperitoneal and visceral injuries.

◈ The use of high-dose IV methylprednisolone in spinal cord trauma is controversial. Discuss with neurosurgical or orthopaedic colleagues first.

Musculoskeletal trauma

Active bleeding from limb injuries should be controlled during the primary survey as part of 'C'. Obvious long bone fractures (especially femoral fractures) should be reduced to an approximate anatomical position and splinted as part of haemorrhage control. Any fractures not reduced at this point should be reduced as an adjunct to the primary survey.

A full assessment of the peripheral musculoskeletal system should be performed during the secondary survey. Full and adequate assessment and appropriate referral is essential in order to avoid missing potentially limb- or life-threatening injuries such as open fractures (📖 p.406), peripheral nerve injuries (📖 p.418), compartment syndrome (📖 p.412), and vascular injuries (📖 p.337).

History
- Mechanism of injury.
- Tetanus immunization history.

Examination
Do a thorough examination of the injured area, and always examine the joint above and below.
- Look: deformity, swellings, wounds, pale extremity.
- Feel: crepitus, tenderness, swellings.
- Move: range of motion (active and passive), joint instability.
- ❶ Actively exclude a compartment syndrome.
- ❶ Perform a thorough neurovascular examination. A hand-held Doppler probe is useful to detect distal pulses in swollen limbs, but proximal vascular injury cannot be excluded.

Investigations
- Plain X-rays: at least 2 views (usually AP and lateral), with the joint above and below included.
  - ❶ Soft tissue injuries are not apparent on X-rays but are a considerable source of morbidity.
- CT/MRI: when X-ray findings are equivocal or for soft tissue injuries (MRI).

Management
- Give adequate parenteral opioid analgesia.
- Fractures or fracture/dislocations with impaired distal perfusion should be reduced **immediately**. Do not delay for X-rays.
- Immobilize all fractured extremities with splints and reduce any dislocations. Check the distal pulses before and after reduction.
- Consider every fracture with an overlying skin wound as being open, even if it is only an abrasion.
- Suspected peripheral nerve injury or compartment syndrome must be referred to an orthopaedic surgeon **immediately**.
- Suspected vascular injury mandates **immediate** referral to a vascular surgeon.

Key points in common musculoskeletal injuries

A detailed description of the management of common musculoskeletal injuries is beyond the scope of this book. Below are some key points on common musculoskeletal injuries in the polytrauma patient, arranged anatomically.

- Sternal fracture.
  - Commonly in the body of the sternum.
  - Always consider myocardial contusion (📖 p.68) as an underlying injury.
  - Fixation is rarely required.
- Sternoclavicular dislocation.
  - May dislocate anteriorly or posteriorly. Posterior dislocation needs urgent reduction due to the risk of vascular compromise.
  - A high-energy injury; consider occult injuries elsewhere, e.g. traumatic aortic rupture.
  - It is difficult to image the sternoclavicular joint with plain X-rays. If suspected, obtain a CT scan of the thoracic inlet and chest.
- Fracture of the clavicle.
  - Check the distal neurovascular status and overlying skin. Urgent surgery is only required if the skin is threatened, or if neurovascular compromise or an open fracture is present.
- Fracture of the scapula.
  - Usually treated non-operatively, unless the fracture involves the glenoid and is displaced.
  - This is a high-energy injury; consider occult injuries elsewhere, e.g. traumatic aortic rupture.
- Dislocation of the shoulder joint.
  - Usually anterior. Check for axillary nerve function (📖 p.420).
  - Posterior dislocations can easily be missed. Have a high index of suspicion, particularly in electrocutions and patients with epilepsy. Patients present with a painful shoulder and reduced external rotation. Get an axillary view radiograph if in doubt—don't accept a poor quality lateral scapular view.
- Fracture of the humeral shaft.
  - Check radial nerve function (📖 p.420). Document function clearly before applying any splints or braces.
  - Most humeral shaft fractures are treated non-operatively unless open or polytrauma is present.
- Supracondylar elbow fracture.
  - Common in children. Check the function of the radial, ulnar, and median nerves (📖 p.420), and perfusion of the hand.
- Dislocation of the elbow joint.
  - Requires urgent reduction. Most reduce with inline traction.
  - Carefully check for radial, ulnar, and median nerve function (📖 p.420) and vascular deficits pre- and post-reduction.
  - Document stability post-reduction. In children, ensure that the medial epicondyle is not stuck in the joint post-reduction (it ossifies at ~ 6–7 years of age).
- Combined fractures of the radius and ulna.
  - Examine closely for compartment syndrome (📖 p.412), ensuring full passive extension and flexion of the fingers.

- Isolated fracture of the radius or ulna.
  - Check median nerve function (📖 p.420).
  - If only one bone in the forearm is fractured look closely to exclude associated dislocation of the proximal or distal radioulnar joint, i.e. Galeazzi (fracture in the distal 1/3rd of the radius with dislocation of distal radioulnar joint) or Monteggia (fracture of the proximal ulna with dislocation of the radial head).
- Fracture of the scaphoid.
  - Feel for tenderness in the anatomical snuff box. Easy to miss in the polytrauma patient.
- Carpal dislocations.
  - Radiocarpal, lunate, or perilunar dislocations may be associated with fractures of carpal bones. They require emergency reduction if median nerve compression is present (📖 p.420).
- Dislocations of metacarpophalangeal and interphalangeal joints.
  - Most interphalangeal joint dislocations will reduce easily with inline traction.
  - Beware of metacarpophalangeal dislocations, as longitudinal traction may tighten the soft tissues and entrap the metacarpal head, or pull the volar plate into the joint. Metacarpophalangeal dislocations are best **pushed** back into place, **not** pulled. Seek orthopaedic advice early. Test and document the stability of the joint post-reduction.
- Pelvic injuries (📖 p.72).
- Hip dislocation.
  - Usually posterior. The leg lies internally rotated and shortened. Often associated with posterior wall fracture. Requires emergency reduction to minimize the risk of AVN. Check sciatic nerve function (📖 p.421).
  - In anterior dislocation, the leg lies externally rotated, abducted, and slightly flexed. A rare injury. Requires emergency reduction. May get femoral vein thrombosis. If reduction is delayed, consider placing an IVC filter prior to reduction.
  - Central dislocation follows a direct blow to side of hip, driving the hip into the pelvis through the floor of the acetabulum. Emergency treatment is with resuscitation and in-line traction.
- Hip dislocation (prosthetic joint).
  - Usually a posterior dislocation after flexion and internal rotation. Check sciatic nerve function (📖 p.421). Reduce by flexing the hip and knee to 90° and then pull up to the ceiling, allowing the hip to rotate freely as it reduces. Alternatively, try in-line traction and hip adduction.
  - Anterior dislocation occurs after extension and external rotation. Reduce with in-line traction or convert to a posterior dislocation and reduce as above.
- Fracture of the femoral neck.
  - Femoral neck fractures in the elderly are **totally different** to those in the young patient. Consider the force/energy involved.
  - ❶ An intracapsular femoral neck fracture in a young patient is an emergency due to the risk of AVN. Involve an orthopaedic surgeon early.

- Fracture of the femoral shaft.
  - Emergency treatment is with resuscitation and temporary splintage (Thomas splint) and in-line traction. Definitive treatment in an adult is a reamed intramedullary nail.
  - Ensure adequate X-rays of the femoral neck; there is a 10–15% incidence of ipsilateral femoral neck fracture.
  - ❶ Blood loss can be > 1000mL. Ensure adequate resuscitation.
- Knee dislocation.
  - A high-energy injury, with a significant risk of injury to the popliteal artery (📖 p.337), common peroneal nerve, and/or tibial nerve (📖 p.421).
  - Requires **emergency** reduction. Check the distal neurovascular status pre- and post-reduction: presence of any neurovascular symptoms or signs mandate an angiogram to rule out an intimal lesion to the popliteal artery. Have a very low threshold to obtain an angiogram even if the pulses are normal. If no angiogram is obtained make sure you constantly re-assess the limb for any signs of vascular injury.
- Fracture of the tibia.
  - Exclude compartment syndrome (📖 p.412). Don't underestimate simple transverse fractures; they too can develop a compartment syndrome.
- Fracture–dislocation of the ankle joint.
  - If the limb is grossly deformed, reduce it with in-line traction and place in a splint **before** getting an X-ray. This takes the pressure off neurovascular structures and helps prevent further soft tissue injury.
- Fracture of the calcaneus.
  - Usually caused by fall from a height with axial load. Actively look for and exclude an injury to the lumbar spine.
- Fracture of the talus.
  - If displaced, urgent open reduction and internal fixation is required. Seek orthopaedic input **early**.
- Fracture–dislocation of the midfoot (Lisfranc injury).
  - X-rays of the midfoot may be difficult to interpret. Look at the foot; it normally swells dramatically.
  - Beware of compartment syndrome (📖 p.412) and vascular compromise. Splint, elevate, and seek orthopaedic input.

Trauma in children

The basic principles underlying the management of polytrauma in children are identical to those in adults. However, multiple injuries are more common due to small body size, and internal organs are more easily damaged due to reduced body fat and incompletely calcified bones.

In addition, specific anatomical and physiological differences need to be taken into account (see later this section and 📖 p.356). Also, be aware of the specific psychological needs of children—the presence of the parent in the resuscitation room may help reduce the child's anxiety.

- ❶ Use a Broselow™ tape to estimate weight and calculate drug doses, tube sizes, fluid boluses, airway sizes, etc.
- ❶ Involve the on-call paediatric team early. Transfer to a specialist paediatric unit may be required for expertise in either paediatric intensive care or paediatric surgery. The on-call paediatric team will be aware of local protocols regarding transfer.
- ❶ Have a high index of suspicion for NAI. If suspected, involve the paediatric team **immediately**.

Airway with cervical spine protection

- Increased size of the cranium relative to the body in infants and toddlers induces passive flexion of the head and neck when lying flat. Place padding under the entire torso to open the airway.
- Oropharyngeal (Guedel) airways should not be rotated within the oropharynx due to the risk of local trauma. Insert directly.
- Endotracheal intubation.
  - Airway anatomy is altered, making endotracheal intubation more difficult.
  - Use uncuffed tubes in children < 10 years old.
  - Inadvertent intubation of the right main bronchus is easier due to the short length of the trachea.
- Cricothyroidotomy should only be performed when the cricothyroid membrane is palpable, usually after 10 years of age. If impalpable, use jet insufflation.
- A distressed child is difficult to immobilize; consider removing the semi-rigid collar, blocks, and tapes and using manual in-line stabilization.

❶ Paediatric airway management requires specialist knowledge and skills. Call for a senior anaesthetist **immediately** if simple measures alone are unable to open the airway.

Breathing

Normal respiratory rates decrease with age (📖 p.357).

Circulation with haemorrhage control

- Normal heart rates, BP, and urine outputs vary with age (📖 p.357).
- Normal blood volume in a child is 80mL/kg.
- ❶ Early signs of shock are masked due to increased physiological reserve.
- Intravenous access can be difficult.
  - If peripheral IV access cannot be obtained in children < 7 years old, consider intraosseous infusion via the proximal tibia or distal femur in an uninjured limb.

- Central venous line placement may also be difficult.
- Give 20mL/kg warmed Hartmann's IV for resuscitation of the shocked child.
- If signs of shock persist after 2 × 20mL/kg boluses:
  - consider non-haemorrhagic shock;
  - if haemorrhagic shock is likely, consider a 10mL/kg bolus of packed RBCs and give a further 20mL/kg Hartmann's bolus.
- Unlike in adults, intracranial haemorrhage **can** result in hypotension in infants due to unfused cranial sutures and fontanelles.

Disability (neurological assessment)

In children < 4 years old, use the paediatric verbal scale for GCS (check with the parents/guardians regarding the best usual response):
- alert, babbles, coos, words or sentences to usual ability, 5 points;
- less than usual ability and/or spontaneous irritable cry, 4 points;
- cries inappropriately, 3 points;
- occasionally whimpers and/or moans, 2 points;
- no vocal response, 1 point.

In pre-verbal children, assess the grimace 'verbal' response:
- spontaneous normal facial/oro-motor activity, 5 points;
- less than usual spontaneous ability or only response to touch, 4 points;
- vigorous grimace to pain, 3 points;
- mild grimace to pain, 2 points;
- no response to pain, 1 point.

Exposure/environment

❶ High body surface area to volume ratio and less body fat lead to rapid development of hypothermia. Use active warming devices.

Trauma in pregnant women

As with trauma in the paediatric population, the basic principles underlying the management of trauma in pregnant women remain unchanged except for the recognition of certain anatomical and physiological differences. Resuscitation of the fetus is best served by adequately resuscitating the mother.

Specific traumatic obstetric pathologies to consider include uterine rupture and placental abruption.

- Uterine rupture can occur after blunt or penetrating trauma and presents with abdominal pain, shock, abdominal tenderness or peritonism, and easy palpation of fetal parts. Extended fetal limbs on X-ray also suggest uterine rupture. **Emergency** laparotomy is required.
- Placental abruption may occur after even relatively minor injuries. The diagnosis is suggested by abdominal pain, shock, uterine tenderness, or irritability. Blood may or may not be seen in the vagina.

❶ Consider the possibility of pregnancy in all females aged 10–50. Obtain urine or blood early for βhCG testing.

❶ In women with significant trauma and confirmed pregnancy, involve the on-call obstetric team early. Emergency Caesarean section may be required for the above conditions. C-section after maternal cardiac arrest due to haemorrhagic shock is unlikely to be successful as prolonged hypotension fatally compromises the fetus.

Primary survey

Breathing In the 3rd trimester the growing uterus compresses the thoracic cavity. Insert intercostal chest drains in the 4th intercostal space rather than the 5th (📖 p.522).

Circulation with haemorrhage control

- Physiological changes to the heart rate and BP may mimic shock:
  - heart rate increases by 10-15bpm.
  - systolic and diastolic BP ↓ by 5–15mmHg in the 2nd trimester, but return to normal at term.
- On palpation of the abdomen, signs of peritonitis may be masked as the gravid uterus displaces and conceals intraabdominal organs.
- Increased plasma volume leads to physiological anaemia of pregnancy.
  - In the 3rd trimester, the mother may not exhibit clinical features of shock until > 1000mL blood lost.
  - Even in seemingly haemodynamically normal women, give bolus resuscitation fluids, as fetal oxygenation may be compromised by small reductions in maternal blood volume.
- Maternal cardiac output can be compromised by the uterus compressing the IVC.
  - Manually displace the uterus to the patient's left.
  - Partially roll the patient to the left using a wedge or pillow under the right hip. If spinal injury is possible, roll on the spinal board.

Adjuncts to the primary survey

- Physiological changes lead to alterations in FBC, U&Es, and ABG results (Box 3.9).

- Delayed gastric emptying leads to a high risk of aspiration. Have a low threshold for insertion of an NG tube.
- Critical radiological investigations should **not** be withheld. Pelvic XR may show physiological widening of the symphysis pubis. Maternal pelvic fracture may result in fetal head trauma in the late 3rd trimester. Check for fetal limb positioning.
- DPL may result in uterine perforation and should **only** be performed by a senior surgeon.
- Trauma may result in fetal blood entering the maternal circulation. In rhesus-negative women this may result in immunization against fetal rhesus D antigen and haemolytic disease of the newborn. Give anti-D immunoglobulin to all Rh-negative mothers with significant trauma. Do **not** rely on the Kleihauer test.

Assessment of the fetus

This should be performed by a member of the obstetric team **before** the secondary survey of the mother.

- For fetuses > 10 weeks' gestation, check for viability by listening for the fetal heart beat with a hand-held Doppler.
- For fetuses > 20 weeks' gestation a cardiotocogram can be used to measure uterine contractions and the response of the fetal heart rate.

Maternal secondary survey

- A vaginal exam should be performed by a member of the obstetric team, looking for bleeding, amniotic fluid in the vagina, and cervical dilatation.
- The uterus and fetus should be palpated looking for tenderness, positioning, and fetal lie.

Box 3.9 Altered laboratory indices in pregnant women

- FBC. Mild ↓ Hb due to the physiological anaemia of pregnancy. Mild ↑ WCC (12–15) is normal.
- U&Es. Decreased creatinine due to ↑ GFR and renal blood flow, therefore ↑ creatinine is a concern.
- ABG. ↑ Tidal volume leads to mildly ↓ $PaCO_2$. A normal $PaCO_2$ in late pregnancy may indicate incipient respiratory failure.

Tetanus

Tetanus is a potentially fatal disease characterized by acute rigidity and spasms of skeletal muscle, caused by the toxin produced by *Clostridium tetani*, an anaerobic, Gram-positive, spore-forming rod. *Clostridium* spores remain present in soil and animal faeces for years. Anaerobic conditions within wounds encourage spore germination and production of toxin (tetanospasmin).

Immunization against tetanus is achieved with a tetanus toxoid vaccine. This is usually given as a combined diphtheria and tetanus vaccine. In the UK, a primary (3 dose) course is given to a pre-school child. Two booster doses are given: the first at 4–5 years of age; the last at 15 years of age. Any adult who has received 5 doses is likely to have lifelong immunity.

Where immediate protection is required, tetanus immunoglobulin can be given. This provides transient protection while tetanus toxoid immunization takes effect.

❶ Good wound management and assessment of tetanus immunization status is essential to prevent tetanus.

Wound management

- Obtain the tetanus vaccination history:
  - group A: fully immunized (i.e. a total of 5 doses of tetanus vaccine received at appropriate intervals);
  - group B: primary course completed, boosters up-to-date, but full 5 doses yet to be given (e.g. a 14 year old yet to receive a final booster);
  - group C: primary immunization incomplete or boosters not up-to-date;
  - group D: non-immunized or vaccination history unknown.
- Clean and debride the wound meticulously.
  - ❶ If this cannot be adequately achieved under LA, refer for debridement under GA.
- Decide if the wound is tetanus-prone (Box 3.10).
- Give tetanus immunization/immunoglobulin as required (see "Tetanus prevention').
  - The standard prophylaxis dose of tetanus immunoglobulin is 250U IM. Give 500U if > 24h since injury or if there is a risk of heavy contamination, or following burns.
  - The tetanus toxoid vaccine can be given to pregnant women and those with HIV. Previous anaphylaxis (extremely rare) is a contra-indication to further vaccination.

❶ Consider giving co-amoxiclav 625mg tds PO or metronidazole 400mg tds PO for 5 days for tetanus-prone wounds.

Box 3.10 Tetanus-prone wounds

- Wounds/burns > 6h old.
- Wounds/burns with a significant degree of devitalized tissue.
- Puncture wounds.
- Wounds where there has been contact with soil or manure.
- Wounds containing foreign bodies.
- Open fractures (📖 p.406).
- Wounds/burns in patients who have systemic sepsis.

Tetanus prevention

Clean wounds
- Groups A and B. Tetanus vaccine or immunoglobulin not required.
- Group C. Give the combined diphtheria/tetanus vaccine. Further doses may be needed to complete the schedule.
- Group D. Give the combined diphtheria/tetanus vaccine. Further doses will be needed to complete the schedule.

Tetanus-prone wounds
- Groups A and B. Tetanus vaccine not required. Give tetanus immuno-globulin if the risk of infection is high (e.g. contamination with manure, or extensive devitalized tissue).
- Group C. Give the combined diphtheria/tetanus vaccine. Further doses may be needed to complete the schedule. Give tetanus immunoglob-ulin.
- Group D. Give the combined diphtheria/tetanus vaccine. Further doses will be needed to complete the schedule. Give tetanus immunoglobulin.

❶ Inject tetanus vaccine and immunoglobulin at different sites.

❶ Patients who are immunosuppressed (e.g. HIV infection, transplant recipients, chemotherapy patients) may not be adequately protected, despite having full tetanus immunization. They should be managed as if they were incompletely immunized (group C).

The acute abdomen

Introduction

The acute abdomen may be defined as abdominal pain of recent onset requiring urgent surgical assessment. The commonest surgical cause is acute appendicitis (Table 4.1), but it is more common for no diagnosis to be made, so-called non-specific abdominal pain. This is a diagnosis of exclusion, and a thorough assessment is necessary before such a diagnosis is made; many such cases re-present in the future with identifiable pathology.

Anatomy and embryology

A knowledge of embryology helps understanding of the differences in visceral and parietal pain, and the different patterns of radiation of pain.

Embryologically, the gut is divided into foregut, midgut, and hindgut.

- The foregut forms the oesophagus, stomach, and the duodenum proximal to the opening of the CBD. Outpouchings of the primitive foregut give rise to the liver, biliary tree, and pancreas.
- The midgut forms the duodenum distal to the opening of the CBD, the rest of the small intestine, caecum, appendix, and right colon to 2/3rds of the way along the transverse colon.
- The hindgut gives rise to the distal transverse colon down to the rectum and upper anal canal. The bladder also derives from hindgut.

The arterial supply to the foregut is from the coeliac trunk, to midgut is from the SMA, and to the hindgut from the IMA.

The kidneys form from the metanephroi, and ascend the retroperitoneum along the aorta to the loins. Failure of ascent gives rise to a pelvic kidney, and fusion of metanephric buds in front of the aorta creates a horseshoe kidney, which appears as a mass lying in front of the aorta. On palpation, this can easily be confused with an AAA, although it is not expansile.

The testes arise from embryological precursors cranial to the kidneys, and descend the abdomen through the inguinal canals into the scrotum.

Abdominal pain

Location of the pain and nomenclature

Although the location of the pain may alter during disease progression, the site of the most severe pain is often the best indicator of which structure is diseased. The abdomen is nominally divided into 9 regions (Fig. 4.1) or 4 quadrants (right and left, lower and upper). Surgical usage tends to mix the two, referring to the right and left upper quadrant in place of the right and left hypochondrium. For this reason we follow common surgical parlance in this chapter, while recognizing that it is not strictly accurate.

Table 4.1 Causes of the acute abdomen

Cause	Approximate incidence (%)
Non-specific abdominal pain	35
Acute appendicitis	20
Intestinal obstruction	15
Biliary pain	10
Urological causes	6
Acute colonic diverticulitis	3
Perforatiion	2
Acute pancreatitis	2
Ruptured AAA	< 1
Mesenteric ischaemia	< 1
Gynaecological emergencies	< 1
Miscellaneous, e.g. primary peritonitis	4

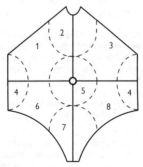

Fig. 4.1 Regions of the abdomen. 1, Right hypochondrium; 2, epigastrium; 3, left hypochondrium; 4, right and left flanks/loins; 5, periumbilical region; 6, right iliac fossa; 7, suprapubic region; 8, left iliac fossa.

Visceral versus parietal pain

- Visceral pain.
  - Arises from stretching, distension, or early inflammation of an organ, the pain being a non-specific ache felt in relation to the embryological origin (Fig. 4.2).
  - Pain from foregut structures is referred to the epigastrium.
  - Pain from midgut structures is referred to the umbilicus.
  - Pain from hindgut structures is referred to the suprapubic region.
  - ❶ Testicular visceral pain is also experienced periumbilically.
- Parietal (somatic) pain.
  - Arises from irritation of the overlying parietal peritoneum.
  - Is perceived to be from the overlying dermatome.
  - Tends to be sharper, more intense, and better localized than visceral pain.
  - Is exacerbated by movement and coughing.
  - Parietal involvement also results in involuntary guarding of the overlying muscles.

With disease progression and involvement of the parietal peritoneum, visceral pain develops a more dominant parietal component, e.g. in appendicitis the initial visceral pain is experienced periumbilically but, as inflammation progresses and involves the parietal peritoneum, the pain becomes localized to the RIF—the parietal component.

Radiation of pain

- Pain radiating from loin to groin is from obstruction of the renal tract (Fig. 4.2). It can be mimicked by an expanding haematoma from an AAA stripping the posterior parietal peritoneum caudally as it increases in size.
- Biliary pain radiates through to the inferior angle of the right scapula.
- Shoulder tip pain implies diaphragmatic irritation by pus, gut contents, or blood (Kehr's sign). This is due to the diaphragmatic somatic innervation coming from C3,4,5. It can be precipitated by tipping the patient head-down—particularly useful in a female where a ruptured ectopic pregnancy is being considered.
- Testicular torsion may present with abdominal pain, rather than testicular pain, particularly in young children.

Onset of pain

- Sudden onset of severe pain implies an abdominal catastrophe, such as a perforated viscus or ruptured aneurysm or ectopic pregnancy.
- Rapid onset pain occurs with acute pancreatitis or torsion of either an ovary or testis.
- Pain from inflammatory conditions usually develops gradually (over hours), e.g. appendicitis, diverticulitis.

Periodicity of pain

- Colicky pain arises from the renal tract (renal or ureteric colic), bowel (intestinal obstruction, early appendicitis), uterus (parturition, ectopic pregnancy), or the ampulla of Vater (ampullary colic—biliary colic with jaundice when a stone impacts in the ampulla).
- Constant pain occurs with most inflammatory conditions, perforation, and ischaemic bowel. Biliary colic is a misnomer—it is also a constant pain.

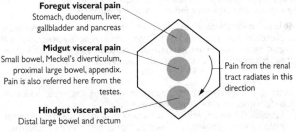

Foregut visceral pain
Stomach, duodenum, liver, gallbladder and pancreas

Midgut visceral pain
Small bowel, Meckel's diverticulum, proximal large bowel, appendix. Pain is also referred here from the testes.

Pain from the renal tract radiates in this direction

Hindgut visceral pain
Distal large bowel and rectum

Fig. 4.2 Referred and radiating abdominal pain.

Assessment of the acute abdomen

The principal objective of the assessment

The principal objective of the assessment process is to answer the following questions.

- Does the patient need an operation?
- If so, when? (📖 p.14)

These questions are usually answered after taking a history, performing an examination, and analysing the results of investigations. Arriving at a diagnosis is sometimes a secondary issue. Repeated assessment over 12–24h is valuable when the need for an operation is initially in doubt.

❶ In polytrauma patients and those with severe shock or sepsis this linear approach may be unsafe (📖 p.4). These patients require resuscitation and urgent senior review with a view to immediate surgery. In such cases, theatre is more likely to save a life than time in CT.

History

Focused history-taking is imperative in assessing the acute abdomen. Carefully document the sequence of events.

- Establish the where, when, what (nature), how long, how bad, and what makes it worse (movement, cough, eating) or better (lying still, leaning forward).
- Check for accompanying features, e.g. rigors, jaundice.

Do a thorough systems review seeking features of GI, urological, and gynaecological disturbance. Specifically consider:

- upper GI symptoms: vomiting (volume, frequency, contents, especially blood), appetite, weight loss, dysphagia, heartburn;
- lower GI symptoms: diarrhoea, constipation, flatus, PR bleeding, change of bowel habit;
- urinary symptoms: frequency, dysuria, haematuria;
- gynaecological symptoms: vaginal bleeding, discharge, LMP, recent menstrual history.

Check for a past history of similar events, surveillance investigations (e.g. USS for AAA), and the past surgical and medical history.

- Document the medications, noting any recent changes.
- Allergies, particularly to antibiotics, iodine, and latex.
- Social history, especially alcohol, tobacco, and recreational drug use.
- Recent travel.
- Have any friends or family been similarly affected?

In most cases a diagnosis should now be apparent.

Examination

While the history should give you the diagnosis, the examination will convey the urgency with which treatment is required. The initial overview of the patient can take place while starting the history taking, with a view to deciding quickly whether to start immediate resuscitation before resuming a more detailed history and examination.

Inspection

Inspect the patient as a whole.
- Do they look ill—are they pale, jaundiced, dehydrated, sweaty, or cachectic? Are they cold and clammy or warm and well-perfused?
- Do they look in pain?
- Are they mobile, or lying as still as possible?
- Patients with peritonitis stay still; it hurts to cough or move.
- Ureteric and ampullary colic patients are restless and walk about, as if they are trying to jolt the stone along.
- Patients with acute pancreatitis sometimes gain relief by sitting forward.
- Are there signs of systemic disease?
- Is the patient mentally bright or confused? Can they respond to questions? If not, is this a new occurrence?

Review the vital signs.
- Pulse—is there a tachycardia or AF (think mesenteric embolus)? Is the pulse volume weak?
- Is the BP normal or low? Is the patient shocked?
- Is tachypnoea present, and is SaO_2 low on pulse oximetry?

Inspect the abdomen.
- Expose the abdomen completely, covering the genitalia until the end of the examination.
- Is the abdomen distended, and is intestinal peristalsis visible?
- Does the abdomen move normally with respiration, or is it still?
- Look for previous scars and determine what surgery caused them.
- Are Cullen's sign or Grey Turner's sign present (periumbilical or flank bruising, respectively, due to retroperitoneal haemorrhage)?
- Are there any hernias? Expose the groins completely to be sure not to miss a femoral hernia.
- Are there any stomas?

❶ Remember, it is better expose the patient now and find the hernia, than later at autopsy because you missed it

Palpation
- Ask the patient to cough—does this cause or exacerbate the pain?
- Ask the patient to point to the site of worst pain.
- Begin palpation at a site remote from the pain, lightly at first before deeper palpation.
- Is there guarding? Guarding may be voluntary or involuntary.
  - Involuntary guarding is a reflex increase in resistance (muscle contraction) to an increasing force of palpation and reflects underlying peritonitis.
  - Voluntary guarding is a conscious contraction of the abdominal muscles and may represent anxiety rather than pathology.
- Is there rigidity (spasm of the abdominal muscles regardless of palpation)?
- Eliciting rebound tenderness by depressing the hand into the abdomen and suddenly releasing it causes extreme pain in patients with peritonitis and should **not** be performed. Evidence of rebound tenderness can be gained by eliciting pain on coughing, or by gentle percussion of

the abdomen. Only if you want to confirm that the patient does **not** have peritonitis is formal testing for rebound tenderness appropriate.

- Difficult patient? When you are unsure whether the patient is anxious and exaggerating pain, try palpating with the stethoscope whilst auscultating. Tenderness or rebound elicited this way is genuine. Also, palpate across the inguinal ligament, from below (extraperitoneal) to above (peritoneal) and, in the presence of peritonitis, pain is experienced as you cross the ligament—difficult to fake.
- Perform the psoas stretch test in suspected retrocaecal appendicitis (📖 p.262).
- Look for hernias, particularly in patients with intestinal obstruction. Careful examination of the inguinal and femoral canals is essential.
- Remember Murphy's (📖 p.228) and Rovsing's signs (📖 p.264).
- If you find a mass determine its size, shape, consistency, and margins.
  • Can you define all around it?
  • Is it pulsatile or expansile?
  • Is it resonant (i.e. overlying bowel gas) or dull?
  • Is it ballotable, implying a mass arising from the kidney?
- In males, examine the external genitalia. Look for scrotal erythema and palpate the testes to exclude torsion, masses, or epididymo-orchitis.
- Remove any stoma bags and inspect the intestinal mucosa—is there ulceration, blood, or is it ischaemic? Perform a digital examination via the stoma if necessary (an ileostomy may be too narrow).

Percussion

- Gentle abdominal percussion reveals rebound tenderness. Loss of dullness on percussion over the liver may indicate free gas from a perforation.
- Percuss the margins of any mass, determine the presence of ascites, and listen for the resonance of any distended gas-filled gut.

Auscultation

- Listen for the presence or absence of bowel sounds, and their character: increased bowel sounds in mechanical obstruction; absent in peritonitis.
- In a patient with vomiting listen for a succussion splash (implying gastric outlet obstruction) on gently rocking the patient from side-to-side.
- In a shocked patient with a possible ruptured AAA listen for the machinery murmur of an aorto-caval fistula.

Digital rectal examination (DRE)

Always consider performing a DRE in adults with acute abdominal pain, especially lower abdominal pain.

- Check for a mass, blood/melaena, tenderness, faecal loading, pale stool.
- Perform a faecal occult blood test.
- In uncertain diagnoses a DRE can help differentiate a possible UTI or gastroenteritis from a pelvic appendicitis, as well as being difficult to fake in the case of an opiate seeker. A finger pressed posteriorly against the sacrum should cause no pain; when moved anteriorly it encounters the peritoneal reflection and is painful in the presence of pelvic peritonitis.

❶ An old surgical aphorism states that there are only two excuses not to do a DRE—no finger, or no rectum! While this may overstate its usefulness, it is often not done when indicated. Obtain consent first.

❶ If appendicitis is thought likely, consider combining your DRE with giving a metronidazole suppository.

Vaginal examination may be indicated in women with lower abdominal pain. Best performed once only and by someone experienced enough to detect the pathology/evidence that is being looked for. Always have a chaperone, and always seek the patient's consent first.

Urine examination

Urine dipstick testing is part of a routine examination. Test for blood, protein, bilirubin, glucose, ketones, nitrites, and leucocytes. Send the urine for microscopy, culture, and sensitivity (M, C, & S) if the dipstick is abnormal. Test for βhCG in all females of child-bearing age.

❶ This is essential to exclude a ruptured ectopic pregnancy

Look again!

If you are uncertain of the diagnosis or severity, go back 2–4h later and review.

❶ The value of repeated examination cannot be underestimated. It gives you a time course for deterioration or improvement following resuscitation, and changing signs and good analgesia may reveal a previously obscure diagnosis. Evidence of unexpected progression of the patient's signs might warrant surgery rather than continued observation.

Munchausen's and hysteria

Lastly, you may think that the patient is hysterical or faking their pain, but take all pain seriously. Infarcted bowel, for example, often gives symptoms out of keeping with signs.

❶ Even hypochondriacs die from something.

Initial investigations

The pace and range of investigation of a patient with acute abdominal pain depends on the condition of the patient. In a sick patient dispatch basic blood tests to the labs while you start resuscitation, history-taking, and seek senior review. In most circumstances, where a diagnosis is more obvious, selective investigation is more appropriate. Indications are as follows.

Blood tests

- FBC, U&Es, CRP: for all cases of acute abdominal pain.
- CBG: all patients. Ketoacidosis may present as an acute abdomen, as well as being the result of an acute abdomen.
- Serum amylase: in all patients with upper abdominal pain, evidence of peritonitis, or when the diagnosis is uncertain.
- LFTs: in all jaundiced patients, and those with upper abdominal pain.
- G&S: if surgery is expected, or if the patient is bleeding. Convert to a cross-match as required.
- PT, APTT, INR: if jaundiced, bleeding, or on warfarin.

- ABG and serum lactate: if ischaemic bowel is possible, or if the patient is shocked or septic (📖 p.482).
- Blood cultures: if the patient's temperature is > 38°C, during a rigor, or in a patient with septic shock.

Radiology

- Erect CXR: in all patients with upper abdominal pain and in those with signs of peritonitis in any area to exclude a pneumoperitoneum.
  - Pneumoperitoneum may be subtle. CT abdomen may be required to diagnose free gas.
  - Lower lobe pneumonia may also cause upper abdominal pain.
  - ❶ Beware of Chilaiditi's sign: a loop of transverse colon between the liver and diaphragm, mimicking pneumoperitoneum. Look for colonic haustra.
- Supine AXR: in all patients where obstruction is suspected (📖 p.268). AXR may also show:
  - signs of free gas, e.g. Rigler's sign (both sides of the bowel wall are visible), gas around the falciform ligament or liver;
  - gas in the biliary tree;
  - calcifications, e.g. ureteric stones, phleboliths, chronic pancreatitis, arterial calcification, and occasionally gallstones.
- ❶ AXR are often requested unnecessarily and, in patients without signs or symptoms of bowel obstruction, have a very low diagnostic yield.
- USS abdomen: for all patients with RUQ pain.
- Transvaginal pelvic USS: may be of use in some women with lower abdominal pain.
- CT abdomen and pelvis: generally requires discussion with a senior first.

Additional tests

- ECG: in all adult patients with upper abdominal pain, to detect myocardial ischaemia.
- Tests may also be requested to determine preoperative fitness (📖 p.13).

Initial management

Initial management steps for patients with an acute abdomen are outlined here. Subsequent sections include additional measures according to the suspected diagnosis.

- Admit: most cases require admission, if only briefly to the acute admissions unit to permit review later in the day or pending results of investigations. It is usually prudent to admit children and the elderly for further evaluation.
- Thromboprophylaxis (📖 p.26): discuss the use of LMWH with the on-call anaesthetist if laparotomy with epidural anaesthesia is likely within a few hours.
- IV fluids: start crystalloid at a rate consistent with the degree of dehydration/hypotension and the risk of fluid overload. Add KCl if ↓ K+ is present.
- NBM: When in doubt, keep NBM and discuss with your senior.
- Analgesia.
  - Prescribe regular paracetamol IV/PR/PO and codeine phosphate PO (unless constipated) and prn morphine/pethidine IV or IM.

- Always prescribe a prn anti-emetic IV/IM as well. Metoclopramide is a prokinetic and should **not** be used in those with possible bowel obstruction.
- Consider an NSAID if contraindications (e.g. GI bleeding, asthma, renal dysfunction) are absent.

❶ Early administration of analgesia before the diagnosis is secure does not affect outcome. Be considerate—**peritonitis hurts**.

Significant organ system dysfunction—the sick patient

- Simultaneous resuscitation and assessment. Call for help early.
- 'ABCDE' approach, as per ATLS® or CCrISP™ (📖 p.4).
- Give O_2 to keep SaO_2 > 97%.
- IV access—2 large bore cannulae; draw blood for labs.
- Start IV fluid resuscitation if volume depleted.
- Insert a urinary catheter (📖 p.504), and aim for a urine output of > 0.5mL/kg/h.
- The patient may require a central venous line for CVP monitoring if predicted severe disease on criteria or if shocked or a history of heart failure is present.
- IV antibiotics: only start if the patient is septic, and culture blood, urine, and other fluids first.
  - Antibiotics can obscure the diagnosis, and should generally be avoided in surgical patients when the diagnosis is uncertain. Once a diagnosis is made, or a decision to operate is taken, appropriate antibiotics can be started.
  - In the immunosuppressed patient, empiric IV antibiotic treatment is often desirable since deterioration with sepsis can be dramatic.
- Arrange early senior review with a view to early intervention if appropriate.
- Consider referral to HDU/ITU for monitoring and organ support.

For the diagnosis of specific causes of the acute abdomen, see the rest of this chapter.

Generalized peritonitis

Generalized peritonitis usually implies widespread peritoneal soiling from pus, intestinal contents, or bile; blood and urine tend not to be so irritant. In non-trauma patients common causes are perforated PU, perforated colonic diverticulum, or perforated appendicitis. Occasionally, GI malignancies may perforate. In patients with generalized peritonitis, establishing a diagnosis of the cause is secondary to resuscitation and an urgent operation.

❶ Pus, faeces, blood, and bile may be contained by adhesions from previous surgery, and not result in generalized peritonitis.

History

- Occurs more often in children and the elderly, where the omentum tends not to localize sepsis.
- Sudden onset, or sudden exacerbation of abdominal pain.
- A history of previous episodes of pain consistent with diverticulitis or PU may be present.
- A recent history of pain in the right iliac fossa (appendix) or left iliac fossa (diverticulitis) may be present.
- Recent NSAID use, heavy alcohol intake, or cigarette use is common in those with PU disease.
- Movement exacerbates pain; reluctant to cough.

Examination

- The patient lies completely still, with shallow respirations due to diaphragmatic splinting.
- Confusion may be present, especially in the elderly.
- The patient may be cold, peripherally shut down, and clammy or sweaty.
- Tachycardia and hypotension are common.
- The presence of pyrexia implies perforation due to appendicitis or diverticular disease; absence of pyrexia suggests PU.
- Generalized abdominal tenderness and involuntary guarding/rigidity.
  - ❶ Rigidity is less common in the very old, in late pregnancy, and following delivery and is difficult to feel in the obese.
- Severe abdominal pain with coughing or moving.
- Scanty or absent bowel sounds.
- Tender anteriorly on DRE.

Investigations

- FBC: ↑↑ WCC (in advanced cases WCC can be ↓); ↓ platelets in DIC.
- U&Es: may reflect dehydration, or early acute renal failure.
- CRP: ↑↑.
- Serum amylase: it is important to exclude acute pancreatitis—a perforated PU can cause a raised amylase, but rarely > 5 x the upper limit of normal.
- G&S.
- Erect CXR: free air under the diaphragm is seen in up to 90% of perforated PU; less following diverticular perforation (Fig. 4.3).

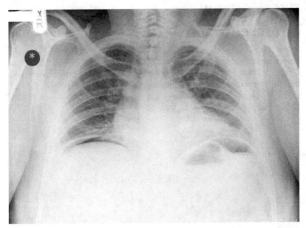

Fig. 4.3 An erect CXR showing free gas under both hemidiaphragms. This has been noted by the radiographer (*).

- Occasionally it can be difficult to distinguish between free gas under the hemidiaphragm and basal lung atelectasis. A lateral decubitus film should be requested, but these can be difficult to interpret.
- ❶ If the patient appears to have generalized peritonitis on examination, but there is no free air on CXR and the amylase is raised, request an urgent CT abdomen to exclude acute pancreatitis.

❶ Inform your senior immediately if generalized peritonitis is present or free gas on erect CXR is suspected.

Management

- Resuscitate aggressively with IV fluids, insert a urinary catheter, and give O_2 and IV analgesia (see 'Assessment of the acute abdomen', 'Initial management').
- Consider HDU/ITU for optimization (📖 p.16).
- Start IV antibiotics according to the local protocol to cover Gram-negative organisms and anaerobes (e.g. benzylpenicillin 1.2g qds, gentamicin 80mg tds, with metronidazole 500mg tds).
- Arrange theatre (📖 p.30).
- Surgery (laparotomy or laparoscopy) should take place as soon as possible after initial resuscitation.
  - Perforated PU is usually treated with an omental patch.
  - Perforated colonic diverticulum requires resection of the diseased segment, usually a sigmoid colectomy + end colostomy (Hartmann's procedure) for sigmoid diverticular disease.
  - Appendicitis requires removal of the appendix.
  - In all cases, thorough peritoneal lavage is mandatory.

Non-operative management is not usually an option unless the patient has a terminal condition (📖 p.13). Get senior help for this assessment.

Differential diagnosis according to site at presentation

In the following sections the differential diagnosis of abdominal pain will be presented according to the typical location of pain due to abdominal conditions **Note that the location of pain for some conditions may be quite variable**. Thus, appendicitis may present with pain in the epigastrium, RIF, or suprapubically. A ruptured AAA may present with central abdominal pain as well as flank and back pain, etc.

Right upper quadrant pain

Anatomy and relevant pathologies

- The right upper quadrant contains the liver and gall bladder, and most pathology relates to these two organs.
- The hepatic flexure of the colon and the duodenum may also cause pain here.

Symptoms and signs

Biliary colic (📖 p.226)

- Pain typically occurs some hours after a fat challenge (e.g. fried food, cheese). Physiologically, this corresponds to cholecystokinin (CCK) release as fat enters the duodenum; CCK causes a sustained contraction of the gall bladder against the obstructing stone(s).
- Typically the patient has had a previous episode. Attacks usually resolve within 4–12h.
- On examination, the patient is afebrile, often with RUQ tenderness. Jaundice is present only if the CBD or CHD are obstructed.
- A stone impacted in the ampulla of Vater causes true colicky pain, with jaundice.

Acute cholecystitis (📖 p.228)

- Presents with severe RUQ pain, nausea, and vomiting.
- On examination, there is pyrexia, tachycardia, with tenderness and guarding over the gall bladder. Murphy's sign may be positive. Patients are more unwell than those with biliary colic.
- Acute cholecystitis may evolve from an episode of biliary colic.
- Mild jaundice is sometimes present.

Acute cholangitis (📖 p.234)

- Presents with sweats and rigors, RUQ pain (less than acute cholecystitis), and obstructive jaundice (Charcot's triad).
- Examination reveals sepsis (pyrexia, hypotension, and tachycardia), jaundice, and mild RUQ tenderness. Confusion is often present, especially in the elderly.

Other conditions

- Acute hepatitis, duodenal ulcer, and right lower lobe pneumonia may present with RUQ pain.
- Appendicitis can cause RUQ pain:
  - in pregnancy, when the appendix is displaced superiorly;
  - if the caecum has failed to descend to the RIF during development;
  - in a long retrocaecal appendix (maximal tenderness is usually in the RIF and right flank).

Initial investigations

- FBC: ↑ WCC with acute cholecystitis and cholangitis.
- U&Es: may reflect dehydration in acute cholecystitis and cholangitis.
- Serum amylase: can be mildly raised (1–4 x the upper limit of normal) in all three major causes of RUQ pain; only very high (> 5 x the upper limit of normal) in acute pancreatitis (📖 p.244).

- LFTs: mild rise in ALP and GGT in biliary colic; rise in ALT, ALP and mild rise in bilirubin in acute cholecystitis; high bilirubin, ALT, ALP in acute cholangitis.
- Blood cultures: usually no growth in acute cholecystitis; often positive in acute cholangitis.
- Erect CXR: to exclude free intraabdominal gas and pneumonia.
- USS RUQ.
  - Discriminates acute cholecystitis (thick-walled GB, stones, Murphy's sign positive with USS probe) from biliary colic (normal size GB wall, with stones in GB ± ducts)
  - Acute cholangitis shows dilated bile ducts, usually with stones in the gall bladder and sometimes with visible stones in the ducts.
  - USS misses lower bile duct stones because the CBD passes behind the duodenum and is obscured by duodenal gas.

Initial management

Significant organ system dysfunction, e.g. acute cholangitis

- Resuscitate with IV fluids, especially if acute cholangitis suspected.
- Give O_2 to keep $SaO_2 > 95\%$.
- Insert a urinary catheter.
- Start IV antibiotics according to local protocol once blood cultures are taken (e.g. ciprofloxacin 200mg bd IV/cefuroxime 1.5g tds IV with metronidazole 500mg tds IV).
- Refer to HDU/ITU if required.
- Arrange biliary drainage as soon as practical—percutaneous (PTC) or endoscopic (ERCP).

Mild presentation, e.g. biliary colic

- IV opioid for analgesia, with an anti-emetic—a single dose usually suffices for biliary colic.
- IV fluids.

Further investigations and management

See the disease-specific treatments in Part 3.

Epigastric pain

Anatomy and relevant pathologies

- Epigastric pain is generally related to the stomach, duodenum, or pancreas.
- ❶ Consider myocardial infarction in the differential diagnosis.
- Inflammatory exudate from the pancreas can track from the lesser sac, through the epiploic foramen of Winslow, and down the right paracolic gutter to produce epigastric pain that appears to move to the RIF. While perforation of a PU usually causes generalized peritonitis, it may cause localized inflammation with gastroduodenal contents also tracking down the right paracolic gutter to produce RIF pain.
  - ❶ The potential thus exists to confuse both presentations with appendicitis.

Symptoms and signs

Acute pancreatitis (📖 p.244)

- Rapid onset of epigastric pain that radiates to the back, with a spectrum of severity, from mild pain to collapse and severe shock.
- The pain is often relieved by sitting forward, and is associated with dry retching and vomiting.
- Hypovolaemia can be severe, with tachycardia, hypotension, and ↓ SaO_2.
- On abdominal examination, findings range from mild epigastric tenderness to generalized peritonitis.
- In delayed presentations, Grey Turner's (flank bruising) and Cullen's signs (periumbilical bruising) may be present.
- In severe cases bowel sounds are absent.

Acute gastritis (📖 p.210)

- Epigastric/LUQ pain, burning in nature, sometimes radiating to back (especially if duodenitis is present).
- A history of alcohol binge/excess or NSAIDs is usual.
- On abdominal examination, epigastric tenderness is present. The patient is apyrexial, with normal bowel sounds.

Initial investigations

- FBC: ↑ WCC with acute pancreatitis; anaemia often seen with gastritis.
- U&Es: may reflect dehydration; disproportionately raised urea if bleeding from gastritis.
- Serum amylase (📖 p.246): if very high, almost always acute pancreatitis. In late presentations amylase is not so high. Don't forget that perforation of a PU and a ruptured AAA can also cause high amylase.
- Erect CXR: mandatory to exclude free intraabdominal gas and pneumonia.
- ECG: detect myocardial ischaemia as a cause or consequence of the pain.
- Bloods for modified Glasgow criteria (📖 p.246) if acute pancreatitis is suspected: WCC, urea, albumin, glucose, calcium, LDH, and ABG on air.
- CT abdomen: confirms the diagnosis of acute pancreatitis where doubt is present; also excludes perforation of PU and other differentials.

Initial management

Significant organ system dysfunction, e.g. acute pancreatitis
- Resuscitate with IV fluids.
- Give O_2 to keep SaO_2 > 95%.
- Insert a urinary catheter and aim for a urine output of > 0.5mL/kg/h.
- Keep NBM and give IV opioids.
- May require central venous line for CVP monitoring if predicted severe disease on criteria, or if shocked.
- Refer to HDU/ITU if required.

Mild presentation, e.g. mild acute gastritis
- IV opioid for analgesia, with an anti-emetic.
- Proton pump inhibitor infusion, e.g. IV omeprazole bolus 80mg, with 8mg/h infusion if severe gastritis/duodenitis.

Further investigations and management

See the disease-specific chapters in Part 3.

Left upper quadrant pain

Anatomy and relevant pathologies

- It is rare for non-trauma patients to present with isolated LUQ pain, as there isn't much in the LUQ apart from the stomach, spleen, and the splenic flexure of colon. Most acute pain will be due to gastritis (📖 p.210).
- Rarely, splenic artery aneurysm rupture and perforation of the splenic flexure can give pain that arises in the LUQ, as can left lower lobe pneumonia. Infectious mononucleosis (glandular fever) can cause splenomegaly with abdominal pain; splenic rupture (📖 p.252) can occur after trivial trauma. Splenic infarcts may occur with sickle cell disease.

Flank pain

Anatomy and relevant pathologies

- The retroperitoneum in the flanks contains the kidneys, and on the left the tail of pancreas.
- Flank pain is generally from the renal tract, and is commonly due to ureteric calculi or infection.
- A ruptured AAA can cause flank pain radiating to the groin.
- Lumbar disc pain does not occur in the elderly, since the discs are desiccated and no longer herniate.
    - ❶ If you think that someone > 60 years old has a prolapsed intervertebral disc, think again and exclude a ruptured AAA.

Symptoms and signs

Renal colic (📖 p.378)

- Colicky flank pain, radiating to the groin and on to the ispilateral scrotum or labia.
- Associated with haematuria (macro- or microscopic).
- On examination the patient is restless. Mild tenderness is present in one flank. Pyrexia is unusual.

Pyelonephritis

- Dysuria and frequency may be present; sweats and rigors are common.
- A history of cystitis and previous UTIs is common.
- On examination, the patient looks unwell, flushed, and septic.
- There is tenderness over the renal angle and urinalysis shows nitrites and leucocytes.

Ruptured AAA (📖 p.326)

- Patients present with severe back or flank pain.
- ❶ Check if the patient is on an AAA surveillance programme.
- There is usually a history of transient loss of consciousness or collapse.
- On examination, the patient is shocked. There is epigastric and flank tenderness.
- ❶ An AAA is **often** not palpable due to obesity, hypotension, and the surrounding haematoma.
- ❶ Renal colic is uncommon in men aged > 65 years old; AAAs are not (5%).

Initial investigations

- FBC: Hb is usually ↓ in ruptured AAA, but may be ↔ in the initial phase. The WCC is ↑ (14–20 x 10^9/L) in pyelonephritis.
- U&E: ↑ creatinine is common in ruptured AAA.
- MSU: leucocytes on microscopy, and positive culture in pyelonephritis; red cells with renal colic.
- X-ray KUB: may show a renal or ureteric calculus; **always** check for a epigastric calcified AAA sac in the elderly.
- USS KUB: request if pyelonephritis suspected and the patient is septic in order to exclude an obstructed infected kidney. This is an indication for urgent nephrostomy.

- USS epigastrium: can be performed in the emergency department if AAA is suspected. Unable to confirm the presence of a retroperitoneal haematoma, indicative of rupture.
- CTU: the investigation of choice in renal colic, this will also detect a ruptured AAA if doubt exists. It is replacing IVU as the investigation of choice.

Initial management

- Emergency theatre: if a ruptured AAA is suspected and surgery is appropriate.
- IV antibiotics: according to local preference if pyelonephritis is suspected.
- Analgesia: (NSAIDs, e.g. rectal diclofenac) if renal colic is present.

Further investigations and management

See the disease-specific chapters in Part 3.

Periumbilical pain

Anatomy and relevant pathologies

- Central abdominal pain is a common presentation of the acute abdomen since it is the visceral referral site for the midgut.
- Testicular torsion may present with periumbilical pain.
- A ruptured AAA occasionally presents with periumbilical pain.

Symptoms and signs

Appendicitis (📖 p.262)

- Presents with central colicky pain, that moves to the RIF as the patient becomes nauseated or vomits (Murphy's triad).
- On examination, there is mild pyrexia with tenderness and guarding in the RIF.

Large or small bowel obstruction (📖 p.268)

- Central colicky pain, often preceded by distension and followed by vomiting, which relieves the pain; absolute constipation is a late feature in small bowel obstruction.
- Distension and hyperresonance to percussion are found on abdominal examination; bowel sounds are variable.

Testicular torsion (📖 p.373)

- Central abdominal pain and vomiting may predominate over local pain in the scrotum.
- On examination, abdominal tenderness is absent, though voluntary guarding is common in young boys unless you distract them—palpating with the stethoscope or with their own hand works well.

❶ It is essential to examine the scrotum of **all** males with ill-defined central abdominal pain.

Mesenteric adenitis (📖 p.264)

- Patients (children) have a history of recent upper respiratory tract infection and may have palpable cervical lymphadenopathy and prominent tonsils.
- Otherwise, symptoms and signs can be very similar to those of appendicitis.
- Lymphoid hyperplasia can occlude the appendix lumen and cause appendicitis, so careful review is required.
- Often the diagnosis can only confidently be made at appendicectomy.

Mesenteric ischaemia (📖 p.284)

- This is characterized by severe pain disproportionate to signs. Pain that is difficult to control with opioids suggests ischaemic bowel.
- Clues include a history of AF or recent angiography (which may dislodge debris into the SMA).
- On examination, the patient is often tachypnoeic due to respiratory compensation for a metabolic acidosis.
- Shock is present and only vague abdominal tenderness may be found.

Initial investigations
- FBC: a ↑ WCC is non-specific, although a ↑↑ WCC (> 20 × 10^9/L) is often found in mesenteric ischaemia.
- U&Es: may reflect dehydration in bowel obstruction or mesenteric ischaemia.
- Serum amylase: may be mildly raised in mesenteric ischaemia.
- ABG: a metabolic acidosis and raised lactate are often present in mesenteric ischaemia.
- AXR: may reveal small or large bowel obstruction (📖 p.270). Check for the presence of a gallstone and/or air in biliary tree, indicating gallstone ileus.

Initial management

Significant organ system dysfunction, e.g. mesenteric ischaemia

- Resuscitate with IV fluids, and discuss with your senior regarding an urgent laparotomy.
- Give O$_2$ to keep SaO$_2$ > 95%.
- Insert a urinary catheter and aim for a urine output of > 0.5mL/kg/h.
- Keep NBM and give IV opioids.
- NG tube if intestinal obstruction to relieve vomiting and reduce risk of aspiration.
- Refer to HDU/ITU if required.

❶ Testicular torsion requires emergency surgery. Discuss with your seniors immediately if this diagnosis is suspected.

Further investigation and management

The investigation and management of the other conditions discussed here are to be found in the disease-specific chapters in Part 3.

Right iliac fossa pain

Anatomy and relevant pathologies

- The appendix, caecum, ascending colon, distal small bowel, right ureter, right common and internal iliac artery, and right ovary and Fallopian tube are the structures to consider.
- In most cases, RIF pain is due to appendicitis, but this can be mimicked by caecal diverticulitis, an ascending urinary infection in a child, ureteric calculus, and gynaecological pathology in a female (e.g. ovarian cyst rupture or torsion, tubo-ovarian abscess).
- Meckel's diverticulitis and mesenteric adenitis may also present with RIF pain. These diagnoses are often only made at appendicectomy. Terminal ileitis due to *Yersinia* or Crohn's disease may also present with acute RIF pain leading to appendicectomy.
- Rupture of a common iliac artery aneurysm or internal iliac artery aneurysm may present with pain in the RIF.

Symptoms and signs

Appendicitis (📖 *p.262*)

- Colicky, central abdominal pain moving to the RIF as a constant pain with nausea and vomiting. This typical history (Murphy's triad) is present in half of all cases.
- Pain in RIF on coughing (localized peritonitis).
- Tenderness and involuntary guarding over RIF; retrocaecal appendicitis is associated with right flank pain and less peritonism; pelvic appendicitis may be associated with diarrhoea or urinary frequency, depending whether the inflamed appendix irritates rectum or bladder.
- Rectal examination elicits pain if pus is in the pelvis.

Gynaecological pathology (📖 *p.126*)

Crohn's ileitis (📖 *p.264*)

- An acute presentation of Crohn's disease is uncommon, with most patients having a past history of abdominal pain, diarrhoea, and weight loss.
- A history of fistula-in-ano or other perianal disease is present in ~ 30%.

Initial investigations

- FBC: moderate ↑ WCC (10–15 x 10^9/L) in appendicitis and Crohn's ileitis.
- Urine dipstick: positive for leucocytes and nitrites in UTI, with leucocytes on microscopy and positive bacterial culture.
- βhCG (urine or blood): positive in ruptured ectopic pregnancy.

Initial management

- Admit, keep NBM, give IV fluids.
- If appendicitis is possible but unlikely, observe and re-examine in 4–6h.
- If the diagnosis of appendicitis is probable, arrange theatre and give antibiotics. In adults, give 1g metronidazole PR at the same time as your DRE. If perforation is possible give IV cefuroxime 1.5g as well.

- Gynaecology referral: if gynaecological pathology suspected or confirmed.
  - ❶ If a ruptured ectopic pregnancy is suspected, refer to the on-call gynaecologist **immediately**; place 2 large-bore IV cannulae and fluid resuscitate.

Further investigations and management

See the disease-specific chapters in Part 3.

Suprapubic pain

Anatomy and relevant pathologies

- The tip of a long appendix, a mobile sigmoid colon, small bowel (including an inflamed Meckel's diverticulum), uterus and Fallopian tubes, and bladder may cause suprapubic pain.
- Presentation with suprapubic pain alone is uncommon, unless bladder pathology such as acute retention or UTI is present. These conditions should both be straightforward to diagnose.

Symptoms, signs, initial investigations, and management

- Exclude UTI/urinary retention by enquiring about lower urinary tract symptoms, examine to exclude an enlarged bladder, and request a urine dipstick.
- See other sections of this chapter on RIF, LIF pain, and gynaecological pathology.

Left iliac fossa pain

Anatomy and relevant pathologies

- The sigmoid colon causes most pathology in the LIF, usually in the form of diverticulitis.
- Gynaecological pathology relating to the left ovary and Fallopian tube may also present with LIF pain. Left ureteric renal colic may cause pain in the LIF, although radiation is usually present.
- Rupture of an AAA or left common or internal iliac artery aneurysm may present with pain in the LIF.

Symptoms and signs

Sigmoid diverticulitis (📖 p.278)

- There is a short history of lower abdominal pain moving to the LIF, associated with a pyrexia and LIF peritonitis.
- Differentiating simple diverticulitis from complicated diverticulitis (abscess formation or perforation) is important and is an indication for urgent abdominal CT.
- Localized LIF peritonitis is assumed to be due to diverticulitis until proven otherwise—unfortunately there is often little haste in providing proof, so where the diagnosis is not correct (~ 25% of cases) the patient is inappropriately treated.

Gynaecological pathology, see (📖 p.126)

Initial investigations

- FBC: ↑ WCC (10–15 x 10^9/L) in diverticulitis.
- Blood cultures: in patients with suspected diverticulitis and T > 37.5°C.
- Erect CXR: in all patients with LIF peritonitis to exclude a free perforation.
- CT abdomen: the most useful imaging test in acute diverticulitis. Excludes an abscess and perforation as well as picking up alternative diagnoses.

Initial management

- IV fluids, analgesia, and keep NBM.
- IV antibiotics: according to local protocol, e.g. ciprofloxacin 500mg bd with metronidazole 500mg tds.
- CT-guided percutaneous drainage: if a diverticular abscess is identified on initial CT abdomen.

Gynaecological causes of the acute abdomen

Lower abdominal pain in women of child-bearing age is often due to a gynaecological cause. Women with confirmed intrauterine pregnancies may present with acute abdominal pain (Box 4.1).

Anatomy and relevant pathologies

- The uterus, Fallopian tubes, and ovaries lie in the pelvis.
- A large ovarian cyst may extend into the iliac fossa, while an ectopic pregnancy commonly implants in the tube or ovary.

Symptoms and signs

Ovarian pathology

- Ovarian torsion occurs in the presence of a large (> 4cm) ovarian cyst, and tends to be a rapid onset iliac fossa pain, with no central component. Pain can be severe. There is no pain on coughing or percussion and no leucocytosis on FBC.
- Rupture of an ovarian cyst has a similar presentation with sudden onset iliac fossa pain, with localized tenderness and little inflammatory response ($\leftrightarrow$ WCC and $\leftrightarrow$/mildly $\uparrow$ CRP). Usually occurs midcycle.
- In older women, ovarian cancer can present with acute iliac fossa pain, although peritonitis is absent and a mass is often palpable.

Ruptured ectopic pregnancy

- Pain is typically sudden in onset in either iliac fossa, and may occur following/during intercourse.
- There may or may not be a history of a missed period. Likewise, vaginal bleeding is a variable finding.
- More common when there is a past history of ectopic pregnancy, with intrauterine contraceptive devices, and in those taking the progesterone-only pill.
- Typically the patient is pale and tachycardic; in severe cases she is hypotensive with significant tenderness in the lower abdomen and signs of shock may be present.
- Shoulder tip pain may be elicited when the patient is tipped head-down (Kehr's sign).
- Do **not** perform a vaginal examination, as this may prompt further haemorrhage.

Pelvic inflammatory disease

- This is an ascending infection of the female genital tract, including endometritis, salpingitis, and tubo-ovarian abscess (pyosalpinx).
- Presentation is usually with bilateral lower abdominal pain and purulent vaginal discharge. Dyspareunia may be present.
- On examination, the patient is usually not systemically unwell, unless a tubo-ovarian abscess has ruptured intraperitoneally. There is mild pyrexia, vague lower abdominal tenderness, and vaginal examination reveals an offensive discharge and pain on cervical excitation. An adnexal mass suggests a tubo-ovarian abscess.

Initial investigations

- FBC: ↑ WCC (10–15 x 10^9/L) in salpingitis and pyosalpinx.
- βhCG (urine or blood): to determine whether pregnant.
  - ❶ Perform in all females of child-bearing age with acute abdominal pain.
- Transvaginal swab: for detection of sexually transmitted diseases causing pelvic inflammatory disease.
- Transvaginal pelvic USS: to diagnose a ruptured ovarian cyst, pyosalpinx, or ovarian cancer. Use IV rather than oral fluids to fill the bladder in case urgent surgery is indicated.

Initial management

- Referral to the on-call gynaecology team: in all cases where gynaecological pathology is suspected.
- Laparoscopy: if pelvic peritonitis is present and the diagnosis is not clear after gynaecological review.
- ❶ Women with acute lower abdominal pain and positive βhCG should be referred immediately to the on-call gynaecology team. A ruptured ectopic pregnancy can be rapidly fatal– always manage aggressively with large-bore peripheral cannulae, IV fluid resuscitation, and blood products as required.

Box 4.1. Acute abdominal pain in pregnant women

Although pregnancy is associated with an increased risk of gallstone-related pathology, acute appendicitis is still common. Pregnant women provide a diagnostic and therapeutic challenge as:

- abdominal organs are displaced as the uterus enlarges, causing atypical presentations, e.g. appendicitis presenting with RUQ pain;
- obstetric emergencies may present with acute abdominal pain, e.g. placental abruption;
- pregnancy itself leads to many physiological changes, e.g. mild tachycardia, neutrophilia;
- ionizing radiation (e.g. CXR, AXR, CT) is best avoided;
- some medications are contraindicated in pregnancy;
- surgery carries a risk of fetal loss, although the 2nd trimester is widely considered to be the safest period.

In order to minimize difficulties do the following:

- have a very low threshold for admission;
- in the 3rd trimester you must check the BP, examine for peripheral oedema, and dipstick the urine for protein—HELLP syndrome, a manifestation of pre-eclampsia, can mimic biliary pain;
- discuss all cases with your senior;
- all pregnant women admitted with acute abdominal pain should be reviewed by the obstetric team. When you think that the pain is due to an obstetric complication a senior member of the obstetric team must be involved immediately.

❶ The mortality from the acute abdomen in pregnancy can be '200%'.

Medical causes of the acute abdomen

Many 'medical' conditions can cause abdominal pain, most being more common than the porphyria beloved of medical students. Common conditions include MI, lower lobe pneumonia, diabetic ketoacidosis, herpes zoster (shingles), meningococcal septicaemia, and rectus sheath haematoma. In addition, constipation, gastroenteritis, ulcerative and pseudomembranous colitis, sickle cell crisis, and Addison's disease, amongst others, may present with abdominal pain.

Assessment and management

Diabetic ketoacidosis (DKA)

- This can cause acute abdominal pain, or may be the result of an underlying pathology causing an acute abdomen. Always treat DKA as a symptom and look for its precipitating cause.
- Patients present with nausea, vomiting, dehydration, and abdominal pain. Most presentations are in patients known to have diabetes, although DKA can be the index presentation of the condition, particularly in children.
- CBG reveals marked hyperglycaemia (> 15mmol/L), with ketones on urine dipstick, and metabolic acidosis on ABG.
- Aggressive IV fluid resuscitation and K^+ replacement is required, along with IV insulin. Discuss with the on-call medical team **immediately**.
- Abdominal symptoms may resolve with blood glucose control, but abdominal CT is essential to exclude other causes of the acute abdomen, particularly appendicitis.

Herpes zoster

- Prodromal dermatomal pain is a feature of zoster, which is generally followed within 48–72h by the appearance of a crop of vesicles in typical distribution. Dermatomes T3–L3 are most commonly involved.
  - ❶ Always examine the back.
- May be mistaken for biliary pain or early diverticulitis.
- Diagnosis is aided by the presence of hyperaesthesia and the absence of ↑ WCC on FBC.
- Start antivirals after discussion with the on-call medical team.

Rectus sheath haematoma

- The rectus sheath contains the rectus abdominis muscles and the superior and inferior epigastric arteries and veins. Bleeding within the sheath, due to damage to the vessels or tearing of the muscles, leads to distension of the rectus sheath and abdominal pain.
- It typically occurs after severe muscle contractions, e.g. with vigorous exercise, coughing, vomiting, or straining. It is much more common in patients on anticoagulant therapy. The onset of pain may be sudden, but usually appears over a few hours. The precipitating cause needs careful retracing of the history.
- Tenderness can be marked, and can convincingly mimic localized peritonitis due to pain with movement/coughing. In slim patients an abdominal mass the shape of the rectus sheath, can be defined. Tensing the abdominal wall, by lifting the head off the pillow, exacerbates the pain and the mass remains palpable—masses below the abdominal wall

disappear on contraction of the abdominal muscles. Patients may be unwell, and may have lost a substantial amount of blood. Low-grade pyrexia is common.

- Resuscitate with IV fluids and correct anaemia and coagulopathies. The diagnosis is confirmed on abdominal CT scanning. Large, expanding haematomas may require embolization of the bleeding vessel using interventional radiological techniques. Surgery is rarely required.

Meningococcal septicaemia
❶ One never to miss.

The patient, often a child, is very sick with a petechial rash that often progresses while you watch. There is generalized abdominal pain and vomiting. The patient is febrile; and examination confirms features of shock, and a non-blanching petechial rash. The conscious level deteriorates as infection progresses.

> ❶ Act **immediately**, as death occurs in hours: take blood for culture and give high-dose IV benzylpenicillin. Seek **urgent** senior help and request ITU admission.

- FBC will reveal a ↑ WCC in early stages, but ↓ WCC as it progresses. Platelets are ↓.
- PT, APTT: both ↑, with ↑ FDPs, indicating DIC.

Conditions you must never forget

There are a few conditions that should always be considered, either because they are rare but treatable, or because they are relatively common but easily overlooked. The following are conditions with high morbidity and mortality that you should **not** miss.

❶ Involve seniors **immediately** if any of these diagnoses are suspected.

Rare, but treatable

Hypoadrenalism/hypopituitarism

- Addison's disease may present with abdominal pain.
- Patients with hypoadrenalism or hypopituitarism may respond to stress with hypotension out of proportion to the nature of the pathology.
- Always consider IV hydrocortisone in someone with unexplained hypotension, particularly in the presence of a low Na^+ and high K^+.
- ❶ Discuss with the on-call medical team **urgently**.

Meningococcal septicaemia See 'Medical causes of the acute abdomen'. Early treatment is simple and can be life-saving.

Relatively common, but easily overlooked

Ruptured AAA (🕮 p.326)

- In patients with small, contained ruptures, the presentation can be subtle and may not include collapse.
- Always consider in patients > 60 years old with abdominal, back, or flank pain, especially in those with cardiac risk factors.
- In obese patients, an AAA is **often** not palpable and, contrary to popular belief, patients with ruptured AAA do **not** lose a femoral pulse.

Acute pancreatitis (🕮 p.244) Can present with a spectrum of severity, and mimic other conditions. Patients with pancreatitis generally do badly if subjected to inappropriate emergency surgery.
- ❶ Request serum amylase in all patients with upper abdominal pain, evidence of peritonitis, or when the diagnosis is uncertain.

Testicular torsion (🕮 p.373) Commonly missed due to failure to appreciate the significance of vague periumbilical pain in young males, combined with incomplete clinical examination.

Mesenteric ischaemia (🕮 p.284)

- Diagnosis can often be difficult due to the paucity of clinical signs.
- Always consider in patients with abdominal pain and dysrhythmias, recent MI, or aortic instrumentation (angiography/plasty).
- In patients with severe pain but minimal signs, always perform an ABG, looking for metabolic acidosis. Can be difficult to diagnose on imaging, including abdominal CT, and thus often only diagnosed at laparotomy.

Ruptured ectopic pregnancy ❶ All females of child-bearing age with acute abdominal pain must have βhCG (urine or blood) as part of their work-up. A positive test mandates immediate referral to the gynaecology team. See 'Gynaecological causes of the acute abdomen', this chapter.

Ward emergencies

Introduction

Surgical patients may develop 'medical' or 'surgical' emergency conditions during their hospital stay. Often the diagnosis is not immediately obvious, and a problem-based approach is necessary.

Whenever an emergency arises in a surgical patient you should assume that it is related to the underlying surgical pathology until proven otherwise. Likewise, 'medical' complications after surgery are **often** the presenting feature of an underlying surgical problem, e.g. an anastomotic leak leading to AF. This is usually not appreciated by juniors, who may contact the on-call medical team without discussions with their senior surgical colleagues. Complications are more likely in those with preoperative co-morbidities, and in patients undergoing long, complex surgery. Delay in the detection of complications leads to high morbidity and mortality.

❶ A **high index of suspicion** is necessary to detect postoperative complications and concerns should be discussed with senior surgical staff **early**.

Most early complications after major surgery are generic (e.g. basal atelectasis, pneumonia, PE) and are dealt with in this chapter. The investigation and management of specific early postoperative complications are dealt with in Part 3 of this book, and the reader should consult the appropriate chapter.

Sick surgical patients are often best approached using the algorithm described in the Royal College of Surgeons of England CCrISP™ course (Fig. 5.1). Less unwell patients do not require ABCDE, and can have a history and examination performed after a chart review.

Immediate assessment and management

As with the approach to the emergency trauma patient (Chapter 3, 📖 p.42), the immediate priority is to examine and manage ABCDE (see 'Airway with cervical spine protection', 📖 p.46; 'Breathing', 📖 p.50; 'Circulation with haemorrhage control' 📖 p.52; 'Disability (neurological assessment)', 📖 p.58; 'Exposure/environment', 📖 p.60). In this initial phase, there are some differences between trauma patients and ward patients.

- Airway. C-spine control is rarely necessary (collapse is an exception).
- Circulation. Give a 20mL/kg bolus of IV crystalloid if hypotension is present and fluid overload or an ACS is clinically unlikely. In patients with a known history of heart failure this fluid challenge should be reduced to a 5mL/kg bolus.
- Disability. Check the CBG—iatrogenic hypoglycaemia is common.
- The additional investigations and procedures required ('adjuncts') often include:
  • FBC, U&Es, amylase, LFTs, PT, APTT;
  • ECG;
  • ABG;
  • portable erect CXR;
  • cross-match (if haemorrhagic shock is likely);
  • insertion of a urinary catheter.

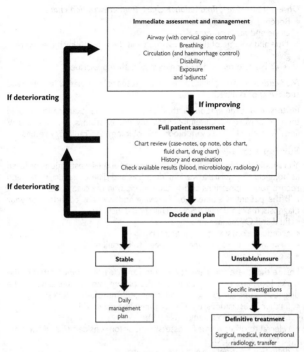

Fig. 5.1 The CCrISP™ approach. (Adapted, with permission, from Anderson, I.D. (ed.) (1999). *Care of the critically ill surgical patient*, p. 8. Arnold, London.)

Full patient assessment

Once the patient has been stabilized, or is improving, review the charts to find out more about the patient and their recent progress.

Case-notes
- History of presenting complaint.
- Co-morbidities, especially IHD, COPD, and organ dysfunction.
- Medication, alcohol, and cigarette history.
- Old ECGs.
- Recent inpatient events.

Operation note Operation performed, intraoperative difficulties, post-operative plan.

Anaesthetic note Type of anaesthetic, estimated blood loss, fluids given, intraoperative events.

Observations chart, fluid balance chart, fluid prescription chart
- Recent trends.
- Urine and drain outputs.
- Type and volume of fluids prescribed and the rate at which they were given.
  - ❶ Fluids often end up running slower than prescribed.

Medication chart Medications given (especially opiates, insulin, and sedatives) or omitted.

History and examination A thorough history and examination should then be performed. Carefully check any drains, stomas, wounds, and IV lines. Also check all relevant blood, microbiology, and radiology results.

Further management

You should then be able to review the results of the investigations ordered as 'adjuncts', formulate a working diagnosis and differential diagnoses, and record your impressions clearly and succinctly in the case notes.

If the patient is stable and improving and you are confident of your diagnosis, make a definitive plan. This should include:
- fluid and O_2 management;
- acceptable physiological parameters;
- clear instructions for when you need to be called;
- a plan for review.

Ensure that these plans are documented and clearly communicated to the nurse looking after your patient. If the patient remains unstable or the diagnosis is unclear, further action is needed. This often includes:
- further investigations, e.g. CT abdomen and pelvis, CTPA;
- discussion with your senior (📖 p.8);
- referral to other teams for assessment, or for consideration of transfer to ITU, CCU, HDU;
- definitive treatment, e.g. return to theatre.

Don't forget:
- ❶ If the patient deteriorates at any point, return to ABCDE.
- ❶ Where the diagnosis is unclear, repeated examination is often invaluable.
- ►► If you need emergency assistance with a very unwell patient, fast-bleep your senior and/or call the resuscitation team.

☼ Collapse

Collapse can be defined as a sudden loss of consciousness and may be due to a very wide variety of causes ranging from the immediately life-threatening to less significant conditions. Every call for collapse must be treated as an emergency. The collapse itself may lead to serious injuries (Box 5.1).

❶ Recognizing unwell patients early is essential in order to prevent subsequent deterioration resulting in collapse.

Box 5.1 Injuries post-collapse

- Cervical spine injury
- Head injury
- Accidental removal of a chest drain, central venous line, operative drain, urinary catheter, etc.
- Long bone fracture, especially fractured neck of femur

Causes

- Airway obstruction (📖 p.47).
- Intracranial haemorrhage (📖 p.427) or CVA.
- Cardiac tamponade (📖 p.474).
- Massive PE, e.g. venous thromboembolism, air embolism from a disconnected central venous line.
- MI with cardiogenic shock.
- Aortic dissection (📖 p.468).
- Anaphylactic shock.
- Cardiac dysrhythmia.
- Tension pneumothorax (📖 p.463).
- Intraabdominal bleed (e.g. ruptured AAA (📖 p.326)).
- Electrolyte abnormalities, e.g. K^+, Ca^{2+}, Na^+.
- Aortic stenosis.
- Addisonian crisis.
- Severe hypoxia or hypercapnia of any cause.
- Vasovagal syncope.
- Permanent pacemaker (PPM) or automatic internal cardiac defibrillator (AICD) dysfunction.
- Drug overdose (e.g. opiates, hypnotics/sedatives, antihypertensives, tricyclic antidepressants, antidysrhythmics).
- Dehydration.
- Hypoglycaemia.
- Epileptic fit.
- Panic attack.

❶ Specific conditions to consider in a surgical patient:
- operative site bleeding;
- anastomotic or suture/staple line leak and septic shock;
- opioid overdose;
- PE (major surgery is a strong risk factor).

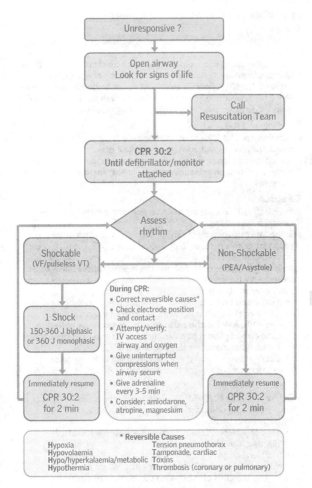

Fig. 5.2 The adult advanced life support algorithm. (Reproduced, with permission, from the European Resuscitation Council (2005). ERC guidelines for resuscitation. *Resuscitation* **67** (Suppl. 1), S1–S190.)

Immediate assessment and management

Airway

- Examination. Look, listen, and feel for movement of air through the airway
- Immediate management. Open the airway with chin lift and jaw thrust. Use simple airway devices (📖 p.47) to maintain airway patency if required. Give high-flow O_2 at 10–12L/min via a non-rebreathing mask.
- ❶ If a fall has occurred, protect the C-spine with manual in-line stabilization and ask for a semi-rigid collar, sandbags/fluid bags, and tape.

Breathing

- Examination. Check for adequate respirations and auscultate the chest. Check the patency and drainage of any chest drains.
- Immediate management. Treat life-threatening thoracic conditions if found, e.g. tension pneumothorax (📖 p.463), massive haemothorax (📖 p.464).

Circulation

- Examination. Check for signs of a cardiac output by palpating the carotid pulse (no more than 10s).
- Immediate management. If signs of a circulation and adequate respiration are both absent, or there is doubt, start CPR, giving 30 chest compressions at a rate of 100/min followed by 2 ventilations with an 'inspiratory' time of 1s. **Ask for the resuscitation team to be called**. Attach a defibrillator and follow the adult advanced life support cardiac arrest algorithm (Fig. 5.2).
  - If the carotid pulse is palpable but there is no breathing (i.e. a respiratory arrest), start ventilations and check for a circulation every 10s. **Ask for the resuscitation team to be called**.
  - If the carotid pulse is palpable, the airway is clear, and respirations are adequate, complete the assessment of 'C'.
  - Get IV access x 2, and give a 20mL/kg bolus of IV crystalloid if hypotension present and fluid overload or ACS clinically unlikely.

Disability

- Examination. Check AVPU or GCS. Observe the pupils for signs of an opioid overdose or intracranial haemorrhage. Check the CBG.
- Immediate management.
  - If hypoglycaemia (CBG < 3mmol/L) present, give 50mL of 50% dextrose IV.
  - If bilateral pinpoint pupils are present, give 200–400mcg of naloxone IV, repeated as necessary (the half-life of naloxone is shorter than that of the opioids causing the overdose).

Exposure

- Examination. Expose the patient and check for haemorrhage in drains. Look for signs of anaphylaxis (Box 5.2).
  - ❶ Surgical drains often block. The absence of blood in a drain does **not** exclude haemorrhage within the same compartment.
- Immediate management. Keep the patient warm.

Box 5.2. Recognition and management of anaphylaxis

Signs of anaphylaxis
- Urticaria, angio-oedema, conjunctivitis, flushing, stridor, and wheeze.

❶ Consider anaphylaxis carefully in those patients receiving antibiotics or a blood transfusion.

Immediate management
- Stop any IV drug infusion or blood transfusion.
- Give 10–12L/min high-flow O_2.
- Give 500mcg adrenaline IM, repeated every 5min as needed to maintain BP. Only give IV adrenaline in life-threatening shock, i.e. if CPR is needed.
- Give 20mL/kg IV crystalloid boluses as needed to maintain BP.
- Also give 10–20mg chlorphenamine slow IV, 100mg hydrocortisone slow IV, and 5mg of nebulized salbutamol.

❶ If hoarseness, stridor, or facial swelling are present, early intubation by a senior anaesthetist is required before airway obstruction occurs.

Adjuncts
- 12-lead ECG. Look especially for signs of myocardial ischaemia (📖 p.143), tachycardia, bradycardia, evidence of aberrant conduction pathways (e.g. the delta wave of Wolff–Parkinson–White syndrome), and a prolonged QT interval.
  - Bradycardia < 40/min, or < 60/min with adverse signs (systolic BP < 90mmHg, signs of heart failure) should be treated with atropine 500mcg IV, repeated as necessary to a maximum of 3mg.
  - Tachycardia > 150beats/min (non-sinus tachycardia) with reduced level of consciousness, chest pain, heart failure, or systolic BP < 90mmHg requires synchronized DC shock.
  - ❶ In a collapsed patient, the presence of ECG abnormalities (apart from sinus tachycardia) requires **immediate** referral to the on-call medical team.
- Send blood for **urgent** FBC, U&Es, Mg^{2+}, Ca^{2+}, LFTs, amylase, PT, APTT. If signs of haemorrhagic shock are present, cross-match at least 4 units of packed RBCs.
- Take blood cultures peripherally, and through all central venous lines present.
- Perform an ABG.
- Request a portable CXR.
- Insert a urinary catheter if one is not already present.

Further assessment

If the patient's haemodynamic state and level of consciousness are improving, further assessment and management are required.

Case-notes, operation note, anaesthetic note
- Look in the case-notes for a past history of collapse, syncope, IHD, PPM, AICD, PE, DVT, epilepsy, and allergies.

- Check the operation and anaesthetic notes for any difficulties, instructions, blood loss, and intraoperative events.
- Recent endoscopy implies oversedation (📖 p.220).

Observations chart, fluid balance chart, fluid prescription chart, medication chart

- Look at the recent trends on the observations and fluid charts: progressive hypotension and tachycardia (haemorrhage), swinging pyrexia and worsening hypotension (sepsis), or sudden deterioration (cardio/neurological event).
- Check the medication chart for recent opioids, benzodiazepines (give flumazenil 200mcg IV to reverse), antibiotics (anaphylaxis), anticoagulants (bleeding), and insulin (hypoglycaemia).

History Take a history of the events surrounding the collapse, asking specifically about recent chest pain, SOB, palpitations, headache, operative site pain, abdominal pain, weakness/altered sensation in arms/legs/face, haemoptysis, haematemesis, PR bleeding, and vertigo.

Examination

Re-examine the patient from head to toe, checking specifically for the following.

- Signs of an intraabdominal cause (bleed, anastomotic leak), e.g. abdominal distension, tenderness, peritonitis, palpable AAA.
- Signs of an aortic dissection (📖 p.468), e.g. hypertension, aortic regurgitation, differential systolic BP > 10mmHg between upper or lower limbs, absent pulses, limb ischaemia, and hemiplegia.
- Signs of a CVA, e.g. dysphasia, facial asymmetry, unilateral limb weakness.
- Signs of C-spine trauma (📖 p.80), head trauma (📖 p.76), and long bone fractures.
- Do a DRE to detect GI bleeding.
- Security of IV lines and drains.

Check available results

- Look for ↓ Hb and coagulopathy (suggesting postoperative haemorrhage) and electrolyte abnormalities.
- Look for hypoxia and hypercapnia on the ABG indicating hypoventilation.
- Check the portable CXR for haemo/pneumothorax, pneumonia, and mediastinal widening (aortic dissection).

Further management

This depends on your working diagnosis and on the response of the patient to your treatment. When the diagnosis is unclear, further assessment and investigations are required. Unstable patients need referral to the on-call medical team for assessment, and the ITU team for HDU or ITU admission. Consider:

- CT abdomen (operative site bleeding);
- CT head (CVA, intracranial haemorrhage);
- CTPA or V/Q scan (PE);
- repeat ECG in 1h + cardiac biomarkers 12h post-collapse (ACS).

Because there are numerous possible causes of a collapse, only the management of relatively common life-threatening conditions is discussed.

Operative site bleeding (📖 p.157)
❶ Inform your senior **immediately** if you suspect bleeding.

Massive PE (i.e. leading to circulatory collapse)
- Give high-flow O_2 via a non-rebreathing mask and 10mL/kg IV crystal-loid boluses. Inotropes may be needed to achieve normotension.
- Start IV unfractionated heparin (e.g. 5000 unit bolus followed by an infusion) before imaging if the clinical probability is intermediate or high.
- CTPA or echocardiography can be used to diagnose massive PE and should be performed as an emergency.
- Consider thrombolysis with 50mg IV alteplase on clinical grounds alone if cardiac arrest is imminent.
- Admission to HDU/ITU is likely; discuss with the on-call ITU team.
- ❶ The decision to anticoagulate or thrombolyse a postoperative patient should only be made after discussion between a senior surgeon and physician.

ACS (📖 p.144)
- Give high-flow O_2, 2 x puffs of sublingual GTN, 300mg aspirin PO + 300mg of clopidogrel, and 2.5–5mg of IV morphine prn.
- Contact the on-call medical team and your senior immediately.
- Admission to CCU/ITU is likely.

Sepsis (📖 p.482)
- Give a 20mL/kg IV crystalloid bolus. If hypotension remains despite further 10–20mL/kg boluses, a central venous line should be placed to guide fluid management. Patients with a history of heart failure require 5mL/kg crystalloid boluses and a lower threshold for central venous line placement.
- Check serum lactate.
- Give high-flow O_2 via a non-rebreathing mask.
- Take blood cultures and start broad spectrum IV antibiotics appro-priate for the suspected source of sepsis. Sputum, urine, wound, drain, and IV line cultures may also be required, depending on clinical suspi-cion. Discuss with the on-call microbiologist.
- HDU or ITU admission is likely. Discuss with your senior and the on-call ITU team.
- Unless the source of the sepsis is obvious, further imaging may be necessary, e.g. CT abdomen. Definitive drainage of the sepsis may require surgery or interventional radiology.

CVA
- Maintain adequate hydration with IV fluids but avoid overhydration due to the risk of cerebral oedema.
- Give O_2 to keep $SaO_2 > 94\%$.
- Keep NBM until the patient's swallowing has been assessed.
- Arrange urgent CT head to exclude a haemorrhagic stroke or intracra-nial haemorrhage (e.g. subdural haemorrhage).
- Discuss with the on-call medical team or stroke team urgently. Thrombolysis is not yet widely practised.

⛭ Chest pain

Patients complaining of acute chest pain require emergency assessment in order to detect potentially life-threatening conditions, e.g. ACS.

The term ACS encompasses unstable angina, non-ST elevation myocardial infarction (NSTEMI), and ST-elevation myocardial infarction (STEMI). Unstable angina is angina present at rest, or with lower levels of activity than previously, or with recently increasing frequency, duration, or intensity. Unstable angina is distinguished from NSTEMI by the absence of elevation in cardiac biomarkers (e.g. troponin I/T, CK, CK-MB, myoglobin). STEMI is distinguished from NSTEMI and unstable angina by the presence of ST elevation on ECG ($\geq$ 0.1mV in $\geq$ 2 adjacent limb leads, or $\geq$ 0.2mV in $\geq$ 2 adjacent chest leads, or new LBBB).

❶ Ask for a repeat set of observations including SaO_2 and an ECG while you are on your way to the ward/HDU.

Causes
- ACS.
- PE.
- Aortic dissection (📖 p.468).
- GORD.
- Pneumothorax (📖 p.458).
- Pericarditis/myocarditis.
- Hospital-acquired pneumonia.
- Oesophageal rupture (📖 p.200).
- Biliary colic/acute cholecystitis (📖 p.226).
- Gastritis (📖 p.210).
- Acute pancreatitis (📖 p.244).
- Asthma.
- Musculoskeletal chest pain.
- Herpes zoster (shingles).
- Panic attack.

❶ *Specific conditions to consider in a surgical patient*
- Anastomotic leak (especially in upper GI surgery).
- Operative site pain, e.g. thoracotomy and upper midline laparotomy incisions.
- ACS due to postoperative anaemia or hypotension due to a bleed.
- Pneumothorax if recent internal jugular vein or subclavian vein central line insertion or thoracic surgery without chest drainage (e.g. thoraco-scopic sympathectomy).
- Major surgery is a strong risk factor for PE.

Immediate assessment and management

Airway
- Examination. Usually intact; if not use airway opening manoeuvres (📖 p.47) and call for the resuscitation team.
- Immediate management. Give high-flow O_2 via a non-rebreathing mask.

Breathing
- Examination. Check carefully for signs of a pneumothorax.
- Immediate management. Treat a tension pneumothorax immediately with needle thoracic decompression (📖 p.516) and then insert an intercostal drain (📖 p.522).

Circulation
- Examination. Look for pallor and poorly perfused peripheries that may indicate haemorrhagic shock. Auscultate the heart carefully for murmurs (e.g. aortic stenosis causing ACS, or aortic regurgitation from aortic dissection) and a pericardial friction rub due to myocarditis or pericarditis.
- Immediate management. Insert 2 peripheral cannulae and take bloods. Fluid boluses may precipitate LVF in ACS and should be avoided unless haemorrhage is the likely underlying cause.

Disability and exposure
- Examination. Usually normal, although ↓ GCS may be due to severe hypoxia or hypotension. If focal neurological signs are present consider aortic dissection. Look at the drains for evidence of bleeding.
- Immediate management: no specific management.

Adjuncts
- 12-lead ECG: look for dysrhythmias and signs of myocardial ischaemia (Box 5.3).
- FBC, U&Es, serum amylase, LFTs, PT, APTT.
- If haemorrhagic shock is present, cross-match 4–6 units of packed RBCs.
- Arrange an urgent CXR (portable if the patient is too unstable to travel to the radiology department).
- If SaO_2 < 95% on air or tachypnoea is present, perform an ABG.

> **Box 5.3 Acute ECG changes in myocardial ischaemia**
>
> Acute ECG changes in myocardial ischaemia are highly variable, but include the following:
> - ST elevation;
> - ST depression (especially horizontal depression, as downsloping depression is associated with LVH and digoxin);
> - T wave changes (tall, flattened, inverted, or biphasic);
> - New LBBB;
> - No changes from previous ECGs;
> - Dysrhythmias ranging from extrasystoles or AF to heart block, VT, and VF.
>
> ❶ Up to 20% of patients with an MI initially have a normal ECG.
>
> ❶ Comparison with old ECGs is essential.

Further assessment

Case-notes, operation note, anaesthetic note
- Look in the case-notes for a past history of IHD, PE, GORD, and risk factors for IHD.
- Check the operation and anaesthetic notes for any difficulties, instructions, blood loss, and intraoperative events.

Observations chart, fluid balance chart, fluid prescription chart, medication chart Look at the recent trends on the observations and fluid charts: progressive hypotension and tachycardia suggest haemorrhage.

History
- Take a history of the pain, checking specifically for localization, intensity, character, duration, referral (e.g. neck, jaw, left or right arm), change with movement/posture, change with food/fluid. Pleuritic pain suggests PE.
- Enquire about a history of IHD or risk factors for IHD.

Examination
- Examination of the patient with ACS is frequently normal. Severe myocardial dysfunction may cause LVF or CHF.
- Examine the abdomen carefully for abdominal tenderness, which may suggest an anastomotic leak.
- Check specifically for aortic regurgitation and unequal pulses and BP in the arms (aortic dissection), and chest wall tenderness (musculoskeletal).

❶ Sharp, stabbing pain, pleuritic or positional pain, or pain reproduced with palpation in a patient with no history of IHD is unlikely to be due to myocardial ischaemia.

Check available results
- Look for ↓ Hb and coagulopathy suggesting postoperative haemorrhage. An ↑ WCC suggests pneumonia or anastomotic leak.
- Check the CXR for haemo/pneumothorax, pneumonia, signs of PE, and mediastinal widening (aortic dissection).

Further management

ACS with no ST elevation or new LBBB on ECG
- Give 2 × puffs of sublingual GTN if systolic BP > 90mmHg.
- Give morphine 2.5–5mg IV boluses, titrated to response.
- Give aspirin 300mg PO + clopidogrel 300mg PO.
- Urgent referral to the on-call medical team is required for consideration of anticoagulation, glycoprotein IIb/IIIa receptor blockers, β-blockers, and GTN infusion. Transfer to CCU may be required.
- Review the patient in 1h with a repeat ECG to detect evolving ST elevation.
- Take blood for cardiac troponin I/T 12h after the onset of chest pain.

ACS with ST elevation or new LBBB
- Give medications as above.
- Refer **immediately** to the on-call medical team for consideration of above treatments and thrombolysis or percutaneous coronary intervention (PCI).
  - ❶ Thrombolysis is contraindicated if major trauma/surgery/head injury has occurred within 3 weeks, or a GI bleed within 4 weeks. PCI may be preferred in this situation.

❶ All patients with suspected ACS should also be discussed with your senior as the use of anticoagulation and potent anti-platelet agents may be contraindicated in the early postoperative period.

PE (📖 p.149)

Hospital-acquired pneumonia (📖 p.150)

:☼: Shortness of breath/low SaO₂

Patients may complain of SOB, or the nursing staff may observe a high respiratory rate or low SaO₂. Although commonly attributable to respiratory disease, these problems may be due to abdominal conditions that reduce the intrathoracic volume, or the respiratory side-effects of opioid analgesia.

Causes
- PE.
- Hospital-acquired pneumonia.
- LVF.
- Pneumothorax (simple or tension; 📖 p.458).
- Asthma.
- Exacerbation of COPD.
- Pleural effusion.
- Atelectasis.

❶ Specific conditions to consider in a surgical patient
- Reduced thoracic volume due to intrathoracic gastric volvulus (📖 p.206), diaphragmatic hernia (📖 p.69), or abdominal distension (e.g. mechanical bowel obstruction (📖 p.268), acute gastric dilatation (📖 p.205), or postoperative ileus (📖 p.295) causing an abdominal compartment syndrome (📖 p.486)).
- Operative site bleeding causing anaemia or shock.
- After oesophageal resection, consider pleural collections due to an intrathoracic anastomotic leak, chylothorax, or haemothorax (📖 p.214).
- Aspiration pneumonia after NG tube insertion, upper GI endoscopy, or with bowel obstruction.
- Acute lung injury (ALI) and acute respiratory distress syndrome (ARDS), e.g. after septic shock, acute pancreatitis, polytrauma, fat embolism syndrome, massive transfusion, or aspiration of gastric contents.
- Operative site pain from thoracotomy and upper midline laparotomy incisions.
- Respiratory depression from opioid overdose.
- High sensory block with an epidural, leading to inadequate ventilation.
- Pneumothorax, if recent internal jugular vein or subclavian vein central line insertion or thoracic surgery without chest drainage (e.g. thoracoscopic sympathectomy).
- Major surgery is a strong risk factor for PE.
- Fat embolism syndrome (📖 p.416) in a trauma or orthopaedic patient.

Immediate assessment and management

Airway
- Examination. Usually intact; if not use airway opening manoeuvres (📖 p.47) and call for the resuscitation team.
- Immediate management. If not on O₂, give 2–4L/min O₂ via a high-flow mask. For those already on O₂, increase by 2–4L/min.

Breathing

- Examination. Check for signs of a pneumothorax and LVF.
- Immediate management. Treat a tension pneumothorax immediately with needle thoracic decompression (📖 p.516) and then insert an intercostal drain (📖 p.522). If LVF is present, stop all IV fluids, and give 40–80mg IV furosemide immediately.

Circulation

- Examination. Look for pallor and poorly perfused peripheries that may indicate haemorrhagic shock. Listen for third and fourth heart sounds (gallop rhythm) associated with cardiac failure, and murmurs.
- Immediate management. Insert an IV cannula and take blood. If haemorrhage is likely, and there are no signs of LVF, give a 10–20mL/kg IV fluid bolus and insert a further cannula.

Disability and exposure

- Examination. Usually normal, although ↓ GCS may be due to severe hypoxia. Check for pinpoint pupils due to opioid overdose.
- Immediate management. If the pupils are pinpoint, give 100–200mcg naloxone IV, repeated as necessary. Stop the PCA or epidural.

Adjuncts

- Send blood for FBC, U&Es, CRP.
- If signs of haemorrhagic shock are present, cross-match at least 4 units of packed RBCs.
- ❶ D-dimers are invariably raised in postoperative patients and are unlikely to be of any help in the diagnosis or exclusion of PE.
- If the patient's temperature is > 37.5°C, take blood cultures peripherally, and through all central venous lines present.
- Perform an ABG.
- 12-lead ECG. Look for signs of myocardial ischaemia (📖 p.143) and PE (sinus tachycardia, AF, S$_I$Q$_{III}$T$_{III}$, right ventricular strain).
- Request a portable CXR.
- Insert a urinary catheter if one is not already present.
- If a productive cough is present, request sputum culture.
- In patients with a history of COPD or asthma, take a PEFR reading and determine the previous best or predicted value.

Further assessment

Case-notes, operation note, anaesthetic note

- Look in the case-notes for a past history of smoking, asthma, COPD, IHD, LVF, DVT/PE, and previous exercise tolerance. Look for PE risk factors and diagnoses associated with ALI/ARDS.
- Check the operation and anaesthetic notes for any difficulties, instructions, blood loss, and intraoperative events.

Observations chart, fluid balance chart, fluid prescription chart, medication chart

- Look at the respiratory rate and SaO$_2$ trends on the observations chart, and look for a grossly positive fluid balance on the fluid chart. Look at the recent chest drain output.
- Check the medication chart for recent opioids, including epidural and PCA. Has VTE prophylaxis (📖 p.26) been prescribed and given?

History

Take a history, including:
- onset of SOB and severity;
- presence and timing of wheeze, cough, purulent sputum, haemoptysis, and pyrexia;
- chest pain and associated features (📖 p.144);
- abdominal pain, distension, vomiting;
- calf pain and leg swelling.

❶ Clinical patterns of PE are variable, but include pleuritic pain and/or haemoptysis (pulmonary haemorrhage syndrome), isolated dyspnoea, or sudden collapse (📖 p.136).

Examination
- Determine the degree of SOB: can the patient complete sentences, or just words?
- Check the level of sensory blockade if an epidural infusion is running.
- Carefully re-examine the chest, looking for chest expansion, dullness/hyperresonance to percussion, wheeze, fine/coarse crepitations, bronchial breathing, and pleural rub.
- Check that any chest drains present are swinging with respiration and look for fresh blood in the drains.
  - ❶ Absence of swing in a chest drain implies blockage, lung re-inflation, or exposure to the atmosphere, e.g. dislodgement from the pleural cavity. Check the chest drain carefully to ensure that the underwater drainage system is set up correctly and that the tube is not clamped, kinked, or has fallen out.
- Examine the abdomen, looking for abdominal distension, tenderness, peritonitis.
- Look for signs of a DVT in the calf (📖 p.322).

Check available results
- FBC: Recent ↑ WCC (or CRP) suggests pneumonia.
- Look for recent sputum culture results.
- Check the portable CXR for haemo/pneumothorax, pneumonia, COPD, and LVF (Fig. 5.3).
  - Radiographic signs of PE are usually non-specific and include focal infiltrate, segmental collapse, raised diaphragm, and small pleural effusion. Wedge-shaped defects are rare, while normal CXRs are common.
  - ALI/ARDS is characterized by bilateral patchy infiltrates on CXR similar to LVF.
- ABG.
  - PEs can cause hypoxia, hypocapnia, or no changes.
  - ALI/ARDS cause severe hypoxia despite high FiO_2.
  - Asthma causes hypoxia and hypocapnia; the presence of normal or ↑ $PaCO_2$ indicates severe/life-threatening asthma.

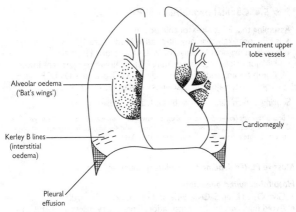

Fig. 5.3 CXR features of LVF. (Adapted, with permission, from Longmore, M., et al. (2007). *Oxford handbook of clinical medicine*, 7th edn, Chapter 4. Oxford University Press, Oxford.)

Further management

Operative site bleeding (📖 p.157)

Suspected PE

- Clinical findings are variable, but tachypnoea, dyspnoea, and pleuritic chest pain are common.
- Investigation findings are also variable; therefore assess and record the clinical probability (Box 5.4).
- If clinical probability is high or intermediate, start treatment dose LMWH (e.g. enoxaparin 1.5mg/kg od SC) or IV unfractionated heparin after discussion with your senior about the risk of haemorrhage.
- Give high-flow O₂ via a non-rebreathing mask to maintain SaO₂ > 94%. If hypotension is present give colloids to maintain BP and refer to HDU/ITU and the on-call medical team. Avoid fluid overload.
- Arrange further imaging, i.e. a V/Q scan if the CXR is normal and the patient has no chronic cardiorespiratory disease; otherwise CTPA.
- If PE is confirmed, start warfarin once bleeding is unlikely, and aim for INR of 2.5. Stop LMWH when INR > 2 for 2 consecutive days.
- An IVC filter can be inserted percutaneously if PEs occur despite therapeutic anticoagulation, or if anticoagulation is contraindicated.
- Continue warfarin for 3 months if temporary risk factors and a low risk of recurrence; 6 months if idiopathic or permanent risk factors.
- ❶ Operative site haematoma due to anticoagulation is a particular concern in orthopaedic patients (📖 p.424). Discuss with the operating surgeon first **before** starting LMWH.

Box 5.4 Clinical probability of PE*

Assuming that PE is a reasonable possibility:
- Is PE more likely than any alternative (if so, score 1)?
- Is there a major risk factor for VTE (if so, score 1)?
  - Major risk factor: recent immobility, major surgery, recent lower limb trauma and/or surgery, clinical DVT, previous DVT/PE, obstetric, major medical illness, metastatic cancer

Scoring: 2, high clinical probability; 1, intermediate; 0, low

* British Thoracic Society Standards of Care Committee Pulmonary Embolism Guideline Development Group (2003). British Thoracic Society guidelines for the management of suspected acute pulmonary embolism. *Thorax* **58**, 470–84.

Massive PE (i.e. leading to circulatory collapse; 📖 p.141)

Hospital-acquired pneumonia

- Give O_2 to keep SaO_2 > 94%, and re-check ABGs regularly.
- Avoid fluid overload and aspiration. If necessary, insert a NG tube to empty the stomach.
- Request urgent chest physiotherapy.
- Start IV antibiotics according to local protocol, e.g. vancomycin 1g bd + ceftazidime 2g tds (add metronidazole 500mg tds if aspiration is likely). If severe sepsis (📖 p.482) or septic shock (📖 p.482) is present, consider giving meropenem 1g tds + vancomycin 1g bd, and discuss with the on-call microbiologist.
- Patients with severe sepsis, septic shock, drowsiness, worsening tachy-pnoea, or deteriorating PaO_2, $PaCO_2$, or pH require urgent referral to the on-call medical team and intensivist to consider HDU/ITU admission and ventilation (non-invasive or invasive).

LVF

- Give O_2 to keep SaO_2 > 94%, and re-check ABGs regularly.
- Repeat furosemide 40–80mg IV and morphine as needed to maintain a good diuresis and clinical improvement.
- Look for the underlying cause (e.g. fluid overload, ACS (📖 p.142), cardiac dysrhythmias, acute valvular regurgitation, sepsis).
- Repeat an ECG in 2h to check for evolving myocardial ischaemia and measure cardiac biomarkers (e.g. troponin I/T) 12h post-LVF.
- Consider central venous line insertion to guide fluid management and transfer to HDU for cardiac monitoring.
- Patients with severe LVF or LVF refractory to initial treatment require urgent referral to the on-call medical team for assessment and consideration of transfer to CCU/ITU for GTN infusion, inotropes, treatment of the underlying cause, and ventilation (non-invasive or invasive).

❶ LVF with cardiogenic shock has a high mortality; refer to the on-call medical team immediately.

❶ Consider ALI/ARDS as a non-cardiogenic cause of pulmonary oedema.

Asthma

- Identify severe/life-threatening asthma early (Box 5.5).
- Correct hypoxia with high FiO_2 to keep SaO_2 > 92%.
- Give nebulized salbutamol 5mg regularly (initially 15–30min intervals), driven by O_2 nebulizer. Nebulized ipratropium (0.5mg qds) should be added for those patients with severe or life-threatening asthma.
- Start oral prednisolone 40mg od, or IV hydrocortisone 100mg qds if the oral route is not available.
- Rehydrate with IV fluids and correct ↓ K^+ caused by salbutamol, but avoid fluid overload.
- Record PEFR before and after nebulized salbutamol.
- Patients with severe or life-threatening asthma and those failing to respond to treatment must be referred immediately to the on-call medical team.
- ❶ LVF may cause wheeze ('cardiac asthma').

Box 5.5 Recognition of severe/life-threatening asthma*

Acute severe asthma

Any one of:
- PEFR 33–50% best or predicted;
- Respiratory rate ≥ 25/min;
- Heart rate ≥ 110/min;
- Inability to complete sentences in one breath.

Life-threatening asthma

Any one of the following in a patient with severe asthma:
- PEFR < 33% best or predicted;
- SaO_2 < 92%;
- PaO_2 < 8kPa;
- Normal $PaCO_2$;
- Silent chest;
- Cyanosis;
- Poor respiratory effort;
- Bradycardia, dysrhythmia, hypotension, confusion.

❶ The presence of ↑ $PaCO_2$ indicates near-fatal asthma.

* British Thoracic Society (BTS)/Scottish Intercollegiate Guidelines Network (SIGN) (2003). British guideline on the management of asthma. *Thorax* **58** (Suppl. I), i1–94.

High sensory block with an epidural, i.e. higher than the nipples (T4)

- Stop the epidural infusion.
- Give O_2 to keep SaO_2 > 94%.
- Contact the on-call anaesthetist immediately to discuss re-starting the epidural at a decreased rate once the block is at T6.

ALI/ARDS (Box 5.6)

- Give high-flow O_2 to maintain SaO_2 > 92%.
- Avoid fluid overload. A central venous line should be inserted.
- Aggressively treat the precipitating cause, e.g. sepsis.
- Most patients require invasive ventilation, although some patients with ALI can be managed with non-invasive ventilation.
- ❶ If ALI/ARDS are suspected, refer to the on-call intensivist.

Box 5.6 ALI/ARDS

ALI can occur as the pulmonary manifestation of the systemic inflammatory response syndrome (SIRS) after severe systemic insults. ARDS is the severe form of ALI. Clinical signs are those of pulmonary oedema. Where risk factors are present, three criteria are required to diagnose ALI/ARDS:

- new bilateral diffuse patchy infiltrates on CXR, consistent with pulmonary oedema;
- no clinical evidence of CCF, LVF, or fluid overload responsible for the radiographic appearances, or pulmonary artery wedge pressure < 18mmHg on Swan–Ganz catheterization;
- PaO_2/FiO_2 < 40kPa (ALI) or < 26kPa (ARDS).

❶ Echocardiography is useful to exclude cardiogenic pulmonary oedema.

Fat embolism syndrome (📖 *p.416*)

Exacerbation of COPD

- Give a precise FiO_2 via a Venturi device and prescribe it on the medication chart. Aim to keep SaO_2 88–92% without increasing $PaCO_2$ or worsening acidosis. Repeat ABGs are essential.
- Avoid fluid overload.
- Request urgent chest physiotherapy.
- Start nebulized salbutamol 2.5mg qds and nebulized ipratropium 250mcg qds. If hypercapnia or acidosis is present on ABG, drive the nebulizer with compressed air (not O_2), giving O_2 via nasal cannulae.
- Start oral prednisolone 30mg od.
- Only give IV antibiotics (e.g. ceftriaxone 2g od + erythromycin 1g qds) if pneumonia is present on CXR and 2 or more of the following are present: ↑ SOB, ↑ sputum volume, development of purulent sputum, or if acute on chronic respiratory failure is present (pH < 7.35). Otherwise give oral antibiotics.
- Patients with drowsiness, worsening symptoms, or deteriorating PaO_2, $PaCO_2$, or pH require urgent referral to the on-call physician and intensivist to consider HDU/ITU admission, IV bronchodilators, and ventilation (non-invasive or invasive).

:O: Hypotension

Hypotension is present when end-organ perfusion is compromised; the systolic BP at which this occurs varies greatly between patients as individuals adapt to their own baseline systolic BP. Inadequate urine output (< 0.5mL/kg/h) is one of the earliest signs of organ hypoperfusion and relative hypotension. In haemorrhagic shock, hypotension indicates severe blood loss (□ p.52).

Operative site bleeding must **always** be considered as a cause of tachycardia/hypotension in a postoperative patient. Bleeding is most common after vascular surgery, pelvic surgery, and upper GI cancer surgery. Immediate postoperative bleeding may occur due to inadequate haemostasis or fibrinolysis (primary haemorrhage); delayed bleeding (5–10 days) is a result of infection (secondary haemorrhage).

Causes
- Haemorrhagic shock:
  - operative site bleeding;
  - trauma;
  - upper or lower GI bleeding.
- Non-haemorrhagic shock:
  - severe sepsis/septic shock;
  - cardiogenic shock, e.g. ACS, dysrhythmias, cardiac tamponade;
  - anaphylactic shock;
  - massive PE;
  - tension pneumothorax.
- Severe hypoxia from any cause.
- Addisonian crisis.
- Drugs, e.g. anti-hypertensives, vasodilators (e.g. GTN), anti-dysrhythmics, opioids.

❶ *Specific conditions to consider in a surgical patient*
- Operative site bleeding.
- Sepsis due to a suture/staple line or anastomotic leak.
- Dehydration.
- Epidural-related hypotension.

Immediate assessment and management

Airway
- Examination. Usually intact. If not use airway opening manoeuvres (□ p.47) and call for the resuscitation team.
- Immediate management. Give 10–12L/min O_2 via a non-rebreathing mask.

Breathing
- Examination. Check for signs of a tension pneumothorax. Severe LVF may lead to cardiogenic shock.
- Immediate management. Treat a tension pneumothorax immediately with needle thoracic decompression (□ p.516) and then insert an intercostal drain (□ p.522). If LVF is present, stop all IV fluids, and give 40–80mg IV furosemide immediately.

Circulation

- Examination. Check for peripheral perfusion (↑ in early septic shock and epidural-related hypotension, ↓ in haemorrhagic shock). Examine the JVP, and auscultate the heart for dysrhythmias and murmurs.
- Immediate management. Insert 2 × large-bore IV cannulae. If haemorrhage is likely, give a 10–20mL/kg IV fluid bolus and insert a further cannula. Avoid if cardiogenic shock is suspected. If cardiac tamponade is suspected, perform pericardiocentesis (◻ p.534).

Disability and exposure

- Examination. Usually normal. Check all operative drains for acute blood loss and ensure that any chest drains are swinging on respiration. Examine the pupils, looking for signs of opioid overdose.
  - ❶ Abdominal drains commonly block or are separate from the site of bleeding. Do **not** rely on them to diagnose operative site bleeding.
- Immediate management. If pin-point pupils are present, give naloxone 100–200mcg IV.

Adjuncts

- Send blood for FBC, U&Es.
- If signs of haemorrhagic shock are present, cross-match at least 4 units of packed RBCs and check PT, APTT, and INR.
- Take blood cultures peripherally, and through all central venous lines present.
- 12-lead ECG. Look for signs of myocardial ischaemia (◻ p.143), dysrhythmias, and PE.
- Request a portable erect CXR if non-haemorrhagic shock or intrathoracic bleeding is suspected.
- Insert a urinary catheter if one is not already present.
- If hypoxia or tachypnoea are present, take an ABG.

Further assessment

Case-notes, operation note, anaesthetic note

- Find the preoperative BP in the case-notes to determine the baseline BP.
- Check the operation and anaesthetic note for any difficulties, instructions, blood loss, and intraoperative events. Look at the recovery chart to see what the immediate postoperative BP was.

Observations chart, fluid balance chart, fluid prescription chart, medication chart

- Progressive hypotension and tachycardia with a falling urine output suggest operative site bleeding. Check drain outputs.
- Look at the fluid prescription chart to see what volume of fluids has been given and whether they have been administered at the prescribed rate.
- Check the medication chart for anti-hypertensives and omit further doses. Stop anticoagulants and LMWH thromboprophylaxis if operative site bleeding is suspected.

History
- Check for symptoms of anaemia, hypoxia, ACS, PE, and upper and lower GI bleeding.

❶ Operative site bleeding can be asymptomatic.

Examination
- Often pale, cold, and clammy with operative site bleeding. After abdominal surgery, overt abdominal signs of bleeding are often absent.
  - Intraperitoneal blood leads to abdominal tenderness, but this is often difficult to distinguish from normal postoperative wound pain.
  - Abdominal distension may be present, but is a late sign.
- Check the level of sensory blockade if an epidural infusion is running.
- Look for features of sepsis and, if present, locate the source, e.g. pneumonia, UTI, intraabdominal abscess, anastomotic or staple/suture line leak.
- Perform a DRE to check for significant GI bleeding (avoid after rectal surgery).

Check available results
- FBC: often shows ↓ Hb with ↑ PT and APTT in operative site bleeding. ↑ WCC suggests sepsis.
- U&Es: ↑ creatinine and urea is common due to renal hypoperfusion.
- PT/INR, APTT: often ↑. This may be the cause or the effect of severe bleeding.

Further management
- Upper GI bleeding (📖 p.190).
- Lower GI bleeding (📖 p.280).
- Severe sepsis/septic shock (📖 p.482).
- ACS (📖 p.144).
- Anaphylaxis (📖 p.139).
- Massive PE (📖 p.141).
- Dysrhythmias.
  - Tachycardia (📖 p.158).
  - Bradycardia < 40/min, or < 60/min with adverse signs (systolic BP < 90mmHg, signs of heart failure) should be treated with atropine 500mcg IV, repeated as necessary to a maximum of 3mg.

❶ Bradycardia in a hypotensive patient requires **immediate** referral to the on-call medical team.

❶ Tachycardic patients with chest pain, hypotension, poor peripheral perfusion, heart failure, or a ventricular rate > 150/min on ECG require **immediate** referral to the on-call medical team for assessment and consideration of electrical cardioversion. This excludes those patients with a sinus tachycardia.

Dehydration
- Give 10–20mL/kg crystalloid fluid boluses, aiming for normotension and urine output of > 0.5mL/kg/h.
- Fluid boluses of 5mL/kg may be necessary in those with a history of cardiac failure or significant cardiorespiratory disease. Consider inserting a central venous line to guide resuscitation.

- Correct electrolyte abnormalities (📖 p.18).
- Search for the underlying cause of the dehydration, e.g. bowel obstruction, poor oral intake.

Operative site bleeding
- Keep the patient NBM.
- Give high-flow O_2 via a non-rebreathing mask.
- Resuscitate with IV fluids and packed RBCs to maintain adequate peripheral perfusion. Avoid excessive resuscitation as this may provoke further bleeding.
- Correct any coagulopathy with FFP and other blood products as required (📖 p.22).
- Operative site bleeding usually requires a return to theatre for haematoma evacuation and haemostasis. Very occasionally, angiographic embolization may be possible.

❶ Inform your senior immediately if you suspect significant postoperative bleeding.

Epidural-related hypotension
- Hypotension occurs due to reduced vascular tone from sympathetic nerve blockade.
- Patients with epidural-induced hypotension are characteristically comfortable, with warm, well-perfused peripheries.
- If systolic BP < 90mmHg, or urine output is poor (< 0.5mL/kg/h), or creatinine is rising, treat by giving fluid boluses (e.g. 250–500mL colloid over 30min–1h). Give O_2 at 4L/min.
- If systolic BP is < 90mmHg after 1000mL colloid, discuss with your senior and the on-call intensivist to consider transfer to HDU, central venous line monitoring, further investigations, and vasopressors (e.g. ephedrine).
- If the level of the sensory block is higher than T4, stop the infusion and discuss further management with the on-call anaesthetist.

❶ Hypotension can only be attributed to an epidural once other causes of postoperative hypotension have been excluded.

❶ Problems with epidurals should be discussed with the on-call anaesthetic team. Reduction in the epidural rate may help reduce hypotension, but with the risk of worsening postoperative pain.

① Tachycardia

Tachycardia (heart rate > 100/min) in a surgical patient is usually a marker of significant systemic upset. As such, it is important to determine the underlying cause, especially a postoperative complication such as an anastomotic or suture/staple line leak. This section deals with the majority of tachycardic surgical patients, who have either sinus tachycardia or AF.

- ►► The management of a pulseless tachycardia is described elsewhere (🕮 p.137).
- ❶ Tachycardic patients with chest pain, hypotension, poor peripheral perfusion, heart failure, or a ventricular rate > 150/min on ECG require **immediate** referral to the on-call medical team for assessment and consideration of electrical cardioversion. This excludes those patients with a sinus tachycardia.
- ❶ Patients with broad complex tachycardias (e.g. ventricular tachycardia) require urgent referral to the on-call medical team.
- ❶ Patients with regular narrow complex tachycardias (excluding sinus tachycardia) can undergo vagal manouevres (e.g. Valsalva) under cardiac monitoring to detect the underlying rhythm. Urgent referral to the on-call medical team is required.
- ❶ Ask for a 12-lead ECG while you are on the way to the ward/HDU.

Causes

- Early haemorrhagic shock (🕮 p.52):
  - operative site bleeding;
  - trauma;
  - upper or lower GI bleeding.
- Tachydysrhythmias, e.g. AF.
- Drugs, e.g. salbutamol.

❶ Specific conditions to consider in a surgical patient

- Operative site bleeding.
- Sepsis, e.g. due an intraabdominal abscess, suture/staple line, or anastomotic leak.
- Pain.
- Dehydration.
- Fat embolism syndrome (🕮 p.416) in a trauma or orthopaedic patient.
- Major surgery is a strong risk factor for PE.

Patients with isolated tachycardias are generally stable enough not to require an ABCDE approach.

Chart review

- Review the case-notes for recent progress and look for a history of IHD, AF, palpitations.
- Check the operation note to see if an anastomosis or suture/staple line has been formed.
- Look at the medication chart to see if any drugs that may cause tachycardia have been given, and what analgesia has been given.
- Examine the observation and fluid charts for evidence of sepsis, e.g. pyrexia and hypotension. Check the pain score.

History

Ask about palpitations, chest pain, SOB, and abdominal pain.

Examination

- General. Is the patient in pain or discomfort? Are signs of sepsis present (🕮 p.482)?
- Chest. Check for signs of pneumonia and LVF. Auscultate the heart.
- Abdomen. Check for signs of an intraabdominal infection.
- Peripheries. Exclude a compartment syndrome.

Investigations

- FBC: look for ↓ Hb.
- U&Es. ↓ K^+ can lead to AF; ↑ creatinine and urea may reflect dehydration.
- ECG: this is essential to diagnose AF and other tachydysrhythmias. Broad complex tachycardias have QRS complexes of > 0.12s duration. Look for evidence of myocardial ischaemia (🕮 p.143).
  - ❶ If you are unsure of the rhythm on ECG, call for assistance from your senior or the on-call medical team.
- Check serum Ca^{2+}, Mg^{2+} if AF is present.
- Erect CXR: look for signs of pneumonia, and free gas. It may be normal to see free gas for the first few days after abdominal surgery or laparoscopy.

Management

All patients with sinus tachycardia or AF should be given O_2 to keep $SaO_2 > 94\%$ and IV access should be inserted.

AF

- Correct hypovolaemia in order to improve myocardial filling, but avoid fluid overload. Insertion of a central venous line may be required.
- Correct ↓ K^+ (🕮 p.18) and ↓/↑ Ca^{2+} and Mg^{2+}, if present.
- AF without haemodynamic instability can be treated with rate-control medications (e.g. digoxin) or pharmacological cardioversion (e.g. amiodarone). Discuss management with the on-call medical team. Anticoagulation may be necessary.

- Check cardiac biomarkers at 12h after the onset to detect NSTEMI.
- Search for an underlying cause, e.g. sepsis due to a suture/staple line or anastomotic leak, ACS, PE, ↓ K$^+$, myocardial contusion. Have a low threshold for CT abdomen and pelvis or water-soluble contrast studies to exclude an intraabdominal abscess or a leak.

❶ Always discuss patients with new-onset AF with your seniors, focusing on detecting the underlying cause and the suitability of anticoagulation.

Pain

- Give regular paracetamol 1g qds (IV, PO, or PR).
- Consider regular NSAIDs PO/PR and oral opioids if no contra-indications are present.
- Ensure that appropriate parenteral opioids are prescribed, e.g. prn morphine 5–10mg IV/IM + an anti-emetic.
- If a PCA is present, consider increasing the bolus dose from 1mg to 2mg.
- If an epidural infusion is running discuss with the on-call anaesthetist about increasing the epidural rate or giving top-up boluses of LA. Review hourly and watch for hypotension. If the epidural is still ineffective, stop it and start a PCA.

❶ Do not prescribe suppositories after rectal surgery.

❶ Do not prescribe oral opioids to patients on a PCA or epidural.

❶ Always search for an underlying cause for the pain, e.g. peritonitis, ischaemic bowel, compartment syndrome.

Dehydration (📖 p.156)
Operative site bleeding (📖 p.157)
Upper (📖 p.190) and lower (📖 p.280) GI bleeding
Sepsis (📖 p.482)
Fat embolism syndrome (📖 p.416)
PE (📖 p.149)

① Pyrexia

A temperature > 37.5°C is considered to be a clinically significant pyrexia. In postoperative patients, the likely causes vary with the time after surgery.

- Lung atelectasis (~ days 0–2).
- Fat embolism syndrome (📖 p.416) in a trauma or orthopaedic patient (~ days 0–2).
- Hospital-acquired pneumonia (~ day 2 onwards).
- DVT/PE (~ day 5 onwards).
- UTI (~ day 5 onwards).
- Infected cannula, line, drain, or epidural site (~ day 5 onwards).
- Wound infection (~ day 5 onwards).
- Operative site infection, e.g. intraabdominal abscess (including subphrenic and subhepatic), suture/staple line or anastomotic leak, parastomal abscess, vascular graft infection (~ day 5 onwards).
- Miscellaneous causes, e.g. infective endocarditis, meningitis, discitis, septic arthritis, pressure ulcers.

When pyrexia is the prime complaint, patients are almost always stable enough not to require an ABCDE approach.

Chart review

- Look in the case-notes for recent progress, and look for a history of smoking (increases the risk of postoperative atelectasis and pneumonia) and DVT/PE.
- Check the operation note to see if an anastomosis or suture/staple line has been formed, or a prosthesis implanted.
- Look at the medication chart to see if prophylactic LMWH has been given.
- Look at the observations and fluid charts: swinging pyrexia implies an intraabdominal abscess; poor urine output may indicate severe sepsis.

History

Ask about localizing signs:

- cough, purulent sputum, chest pain, SOB;
- abdominal pain, vomiting, diarrhoea;
- calf pain or leg swelling;
- dysuria, frequency, suprapubic pain (if not catheterized);
- pain around a cannula, line, or drain;
- increasing pain around the wound, wound discharge;
- back pain, joint pain, headache, rash, photophobia.

Examination

- General. Systemically well, or signs of severe sepsis (confusion, hypotension, poor urine output)?
- Chest.
  - Check for signs of pneumonia (coarse crepitations, bronchial breathing).
  - Auscultate the heart for new murmurs suggesting infective endocarditis.

- Abdomen.
  - Check for signs of an intraabdominal infection (abdominal distension and prolonged ileus, localized tenderness or peritonitis, pelvic abscess palpable on DRE).
  - Remove the wound dressings and look for redness and wound discharge.
  - Look around the catheter for purulent discharge.
- Peripheries.
  - Carefully check the epidural site, and any cannulae, IV lines, and drains looking for erythema, tenderness, or pus.
  - Check the thighs and calves for signs of a DVT (swelling, erythema, tenderness).
  - Look at pressure areas for ulcers.

Investigations

Patients within 48h of surgery who are systemically well with no localizing signs are likely to have lung atelectasis and do not require investigation. In other patients, the following should be performed.

- FBC and CRP. Usually ↑, but non-specific, and WCC and CRP are often ↑ after major surgery anyway. Progressive ↑ in WCC/CRP implies a significant infection (e.g. anastomotic leak, pneumonia).
- U&Es. Check for renal dysfunction caused by sepsis.
- Blood cultures. Take peripherally, and through the central venous line, if present.
- Erect CXR. Look for signs of pneumonia and free gas (implying a suture/staple line or anastomotic leak).
- MSU/CSU and urine dipstick. Check for leucocytes and nitrites consistent with UTI, and send for M, C & S.
- ABG and serum lactate. If signs of severe sepsis are present or SaO_2 < 95% on air.
- Leg USS (duplex venography). If lower limb DVT is suspected. D-dimers are invariably raised in postoperative patients and are not helpful.

Management

This depends on the how unwell the patient is.

Significant organ system dysfunction (severe sepsis) (📖 p.482)
General management

- If hypotension is present, give a 2mL/kg IV crystalloid bolus. If hypotension remains despite further 10–20mL/kg boluses, a central venous line may need to be placed to guide fluid management. Patients with a history of heart failure require 5mL/kg crystalloid boluses and a lower threshold for central venous line placement.
- Give high-flow O_2 at 10–12L/min via a non-rebreathing mask.
- Start broad spectrum IV antibiotics appropriate for the suspected source of sepsis. Discuss with the on-call microbiologist.
- HDU or ITU admission may be needed. Discuss with your senior.
- Unless the source of the sepsis is obvious, further imaging may be necessary, e.g. CT abdomen and pelvis, white cell nuclear medicine scan.

Hospital-acquired pneumonia (📖 p.150).

Intraabdominal abscess (📖 p.294)

Suture/staple line or anastomotic leak (see the disease-specific chapters in Part 3)

Vascular graft infection (📖 p.346)

PE (📖 p.149)

Severe UTI
- Fluid resuscitate.
- Start IV antibiotics (e.g. gentamicin according to local dosage protocols) and monitor renal function carefully.
- If a urinary catheter is present, remove or replace it, as long as there are no urological contraindications (e.g. recent bladder, prostate, or urethral surgery).

Mild presentation

Lung atelectasis
- Prescribe saline nebulizers (5mL qds).
- Encourage mobilization.
- Ensure that analgesia is adequate.
- Request urgent chest physiotherapy.

Infected IV cannulae
- Remove the cannula and send the tip for M, C, & S.
- Start oral antibiotics (e.g. flucloxacillin 500mg qds).

Infected central venous line
- Take both peripheral and central blood cultures.
- Discuss removal with your senior first, as line salvage may occasionally be attempted in patients with poor central venous access and long-term lines.
- If the catheter is to be removed, send the tip for culture.
- Begin IV antibiotics (e.g. vancomycin 1g bd + gentamicin according to local dosage protocols) only after discussion with the on-call microbiologist.

Infected epidural
- Redness and pain around the epidural site suggests infection and the epidural should be removed.
- An epidural abscess can produce severe back pain with a neurological deficit (e.g. limb weakness or paraesthesia, loss of anal sphincter tone, altered bladder control) with pyrexia and ↑ WCC.
- Discuss antibiotic treatment with a microbiologist.

❶ Inform the on-call anaesthetic team of any epidural problems.

Parastomal abscess (📖 p.298)

Superficial wound infection and wound abscess (📖 p.502)

Mild UTI
- If there are symptoms of UTI with an abnormal urine dipstick, start an oral antibiotic (e.g. norfloxacin 400mg bd) and encourage oral fluids.
- If a urinary catheter is present, remove or replace it, as long as there are no urological contraindications (e.g. recent bladder, prostate, or urethral surgery).

DVT (📖 p.322, 424)

Fat embolism syndrome (📖 p.416)

No obvious source
- Take blood cultures whenever the temperature is > 37.5°C.
- Swab all wounds, cannula, and line sites, take MSUs, and consider investigations for occult sources of infection (e.g. CT abdomen for sub-phrenic abscess, echocardiography for infective endocarditis).
- Discuss IV antibiotics with the on-call microbiologist and your senior.

Acute wound problems: introduction

Wound problems can occur after any type of surgery and can lead to potentially significant morbidity, or even mortality. Common acute wound problems include infection, bleeding, and dehiscence.

An understanding of the anatomy of the wound and important underlying structures is essential in order to assess and manage the wound correctly. The majority of midline laparotomy wounds are closed in two layers. The deep wound layer consists of a continuous absorbable or nonabsorbable suture passing through the anterior and posterior layers of the rectus sheath (mass closure technique). The superficial wound layer only closes the skin, either with staples or a continuous subcuticular absorbable suture.

❶ Stoma problems are dealt with elsewhere (📖 p.298).

:☺: **Laparotomy wound dehiscence**

Dehiscence of a laparotomy wound is the spontaneous opening of the deep suture layer, with or without a defect in the superficial layer. Some surgeons use the term 'superficial dehiscence' to describe opening of the superficial layer alone, although this can create confusion. The traditional understanding will be followed here. Dehiscence is a serious complication that extends hospital stay, and substantially increases morbidity and mortality. Dehiscence occurs because of:

- technical factors, e.g. poor surgical technique, knot failure, suture breakage;
- patient factors, e.g. poor nutritional state, abdominal distension, coughing, deep wound infection.

Clinical features

- If the superficial suture layer stays intact, the first sign of a dehiscence is often a sero-sanguinous discharge from the wound around days 7–10 postoperatively.
- ❶ Never ignore a wound discharge. If bowel contents or an abdominal wall defect are palpable contact your senior immediately.
- If the dehiscence goes unrecognized, disruption of the superficial layer leads to a dramatic prolapse of small bowel out of the wound. This is very distressing for both the patient and the nursing staff.

Investigations

Diagnostic investigations are unnecessary and waste time.

Management

- ❶ Contact your senior immediately.
- Cover the wound and prolapsed bowel in a large sterile abdominal pack soaked in sterile saline (trying to return the bowel into the abdominal cavity is futile).
- Give IV morphine 5–10mg for analgesia and as an anxiolytic.
- Keep NBM, start IV fluids, and insert a urinary catheter.
- Arrange for emergency theatre to enable the bowel to be returned to the abdominal cavity, washout, and re-suturing of the abdominal wound.

☼ Wound bleeding

Bleeding from wound edges after surgery is usually minor and settles spontaneously. When blood is soaking through multiple dressings, urgent assessment is needed and intervention may be required.

Clinical features
- Wound haemorrhage causing haemodynamically significant bleeding is rare, but check the pulse (📖 p.158), BP (📖 p.154), and urine output and manage accordingly.
- Gently remove the dressing and inspect the wound, looking for active bleeding, general wound ooze, and a wound haematoma (implying a deep bleed).

❶ Use sterile technique at all times when assessing or treating the wound.

Investigations
- Unless symptoms or signs of haemodynamically significant bleeding are present, these are unnecessary.
- If there is severe general wound ooze, check FBC and PT, APTT to detect a coagulopathy.

Management
- For minor ooze, try gentle firm pressure for 5min.
- For persistent bleeding from a single point, infiltrate 5–10mL of 1% lidocaine subcutaneously and insert non-absorbable sutures (e.g. 3/0 polypropylene or nylon as required to control the bleeding (📖 p.510).

❶ Ongoing bleeds or large wound haematomas require emergency return to theatre. Speak to your senior.

① Superficial wound infection and wound abscess

Fluid between the deep and superficial suture layers commonly becomes infected, leading to a wound abscess and a superficial wound infection. The diagnosis is usually obvious and management is often straightforward. It is important to exclude severe invasive soft tissue infections (📖 p.478) and wound dehiscence (see 'Laparotomy wound dehiscence', this chapter).

Clinical features

- Wound pain, pyrexia.
- Discharge of pus-like fluid from the wound, wound erythema, wound tenderness.

Investigations

- These are usually unnecessary.
- If temperature > 37.5°C or significant upset are present, take blood cultures, FBC, CRP, and U&Es.

Management

- Most superficial wound infections respond rapidly to drainage of the wound abscess (📖 p.502) alone and antibiotics are **not** required. Ensure that a wound swab is sent for M, C, & S.
- If there is significant systemic upset or spreading cellulitis, give IV antibiotics, e.g. vancomycin 1g bd + gentamicin (using local dosage protocols) + metronidazole 500mg tds.

❶ A bowel fistula may present as a wound abscess initially. Ongoing foul-smelling wound discharge despite drainage should alert you.

Part 3

Disease-based emergency surgery

Abdominal wall hernias

Introduction

A hernia is defined as a protrusion of an organ, part of an organ, or tissue through a defect in the wall containing it, into an abnormal position. Hernias of the abdominal wall are common and often present as an emergency. Common types of abdominal wall hernias include:
- inguinal;
- paraumbilical;
- femoral;
- incisional;
- epigastric.

There are also a number of rare abdominal wall hernias. Parastomal hernias are common, but only rarely present as an emergency.

Classification

These hernias can be further classified based on the degree of fixity of their contents, their viability, and whether or not there is bowel obstruction.
- Reducible. Hernia contents can be easily (or spontaneously) reduced back into the abdominal cavity.
- Irreducible (incarcerated). Adhesions between the components of the hernia, or the size of contents in relation to the neck, prevent reduction of sac and/or its contents. Irreducible hernias are particularly prone to obstruction and strangulation.
- Obstructed. Bowel within an irreducible hernia can become obstructed. This may eventually result in strangulation. Small bowel is much more likely than large bowel to enter a hernial orifice.
- Strangulated. Constriction of the hernia contents at the neck occludes the blood supply to the contents (usually small bowel or omentum). Initially venous return is impaired, but oedema results in arterial occlusion and eventually necrosis. Bowel within the hernia will eventually perforate.
  - ❶ A Richter's hernia is where only part of the intestine herniates and becomes strangulated. This can result in intestinal ischaemia and perforation but, because bowel obstruction does not occur, it is easily overlooked. It is usually associated with a femoral hernia or a laparoscopic port site hernia.
  - ❶ Strangulation is a life-threatening complication.

Assessment and management of strangulated hernias

Whereas hernias that are reducible and those that have become irreducible do not usually present as an emergency, an obstructed or strangulated hernia is a serious emergency condition. Urgent resuscitation and surgery are required. Because they often occur in the elderly, major co-morbidity is common and substantially increases the risk of complications and death. Mortality may approach 10%.

History
- May be a history of a known hernia.
- Sudden severe pain in the hernia.
- Central abdominal colicky pain.
- Abdominal distension.

- Vomiting.
- Constipation.

❶ A small hernia (especially a femoral hernia in an obese patient) is easily overlooked as a cause of small bowel obstruction. All patients presenting with obstruction should undergo careful examination of potential hernia sites (Fig. 6.1).

Examination
- Dehydration may be present.
- Tender, irreducible hernia with no cough impulse.
  - ❶ These features are the hallmark of a strangulated hernia.
- Overlying skin may be oedematous and inflamed.
- Abdominal distension.
- Increased bowel sounds.

❶ Strangulation of omentum or extraperitoneal fat may also occur, giving a tense, tender irreducible hernia, but without features of bowel obstruction. This also requires emergency surgery.

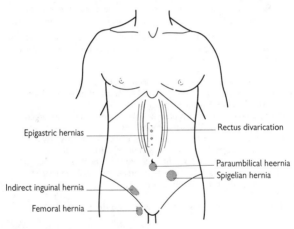

Epigastric hernias

Rectus divarication

Paraumbilical heernia
Spigelian hernia

Indirect inguinal hernia

Femoral hernia

Fig. 6.1 Sites of common abdominal wall hernias. Commonly seen, a rectus divarication is a widening of the rectus muscles and is not a hernia.

Investigations
- FBC: ↑ WCC may indicate strangulation.
- U&Es: ↑ creatinine and urea reflect dehydration.
- ABG and serum lactate: strangulation may lead to a metabolic acidosis.
- Erect CXR: even with bowel perforation, free gas under the diaphragm is rare, as the perforation is usually contained within the hernia sac.
- Supine AXR: evidence of bowel obstruction is seen. This is **not** present with a Richter's hernia, or if omentum/extraperitoneal fat is being strangulated.

- Abdominal CT or USS: helpful when the diagnosis is not clear.

Management

Where strangulation is suspected, prompt surgery (Box 6.1), following a brief period of intensive resuscitation to correct dehydration and electrolyte disturbance, is essential to avoid high mortality.

- Give IV opioid analgesia.
- Give O_2 to keep SaO_2 > 95%.
- Begin IV fluid resuscitation and correct electrolytes, especially K^+.
- Insert a urinary catheter (📖 p.504).
- Insert a NG tube (📖 p.498).
  - ❶ Beware of aspiration during insertion of a NG tube.
- A central venous line line may be useful if significant cardiovascular co-morbidity is present.
- Give broad spectrum IV antibiotics (e.g. cefuroxime 750mg tds + metronidazole 500mg tds).
- Start thromboprophylaxis (📖 p.26). Check with the on-call anaesthetist before giving LMWH, as this may prevent epidural or spinal anaesthesia.
  - ❶ Close liaison between senior surgical and anaesthetic staff is required, especially in elderly patients with multiple co-morbidities

When features of strangulation (e.g. severe pain, overlying erythema, ↑ WCC) are absent, gentle manual reduction (taxis) of a seemingly incarcerated hernia can be attempted.

- Give IV opioid analgesia first.
- Place the patient in a gentle head-down position.
- Put firm, constant pressure over the hernia, directing the contents towards the neck. Patience is essential.
- If reduction is successful, repair should be carried out on an urgent basis, usually the next available elective list.
- ❶ Reduction-en-masse is a risk. The sac and its contents may be returned through the abdominal wall defect. However, the contents may remain constricted by a fibrous ring at the neck of the sac. Therefore, patients should be observed after manual reduction for continuing evidence of intestinal obstruction requiring emergency surgical intervention.
- If reduction is unsuccessful, proceed as for a strangulated hernia.

Box 6.1 Principles of surgical repair of strangulated hernias

Surgery is best performed under GA. Exceptionally, it may be undertaken under regional (or even LA) in those with multiple co-morbidities. The open approach is used; the laparoscopic technique is generally regarded as unsuitable.

• After opening the hernia sac, the viability of the contents is determined. The constricting fascial margins at the neck of the sac may need to be incised to allow full delivery and inspection of the contents. The strangulated sac contents should not be allowed to slip back into the peritoneal cavity as they may be very difficult to retrieve.

• If the viability of any bowel within the hernia is in doubt, resection and anastomosis is performed. If better surgical access is required, an additional midline laparotomy incision is often the best strategy.

• Hernia contents are returned to the abdominal cavity and the defect repaired.

• A standard tension-free repair incorporating a prosthetic mesh can often be performed. Use of prosthetic mesh is best avoided if gross contamination is present, due to the high risk of chronic wound infection.

• Continue broad spectrum IV antibiotics for several days after surgery.

:✪: Inguinal hernias

These account for > 90% of all groin hernias and over 95% occur in males. Up to 5% of inguinal hernias become strangulated. Inguinal hernias in children are covered elsewhere (📖 p.362).

Anatomy

In adults, the inguinal canal is ~ 4cm long and passes obliquely through the abdominal wall superior to the inguinal ligament. The spermatic cord in the male, and the round ligament in the female, passes through the inguinal canal. The ilioinguinal nerve and the genital branch of the genitofemoral nerve also run in the canal. The spermatic cord/round ligament:
- enters the canal via the internal ring just lateral to the inferior epigastric vessels and 1–2cm superior to a point midway between the pubic tubercle and the anterior superior iliac spine;
- exits via the external ring in the external oblique aponeurosis, just superior and lateral to the pubic tubercle.

Inguinal hernias can either be direct or indirect, depending on their origin with respect to the internal ring and inferior epigastric vessels.

Indirect inguinal hernias
- Most common (65% of inguinal hernias in adults).
- They pass through the internal ring, lateral to the inferior epigastric vessels. Large indirect hernias exit through the external ring and may enter the scrotum (inguinoscrotal hernia).
- They have a narrow neck and may strangulate.

Direct inguinal hernias
- They pass through the posterior wall of the inguinal canal medial to inferior epigastric vessels and medial to the internal ring.
- Large direct hernias rarely enter the scrotum.
- They have a wide neck and **rarely** strangulate.

Assessment and management of strangulation

Clinical features
- History and examination as for any strangulated hernia.
- A tender swelling superior to the inguinal ligament that may lie anterior to the pubic tubercle and sometimes extend into the scrotum.

The differential diagnosis of a tender lump in the groin includes the following.
- Lymphadenopathy: usually just inferior to the inguinal ligament, often with lymphadenopathy elsewhere.
- Femoral artery aneurysm: pulsatile and expansile, sometimes coexistent with popliteal or abdominal aortic aneurysms.
- Groin abscess: usually inferior to the inguinal ligament, often at the site of injection in an intravenous drug user.
- ❶ A sigmoid diverticular abscess tracking through the left inguinal canal can be difficult to distinguish from a strangulated inguinal hernia, although features of bowel obstruction will be absent.

- Torsion of a maldescended testis: **always** check for the presence of both testes in the scrotum to exclude this.

Investigation and management
- As for any strangulated hernia (☐ p.175).

Surgery
- Repair using a standard open tension-free hernioplasty using a mesh to strengthen the posterior wall of the inguinal canal.
- Mesh is not advisable if bowel perforation or gangrene has occurred. Simple suture repair (or no repair) may be best if bowel perforation or gangrene has occurred. A definitive repair can be performed 1–2 weeks later once the sepsis and inflammation have resolved.

⚙ **Paraumbilical hernias**

Paraumbilical hernias are less common than groin hernias and usually occur in obese patients.

- The hernia passes through a weakness in the linea alba immediately superior (or occasionally inferior) to the umbilicus. This distinguishes them from congenital umbilical hernias where the defect is directly posterior to the umbilicus.
- They have a narrow neck and are at high risk of incarceration (and hence strangulation).

❶ On occasion, they may be difficult to distinguish from umbilical abscesses. Exploratory surgery or USS may be required.

- Strangulated paraumbilical hernias should be investigated and managed as for any strangulated hernia (📖 p.175).

Surgery

- Strangulated hernias are approached via a transverse incision immediately above or below the umbilicus.
- The hernia sac is opened, the hernial defect enlarged, and ischaemic omentum or bowel excised.
- If small (< 2cm diameter) the hernial defect can closed by simple sutures. Larger defects require prosthetic mesh, though this should be avoided if gross contamination is present.

⚙ **Femoral hernias**

Femoral hernias make up < 10% of groin hernias but commonly present with strangulation (> 40% of cases). They most often occur in the elderly and ~ 75% occur in females.

Anatomy

Femoral hernias pass through the femoral canal bounded:
- anteriorly by the inguinal ligament;
- posteriorly by the pectineal (Cooper's) ligament at its attachment to the pubis;
- medially by the lacunar ligament;
- laterally by the femoral vein.

Assessment and management of strangulation

Clinical features
- History and examination as for any strangulated hernia.
- ❶ Bowel obstruction may be absent, as the small size of the defect makes Richter's hernias more common.
- A tender swelling inferior and lateral to the pubic tubercle.
- ❶ The hernia sac extends through the femoral sheath and may extend upwards, crossing the inguinal ligament. The position of the fundus of the sac superior to the inguinal ligament may lead to misdiagnosis as an inguinal hernia.
- Consider other causes of a tender lump in the groin (📖 p.178).

❶ Femoral hernias are easy to miss if the patient is not exposed appropriately or if the diagnosis is not considered (Fig. 6.2).

Investigation and management
- As for any strangulated hernia (📖 p.175).
- ❶ Suspected strangulation of a femoral hernia should not be treated by manual reduction since a Richter's hernia with necrotic intestine may be returned to the peritoneal cavity, leading to generalized peritonitis. An open surgical repair should instead be undertaken.

Surgery
- The low approach (crural operation) used for elective repair of femoral hernia is best avoided if strangulation is suspected as this provides inadequate exposure for assessment, resection, and anastomosis of small bowel.
- The inguinal approach through the posterior wall of the inguinal canal allows better access but has the disadvantage that use of mesh to repair the posterior wall may be contraindicated in the presence of significant contamination.

- An extraperitoneal (high) approach is best when strangulation is suspected, since this gives good access for bowel resection and does not require use of mesh. After opening the hernia sac and dealing with the strangulated contents, the empty sac is closed and excised and the femoral canal closed by sutures.
- ❶ Particular care must be taken not to damage or permanently constrict the femoral vein, which lies immediately lateral to the hernia.

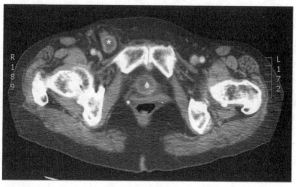

Fig. 6.2 Abdominal CT of an elderly woman with small bowel obstruction showing an obstructed right femoral hernia (*). The groins had not been examined.

⚙ Incisional hernias

Incisional hernias are a common complication after abdominal surgery. They may occur as a result of poor surgical technique, impaired wound healing, or following wound infection. They commonly have a wide neck so are unlikely to strangulate, but those with small necks and complex hernias with multiple defects often present with incarceration and strangulation.

> ❶ Surgery is often complex. The repair of a large incisional hernia may result in respiratory compromise due to increased intraabdominal pressure following return of the hernia contents to the abdominal cavity. Involve senior surgeons and anaesthetists early.

Laparoscopic port sites may give rise to incisional hernias with small necks that are likely to result in a Richter's hernia. These may be difficult to differentiate from a wound abscess or strangulated paraumbilical hernia. USS may be required if the diagnosis is unclear. The principles of management are the same as for other types of strangulated hernia.

☼ Epigastric hernias

These account for ~ 5% of abdominal wall hernias. They occur through a small defect in the linea alba between the umbilicus and the xiphisternum, and are often multiple. They present as a small midline swelling usually comprising extraperitoneal fat that readily strangulates resulting in severe localized abdominal pain. There may also be an associated peritoneal sac containing omentum. Surgical repair is through a small midline incision.

:☼: Rare hernias

There are several well described but uncommon types of hernia, all of which may present acutely with strangulation and intestinal obstruction.

❶ Uncommon hernias can be difficult to diagnose and may only be revealed by radiological imaging (usually CT) or at laparotomy for intestinal obstruction of unknown cause.

Spigelian hernias

- Caused by a defect in the lateral border of the rectus sheath, usually in the lower abdomen.
- Most common in those > 50 years old.
- Often lie between the external oblique and internal oblique muscles, spreading out like a mushroom (Fig. 6.3), forming a palpable lump.

Obturator hernias

- Pass through the obturator foramen of the pelvis with the obturator nerve and vessels.
- Seen most often in elderly emaciated females.
- Pressure on the obturator nerve causes acute medial groin pain, radiating inferiorly to the knee.
- Difficult to diagnose clinically, and are usually diagnosed on CT or at laparotomy.

Lumbar hernias

- Pass through the inferior lumbar triangle immediately above the iliac crest.
- Rarely strangulate, due to their usually broad neck.

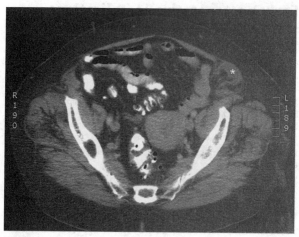

Fig. 6.3 Abdominal CT showing a left-sided Spigelian hernia (*).

Early postoperative complications

Most straightforward abdominal wall hernias are repaired electively as day cases and the incidence of significant emergency complications is very low. Since elective repair of many types of hernia is often undertaken laparoscopically, the general complications of laparoscopic surgery (including injury to an intraabdominal viscus or intraperitoneal haemorrhage from vascular injury) should be kept in mind.

Bruising Common after all types of hernia repair and not usually of importance, but can be alarming for the patient. After surgery for groin hernias it may gravitate to the scrotum and be associated with scrotal oedema. Reassurance is usually all that is needed.

Urinary retention is common, especially after groin hernia repair in elderly men. Insert a urinary catheter (📖 p.504).

Wound haematoma predisposes to infection and, if substantial, may require semi-urgent surgical evacuation.

Wound bleeding Minor haemorrhage usually stops with application of direct pressure. Wound edge bleeding can be controlled with a sutures placed under LA. Moderate and severe haemorrhage require urgent surgical exploration and suture/diathermy of the bleeding point.

Seromas in the residual sac, or in the space the sac used to occupy, is common, particularly after laparoscopic repair (inguinofemoral and ventral). USS is required to exclude recurrence or haematoma. Aspirate if large and symptomatic.

Nerve entrapment or injury

Repair of groin hernias may result in injury to the genitofemoral, lateral cutaneous nerve of thigh, ilioinguinal, or iliohypogastric nerves, causing pain or paraesthesia over the cutaneous distribution. Treat with analgesia in the emergency setting.

❶ Some anaesthetists place nerve blocks in the groin before inguinal hernia repair. This may lead to inadvertent femoral nerve block and leg weakness postoperatively. Inform the anaesthetist, and reassure the patient that leg strength will return over 12–24h.

Early recurrence (technical failure) requires re-operation, but not necessarily as an emergency.

Intraperitoneal haemorrhage (📖 p.157) may occur after open repair of incisional or umbilical hernias and after laparoscopic repair. Standard evaluation and resuscitation for haemorrhage is required. If substantial, emergency re-operation may be indicated.

Damage to an intraabdominal viscus presents with severe abdominal pain, progressing to peritonitis. Emergency surgery is required.

Prolonged ileus (📖 p.295) is uncommon. Suspect intestinal ischaemia.

Testicular ischaemia is rare, but can occur as a result of inadvertent damage to the testicular vessels. It presents with testicular pain and the diagnosis is confirmed with a Doppler USS. Surgical intervention is seldom required.

Oesophagus and stomach

:❂: **Acute upper GI bleeding**

This is a potentially life-threatening condition that requires prompt attention and action. Although in many hospitals patients with acute upper GI haemorrhage are cared for by the on-call medical team, it is essential that junior surgeons are able to manage this condition, as some of these patients will eventually require emergency surgery. Acute upper GI bleeding is a relatively common problem in postoperative patients.

The upper GI tract is defined as being proximal to the duodenal–jejunal flexure. Acute lower GI bleeding is discussed elsewhere (📖 p.280). The main causes of acute upper GI haemorrhage are listed here but, whatever the cause, the initial treatment is urgent resuscitation.

Causes

Common causes

- Peptic ulcer disease (PUD).
- Gastric erosions.
- Oesophageal varices.
- Mallory–Weiss tear (a longitudinal lower oesophageal mucosal tear occurring after forceful vomiting).

Less common causes

- Severe oesophagitis.
- Tumours of the oesophagus, stomach, or duodenum.
- Gastric varices/portal hypertensive gastropathy.
- Dieulafoy's lesion (gastric arteriovenous malformation).
- Aorto-enteric fistula (usually after AAA repair).

History

- Usually haematemesis and/or melaena.
  - Haematemesis may be fresh or 'coffee-ground'. Haematemesis after a forceful vomit suggests a Mallory–Weiss tear.
- ❶ Very heavy upper GI bleeding may present with bright red or dark red PR bleeding (📖 p.280).
- Symptoms of anaemia and/or hypotension are common.
- ❶ Occasionally these patients present with collapse without apparent bleeding.
- A history of upper abdominal pain suggests PUD.
- A history of NSAID or oral steroid use may point to PUD, while heavy alcohol intake or chronic liver disease should raise the possibility of varices.

Examination

- Often pale and clammy, occasionally confused.
- Haematemesis or melaena may be seen (or smelt).
- Stigmata of chronic liver disease: palmar erythema, leuconychia, hepatic flap, jaundice, ascites, or spider naevi suggest oesophageal or gastric varices.
- Tachycardia, hypotension, or narrowed pulse pressure.
  - ❶ The physiological response to blood loss may be altered by cardiac disease or medications.

- Upper abdominal tenderness: PUD or gastric erosions usually cause mild tenderness only.
  - ❶ Peptic ulcers tend either to bleed or perforate (📖 p.196). It is rare for a perforated peptic ulcer to bleed significantly.
- Melaena may be found on DRE.

Initial investigations

❶ Shocked patients require immediate resuscitation that should not be delayed while waiting for investigations.

- FBC: ↓ Hb is frequent and may be severe.
- U&Es: ↑ urea with a ↔ creatinine may indicate an acute gut protein load due to an upper GI bleed.
- LFTs: look for evidence of chronic liver disease.
- Serum amylase: if abdominal pain is present, exclude acute pancreatitis.
- PT, APTT, and INR: in all patients. Repeat if bleeding continues as coagulation factors will be consumed.
- G&S: in all patients. Cross-match 4–6 units of packed RBCS if Hb is ↓ or bleeding is severe.
- ECG and CXR: request in the elderly and in those with cardiorespiratory co-morbidities.
- Supine AXR: rarely needed. Occasionally, 'coffee-ground' vomiting can be confused with faeculent vomiting of bowel obstruction.

Initial management

❶ Consider the diagnosis of aorto-enteric fistula in any patient who has had previous AAA repair or untreated AAA. Discuss with your senior **immediately** and consider emergency abdominal CT.

- Protect and maintain the patient's airway.
- Fluid resuscitation.
  - Insert 2 large-bore (14–16G) peripheral IV cannulae.
  - Start aggressive IV fluid resuscitation with crystalloids or colloids, appropriate to the degree of shock.
  - If shock is present, or Hb < 10g/dL with ongoing bleeding, packed RBCs will be needed. O negative or type-specific blood can be given in life-threatening situations until cross-matched blood arrives.
- Give high-flow O_2 via a non-rebreathing mask.
- Correction of abnormal coagulation.
  - Stop warfarin and anti-platelet agents. Do not give LMWH.
  - If INR > 1.5 give 10–15mL/kg FFP and consider giving 1mg of IV vitamin K. Patients with severe bleeding with abnormal coagulation should be discussed with the on-call haematologist.
  - Platelet transfusions should be considered for patients on clopidogrel or aspirin.
  - Desmopression infusion (e.g. DDAVP® 0.4mcg/kg over 30min) should be given in renal failure where uraemia affects platelet function.
  - Consider cryoprecipitate if fibrinogen levels are depleted.
- Monitoring.
  - Insert a urinary catheter, and aim for hourly urine output of > 0.5mL/kg/h.

- In those with significant cardiorespiratory co-morbidities and heavy bleeding, consider inserting a central venous line to guide resuscitation.
- Patients with severe bleeding may require HDU/ITU admission for monitoring and ongoing resuscitation.
- Keep NBM.
- The Rockall score (Box 7.1) estimates predicted mortality and is used in some hospitals to guide management.
- ❶ Patients with significant bleeding or co-morbidities should be discussed with your senior and the ITU team urgently. Those with known or suspected chronic liver disease should be discussed with the on-call medical team.

Further investigations

- Upper GI endoscopy: this is diagnostic, and is frequently therapeutic.
  - Perform as an emergency in those with ongoing significant bleeding.
  - Patients who respond rapidly to fluid resuscitation and do not appear to have ongoing bleeding can have endoscopy performed the following morning.
  - Bleeding from peptic ulcers may be stopped with injection sclerotherapy, laser coagulation, or application of haemostatic clips.
  - Oesophageal variceal bleeding can be treated with endoscopic banding or injection sclerotherapy. Gastric varices are more difficult to treat endoscopically.
- ❶ Endoscopy itself is not without risk. Ensure that the patient is optimally resuscitated and that the endoscopy team is fully informed of the patient's co-morbidities, recent blood results, and available blood products.
- When no cause for active bleeding is found at endoscopy, consider mesenteric angiography. Emergency laparotomy is rarely diagnostic as localization of the bleeding point is difficult.

Further management

- PPIs have no beneficial effect pre-endoscopy. Give IV PPIs (e.g. 80mg omeprazole IV followed by an 8mg/h infusion) after endoscopy if therapeutic endoscopic intervention is needed, or if there are major stigmata of recent haemorrhage.
- Tranexamic acid 1g IV tds for 3 days can be given after endoscopy in patients with confirmed PUD at high-risk of re-bleeding.
- Oesophageal variceal bleeding.
  - First-line management is with endoscopic banding.
  - An IV infusion of vasopressin or octreotide can be used to reduce portal venous pressure.
  - Give phosphate enemas bd to prevent/treat hepatic encephalopathy.
  - Indications for a Sengstaken–Blakemore tube include failed endoscopic control of oesophageal varices and bleeding gastric varices.
  - Ongoing bleeding may require TIPSS to reduce portal venous pressure, although this is only available in specialist centres.

Box 7.1 The Rockall score*

Variable	Score
Age	
< 60 years	0
60–79 years	1
≥ 80 years	2
Shock	
HR < 100/min + systolic BP ≥ 100mmHg	0
HR > 100/min + systolic BP ≥ 100mmHg	1
Systolic BP < 100mmHg	2
Co-morbidity	
No major co-morbidity	0
Cardiac failure, IHD, any other major co-morbidity	2
Renal failure, liver failure, or disseminated malignancy	3

The top table gives an initial (clinical) score, with maximum of 7. Predicted mortality for score 0 = 0.2%, 3 = 11%, 7 = 50%

Variable	Score
Endoscopic diagnosis	
Mallory–Weiss tear, or no lesion and no sign of bleeding	0
All other diagnoses	1
Upper GI malignancy	2
Major stigmata of recent haemorrhage	
None, or dark spot only	0
Blood in upper GI tract, adherent clot, visible or spurting vessel	2

The two tables combined give the final score, with a maximum of 11. Predicted mortality for score 0 = 0%, 3 = 2.9%, 7 = 27%, > 7 = 41.1%.

* Rockall, T.A. et al. (1996). Gut **38**, 316–21; Vreeburg, E.M. et al. (1999). Gut **44**, 331–5.

- Bleeding from a Mallory–Weiss tear usually settles spontaneously, but can be controlled endoscopically.
- Although the majority of patients with upper GI bleeding can be managed non-operatively, emergency surgery may be required (Box 7.2).
- Once bleeding from a peptic ulcer has been controlled and oral intake is resumed, give triple therapy to eradicate *Helicobacter pylori* (e.g. omeprazole 20mg bd + amoxicillin 1g bd + clarithromycin 500mg bd, all for one week) if the CLO test is positive. Gastric ulcers require repeat endoscopy in 6–8 weeks to exclude gastric cancer.

❶ The management of severe acute upper GI bleeding requires close co-operation between gastroenterologists, surgeons, and intensivists. Patients with portal hypertension may require transfer to a specialist liver centre.

Box 7.2 Indications for emergency surgery

- Failed endoscopic control.
- Ongoing transfusion requirements, e.g. > 8 units of packed RBCs in 24h if age < 60 years; > 4 units if over 60 years old.
- Re-bleeding after initial endoscopic control.

❶ The threshold for emergency surgery in the elderly should be lowered, as they tolerate re-bleeding poorly.

❶ Emergency surgery for variceal bleeding has a high mortality due to the underlying liver disease, but may occasionally be necessary.

☼ Perforated peptic ulcer

PUD most commonly affects the 1st part of the duodenum, the pylorus, and the lesser curve of the stomach. Risk factors for PUD include *Helicobacter pylori* infection, NSAIDs, steroids, and smoking. PUD is occasionally caused by gastrin-producing pancreatic tumours (Zollinger–Ellison syndrome). The incidence of PUD has declined over the last few decades due to the widespread use of H_2-receptor antagonists, PPIs, and *H. pylori* eradication regimens.

The main complications of PUD are perforation, bleeding, and gastric outlet obstruction. Bleeding and gastric outlet obstruction are discussed elsewhere (📖 p.190, p.208). A peptic ulcer that perforates anteriorly (usually in the 1st part of the duodenum) almost always presents with symptoms and signs of generalized peritonitis (📖 p.108). Contained perforations or perforations posteriorly into the lesser sac may present in more subtle ways.

History
- Sudden onset, severe generalized abdominal pain, exacerbated by movement or coughing.
- A history of NSAID or steroid use may be present.

Examination
- The patient lies still, cold, and clammy, with dehydration.
- Pyrexia develops some hours later.
- Tachycardia, hypotension.
- Generalized abdominal tenderness with signs of peritonitis.
- Bowel sounds are diminished, or absent.
- ❶ Sealed perforations or perforations contained by adhesions or omentum may present with upper abdominal signs only.
- ❶ Peptic ulcers that perforate posteriorly into the lesser sac may present with minimal abdominal signs.
- ❶ Localized RIF peritonitis may occur if gastroduodenal contents track down the right paracolic gutter, mimicking appendicitis.

Investigations
- FBC: ↑↑ WCC; in advanced cases WCC can be ↓
- U&Es: may reflect dehydration, or early acute renal failure.
- CRP: ↑↑
- Serum amylase (📖 p.246): it is essential to exclude acute pancreatitis—a perforated PU can cause a raised amylase, but rarely > 5 × the upper limit of normal.
- G&S.
- ECG: as a preoperative baseline investigation.
- Erect CXR: free gas is seen under the diaphragm in up to 90% of perforated PU (Fig. 7.1).
    - ❶ It is often difficult to distinguish between a perforated peptic ulcer and other common causes of perforations (i.e. diverticular disease and appendicitis). Where generalized peritonitis is present, inform your senior **immediately**.

- Urgent CT abdomen and pelvis.
  - Consider if there is generalized or localized upper abdominal peritonitis with no free gas seen on plain X-rays and the serum amylase is ↑.
  - Shows small amounts of free intraperitoneal air and fluid, and can detect acute pancreatitis. CT can often also help identify possible alternative sites of perforation such as colonic diverticular disease.

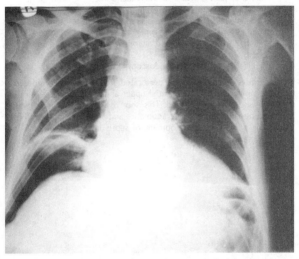

Fig. 7.1 Erect CXR showing large amounts of free gas under both hemidiaphragms.

Management

Laparotomy/laparoscopy should be performed as soon as possible once the patient has been adequately resuscitated.
- Give high-flow O_2 via a non-rebreathing mask.
- Give parenteral opioid analgesia.
- Insert 2 large-bore peripheral cannulae and begin aggressive IV fluid resuscitation.
- Insert a urinary catheter (◻ p.504).
- Keep NBM.
- Insert a NG tube, aspirate, and leave on free drainage.
- Start thromboprophylaxis (◻ p.26). Check with the on-call anaesthetist before giving LMWH, as this may prevent epidural or spinal anaesthesia.
- Give broad spectrum IV antibiotics according to the local protocol (e.g. cefuroxime 750mg tds + metronidazole 500mg tds).

- Laparotomy/laparoscopy.
  - Perforated duodenal ulcers are usually repaired with an omental patch followed by an extensive peritoneal washout.
  - Gastric ulcers should have biopsies taken from the edge to exclude a perforated gastric cancer. Small ulcers can be repaired as for a duodenal ulcer.
  - Large duodenal or gastric ulcers that cannot be closed safely with an omental patch require gastric resection.
- Postoperatively, give an IV PPI, e.g. omeprazole 40mg od.
- Once oral intake is resumed, give oral triple therapy to eradicate the presumed *H. pylori* infection, e.g. omeprazole 20mg bd + amoxicillin 1g bd + clarithromycin 500mg bd, all for 1 week. PPIs should be continued.
- Gastric ulcers require repeat endoscopy after 6–8 weeks.

Non-operative management of perforated PUD can be considered if the pain is mild and localized to the upper abdomen, as the perforation may have spontaneously sealed. This should be verified with a water-soluble contrast study. Begin IV antibiotics and an IV PPI and keep NBM. Worsening pain or the development of sepsis indicates failure of non-operative management.

☼ Oesophageal perforation

Perforation of the oesophagus most commonly occurs during upper GI endoscopy, especially if oesophageal dilatation or stenting is being performed or if the patient has an unrecognized pharyngeal pouch. The location of the perforation is variable. Iatrogenic perforation may also occur during transoesophageal echocardiography and antireflux or thoracic surgery.

Perforation may also occur as a result of vomiting against a closed glottis, leading to a sudden increase in oesophageal intraluminal pressure (Boerhaave's syndrome). The rupture usually occurs in the lower 1/3rd of the oesophagus, leading to the spillage of highly irritant oesophago-gastric contents into the mediastinum and widespread chemical and bacterial mediastinitis. Occasionally the site of perforation can be intraperitoneal.

Other causes of oesophageal perforation, such as ulcerating oesophageal carcinomas or gunshot/knife injuries, are much less common.

❶ Oesophageal perforation carries a high morbidity and mortality and an early diagnosis can be life-saving.

History

Symptoms vary, depending on the mechanism and site of perforation.
• Post-endoscopy.
  • Cervical oesophageal perforations can present with localized neck pain, suprasternal dysphagia, and hoarseness.
  • More distal perforations present with retrosternal chest pain and SOB. Severe abdominal pain may be a feature.
• Boerhaave's syndrome.
  • Vomiting or attempted vomiting on a full stomach, followed by severe chest pain (usually retrosternal).
  • Severe abdominal pain may also be present.

Examination

• Pale, clammy, tachypnoea.
• Low-grade pyrexia.
• Tachycardia or dysrhythmia, hypotension.
• Signs of a pleural effusion may be present.
• Distal perforations may cause epigastric tenderness.
• Subcutaneous ('surgical') emphysema in the neck or chest. This may take more than an hour to develop.

❶ Mackler's triad describes the classical features of Boerhaave's syndrome (vomiting, followed by severe chest pain and subcutaneous emphysema).

❶ Delayed presentation may result in collapse, with features of severe sepsis (🕮 p.482).

Initial investigations

• FBC: Hb is ↔, while a moderately ↑ WCC is common.
• U&Es: usually ↔.
• LFTs: usually ↔.
• Serum amylase: ↔ or slightly ↑. Helps to excludes acute pancreatitis in those with severe epigastric pain.

- G&S: in all patients with suspected oesophageal perforation.
- Blood cultures: take if febrile.
- ABG: perform if tachypnoea or hypoxia is present.
- ECG: to detect myocardial ischaemia as a possible cause of chest pain and to identify dysrhythmias (commonly AF).
    - ❶ The ECG is often abnormal and cardiac biomarkers may be needed to exclude NSTEMI.
- Erect CXR.
    - Pneumomediastinum is pathognomonic, but may be difficult to identify (Fig. 7.2).
    - A pleural effusion or pneumothorax (both usually left-sided) and/or subcutaneous emphysema are commonly seen.
    - Less commonly, lung collapse or consolidation is present.
    - Perforation of the intraabdominal oesophagus results in free gas under the diaphragm.
    - ❶ It may be difficult to distinguish between a perforated peptic ulcer and a perforated intraabdominal oesophagus.

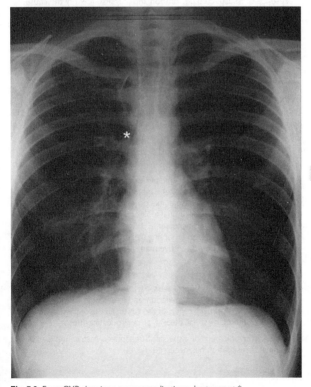

Fig. 7.2 Erect CXR showing a pneumomediastinum, best seen at *.

Immediate management

- Give high-flow O_2 via a non-rebreathing mask.
- Insert 2 large-bore IV cannulae; begin aggressive IV fluid resuscitation.
- Insert a urinary catheter (📖 p.504).
- Start thromboprophylaxis (📖 p.26).
- Give parenteral opioid analgesia.
- Start broad spectrum IV antibiotics (e.g cefotaxime 1g bd + metronidazole 500mg tds, or as per the hospital's protocol) and IV antifungal therapy (e.g. fluconazole 200mg od).
  - ❶ Advice should be sought from the microbiology department.
- Begin an IV PPI (e.g. omeprazole 40mg od).
- Keep NBM.
- ❶ If oesophageal perforation is suspected, contact your senior **urgently**. Do **not** attempt to insert an NG tube.

Further investigations

- CT thorax and abdomen with oral contrast: this can confirm the presence of a suspected perforation and may also identify the cause, e.g. mediastinal pathology. Signs of a perforation include extraluminal contrast, air in the mediastinum, and pleural effusions.
- Upper GI endoscopy: this can be used intraoperatively or if CT is inconclusive. Because air insufflation can worsen the perforation, it should only be performed by an experienced endoscopist.
- Contrast swallow: a water-soluble contrast swallow can be useful in making the diagnosis, but has a 20–30% false negative rate.

Further management

This depends on the mechanism of injury, location of the perforation, the degree of mediastinal contamination, and the haemodynamic stability of the patient.

❧ The management of oesophageal perforation is controversial.

Non-operative management

- Consider in those with iatrogenic perforations, cervical oesophageal perforations, minimal mediastinal contamination, and in stable patients.
- Begin enteral feeding via nasojejunal or jejunostomy route.
- Insert an intercostal chest drain if a pleural effusion is present.
- ITU or HDU level care is necessary.
- Oesophageal stenting is an emerging treatment modality.
- Deterioration with non-operative management is an indication for operative repair.

Operative management

- Consider in those with Boerhaave's, perforation of the abdominal oesophagus, extensive contamination, and in unstable patients.
- Surgery involves primary repair of the ruptured oesophagus, with washout of the mediastinal, pleural, or peritoneal cavities.

❶ The early involvement of a specialist oesophago-gastric unit is essential once initial resuscitation has occurred.

✸ Corrosive oesophageal injuries

This uncommon but serious injury tends to occur in young children who accidentally ingest corrosive substances and in adults who deliberately ingest them. Oesophageal mucosal necrosis is followed by fibrosis and stricturing. The depth of the oesophageal burn is a prognostic factor for outcome and ranges from a first-degree (superficial mucosa only) to a third-degree burn (full thickness injury with extension into perioesophageal tissues). Injuries to the mouth, oropharynx, laryngopharynx, and stomach can also occur.

Clinical features

- History of ingestion of corrosive with dysphagia and odynophagia.
- Drooling and burns to the mouth and oropharynx may be seen on examination.
- ❶ Retrosternal pain and respiratory distress suggest a third-degree injury.
- ❶ Stridor or noisy breathing indicate airway compromise. Call for anaesthetic assistance **immediately**.

Investigations

- ABG: if SaO_2 < 95% on air.
- Erect CXR: useful if oesophageal perforation or aspiration is suspected.
- Upper GI endoscopy: should be performed early to evaluate the extent of the oesophageal and gastric injuries.

Management

The priority is protection of the airway. If this is secure:
- give high-flow O_2 via a non-rebreathing mask;
- begin IV fluids;
- keep NBM;
- start thromboprophylaxis (📖 p.26);
- avoid induced emesis, gastric lavage, and NG aspiration.
- consult with a poisons unit;
- contact a specialist oesophago-gastric centre.
  - first-degree injuries may resolve with no long-term sequelae;
  - surgical intervention, including oesophagectomy, may be required in third-degree oesophageal burns.

☛ The use of steroids and antibiotics is controversial.

:✪: **Acute gastric dilatation**

This is a failure of gastric peristalsis (ileus) leading to massive gastric distension in the absence of any mechanical obstruction. It is associated with abdominal surgery (particularly on the stomach or spleen), severe trauma, electrolyte abnormalities, severe systemic illness, and eating disorders. It is a potentially fatal condition, that left untreated may result in gastric necrosis and perforation.

Patients may present with shock, acute epigastric pain, or vomiting. On examination a distended abdomen is found, and a succussion splash may be present. Chest and abdominal X-rays may show a grossly distended air-filled stomach, although CT is required to make the diagnosis if the stomach is completely fluid-filled. Emergency treatment is with decompression of the stomach via a NG tube, aggressive IV fluid resuscitation, and correction of any electrolyte abnormalities. Gastric necrosis requires emergency gastrectomy, with an estimated mortality of > 50%.

:O: **Gastric volvulus**

Volvulus of the stomach is an uncommon condition that may present acutely, or chronically with intermittent symptoms. It can be classified according to:

- location:
  - abdominal (subdiaphragmatic);
  - thoracic (supradiaphragmatic);
- axis of rotation:
  - organoaxial (~ 60% of cases), i.e. about an axis of rotation through the gastric cardia and pylorus;
  - mesenteroaxial, i.e. about an axis of rotation through greater and lesser curvatures of the stomach.

Supradiaphragmatic volvulus is associated with a diaphragmatic defect due to a rolling (paraoesophageal) hiatus hernia, surgery, or trauma. Congenital diaphragmatic defects can lead to gastric volvulus in children, but the majority of cases occur in 40–60 year olds. Organoaxial volvulus is often associated with diaphragmatic defects, and the risk of strangulation and subsequent gastric necrosis is higher than with mesenteroaxial volvulus.

Only the acute presentation of gastric volvulus is dealt with in this section. The clinical features and radiological findings are dependent primarily upon the location of the volvulus.

History

- Abdominal gastric volvulus: sudden onset of epigastric and LUQ pain.
- Thoracic gastric volvulus: sudden onset of left-sided chest and arm pain with severe dyspnoea.
- Severe retching, without vomiting, is associated with both types.

Examination

- Pale, sweaty.
- Tachycardia, hypotension may be present.
- Abdominal gastric volvulus: upper abdominal distension and tenderness.
- Thoracic gastric volvulus: tachypnoea, occasionally with decreased air entry in the left chest.
  - ❶ Abdominal signs are often minimal with a thoracic gastric volvulus, and patients with a thoracic gastric volvulus are often initially assessed by the on-call medical team. Diagnosis is difficult and is often delayed.

Initial investigations

- FBC: ↑ WCC is a sign of gastric strangulation.
- U&Es: usually normal.
- G&S.
- ABG: if tachypnoea is present or SaO_2 < 95% on air.
- ECG: to look for evidence of a myocardial ischaemia, which thoracic gastric volvulus can closely mimic.
- Erect CXR: may show an intrathoracic stomach, or free gas under the diaphragm if an abdominal gastric volvulus has perforated.

- Supine AXR: may show a dilated stomach with an abdominal gastric volvulus, but can be very difficult to interpret due to the abnormal anatomy.

Initial management

- Give high-flow O_2 via a non-rebreathing mask.
- Begin aggressive IV fluid resuscitation.
- Insert a urinary catheter (📖 p.504).
- Give parenteral opioid analgesia.
- Start thromboprophylaxis (📖 p.26).

❶ Insertion of a NG tube characteristically fails.

❶ Significant cardiorespiratory compromise may require intubation and ventilation with ITU care.

Further investigations

If free gas is present on erect CXR, further investigations are inappropriate, and emergency surgery should be arranged.

When free gas is absent and the diagnosis is in doubt, consider the following.
- CT chest and abdomen with oral and IV contrast: the investigation of choice, especially for thoracic gastric volvulus, when diagnosis is difficult.
- Upper GI endoscopy: risks perforating a necrotic stomach, but occasionally can be successful in gastric decompression. Interpretation can be difficult.
- Water soluble contrast swallow: helpful for anatomical clarification.

Further management

❶ This is an uncommon and complicated emergency. An oesophago-gastric surgeon should be involved early. Advice from a specialist centre may be necessary, and transfer should be considered.
- Emergency surgery (open or laparoscopic). This involves reduction and/or untwisting of the stomach, assessment of gastric viability ± gastrectomy, and repair of any diaphragmatic defect. If the stomach is viable, anterior gastropexy is usually performed to prevent recurrence, e.g. with a gastrostomy.
- Occasionally, gastric decompression can be achieved endoscopically or via an NG tube, allowing surgery to be performed once the patient has recovered sufficiently.

☼ Gastric outlet obstruction

The two common causes of gastric outlet obstruction (GOO) in adults are malignancy (gastric or pancreatic cancer) and stenosing PUD of the 1st part of the duodenum. The patient becomes increasingly dehydrated and loses considerable amounts of weight as progressively smaller amounts of food and fluid are able to pass into the small intestine.

❶ Aspiration pneumonia can also occur.

History

- Large volume vomiting. Bile is absent.
- Upper abdominal pain may or may not be present.
- The patient may complain of weight loss.

Examination

- The patient appears unwell, underweight, and dehydrated.
- Abdominal distension and a succussion splash are common.
- Supraclavicular fossa lymphadenopathy may be present.

Initial investigations

- FBC: mild ↓ Hb may be due to malignancy or malnutrition, but is initially disguised by dehydration. Check haematinics.
- U&Es and serum chloride: ↓ K^+, ↓ Cl^-, due to loss of gastric juices and metabolic effects.
- Serum amylase and LFTs: if significant upper abdominal pain or tenderness is present, to exclude acute pancreatitis and hepatobiliary pathologies.
- ABG: metabolic alkalosis with respiratory compensation may be present due to loss of gastric acid.
  - ❶ Although corrected serum Ca^{2+} is usually ↔, the alkalosis results in ↓ ionized Ca^{2+} and tetany may result.
- Erect CXR: may show a large bubble in the gastric fundus.
- Supine AXR: the absence of small bowel distension assists in excluding small bowel obstruction.

Initial management

The priority is to correct the fluid, electrolyte, and metabolic abnormalities.
- Keep NBM.
- Give O_2 if SaO_2 < 95%.
- Start IV fluid resuscitation; replace lost fluids initially with normal saline + KCl.
- Insert a urinary catheter and keep the urine output > 0.5mL/kg/h.
- Insert a large-bore NG tube, aspirate, and keep on free drainage.
- Transfuse with packed RBCs if Hb < 8g/dL.
- Begin an IV PPI (e.g. 40mg omeprazole od).
- Start thromboprophylaxis (📖 p.26).
- Check for *Helicobacter pylori* infection with serology or faecal antigen tests.

Further investigations

- Upper GI endoscopy: to identify the cause and obtain biopsies (histology and CLO). Gastric contents may obscure the obstruction.
- Water-soluble contrast meal: helpful to distinguish between mechanical GOO and acute gastric dilatation (📖 p.205) when upper GI endoscopy fails.
- Thoracic and abdominopelvic CT: delineates the anatomy of the obstruction, and detects any associated masses, lymphadenopathy, and metastases.

Further management

Definitive management depends on the cause of the GOO. With both benign and malignant GOO, adequate nutrition is essential, e.g. via percutaneous jejunostomy or TPN.

Benign GOO

- Give triple therapy to those with *H. pylori* . Occasionally, triple therapy and PPI treatment lead to GOO resolution.
- Endoscopic dilatation can be successful in some benign cases.
- When these treatments fail, there are a number of surgical options, e.g. gastrojejunostomy.

Malignant GOO

- Treatment depends on the resectability of the tumour and the patient's fitness for surgery.
- Occasionally, curative surgical resection is possible, e.g. Whipple's pancreaticoduodenectomy or gastrectomy.
- More commonly, the tumour is not resectable. In patients with a very poor short-term prognosis, options include palliative care or endoscopic stenting. Gastrojejunostomy (open or laparoscopic) can be performed in those fit enough for surgery.

① Gastritis

Gastritis is a clinical description that is loosely applied to a collection of upper GI pathologies that present acutely with epigastric/RUQ pain and vomiting but without significant systemic upset. These include:
- severe gastro-oesophageal reflux disease (GORD);
- erosive gastritis, commonly due to NSAIDs and/or alcohol;
- uncomplicated PUD;
- stress gastritis, e.g. after major surgery.

Clinical features
- Epigastric/RUQ pain and vomiting.
- Occasionally there may be symptoms of GORD (e.g. retrosternal pain, waterbrash, odynophagia).
- On examination, localized epigastric tenderness (sometimes marked) is present, but the patient is haemodynamically stable and afebrile.
- ❶ If haematemesis or melaena are present, investigate and manage as for an acute upper GI bleed (📖 p.190).

Investigations
Investigations are usually unremarkable.
- FBC: WCC is usually ↔, but may be mildly ↑.
- U&Es and LFTs: typically normal.
- Serum amylase: to exclude acute pancreatitis.
- ECG: to detect myocardial ischaemia.
- Erect CXR: exclude free gas under the diaphragm.
- USS RUQ: to exclude biliary colic and acute cholecystitis.
- Upper GI endoscopy: is diagnostic. Biopsies should be taken for histopathology and for the urease test (e.g. CLO test) for *Helicobacter pylori*.

Management
- Many patients require admission for analgesia and for investigations (i.e. USS, OGD) to exclude other pathologies.
- Keep NBM.
- Start IV fluids.
- Start IV PPI (e.g. omeprazole 40mg od) and analgesia (parenteral opioids may be required).
- Begin thromboprophylaxis (📖 p.26).
- After the diagnosis has been confirmed by upper GI endoscopy:
  - resume normal oral intake;
  - treat according to the pathology encountered, e.g. oral PPI and/or sucralfate, triple therapy for *H. pylori* infection (📖 p.198);
  - give advice on avoidance of causative agents, e.g. NSAIDs, alcohol, cigarettes.

Early postoperative complications: gastrectomy

Gastrectomy (total or subtotal) is most commonly performed for gastric cancer. Radical gastrectomies may include a splenectomy and distal pancreatectomy, adding to the risk of postoperative complications. After a total gastrectomy, a Roux-en-Y reconstruction is created (Fig. 7.3).

Operative site bleeding (📖 p.154)
Duodenal stump leak

Manifests as leakage of duodenal contents (i.e. large volume of amylase-rich, bile-stained fluid) from abdominal drains. If the leak is localized and draining well, clinical signs may be minimal. If no drains were placed during surgery, or if they have been removed, then the patient may present with non-specific clinical deterioration, signs of intraabdominal sepsis, ileus, or peritonitis. Early leaks (within 24h of surgery) should be re-explored surgically, whereas a late leak (if drains are still in situ) can be managed conservatively in a stable patient by continued drainage, broad spectrum IV antibiotics (as per local protocol, or on microbiology advice) and parenteral nutrition.

Anastomotic leak

This usually presents with sudden change to the patient's clinical state, e.g worsening abdominal pain and pyrexia or new onset AF. Occasionally the presentation may be more subtle, e.g. with prolonged ileus or rising WCC. Leaks most commonly occur from days 2–10 postoperatively. After IV fluid resuscitation, diagnosis can be proven by contrast radiology (e.g. swallow study). Early leakage usually requires re-operation, whereas late leaks (> 1 week postoperatively) with minimal systemic upset can sometimes be managed non-operatively with IV antibiotics and nutrition. Failure of non-operative management requires re-operation.

Pancreatic fistula (📖 p.256)
Post-splenectomy infection (📖 p.258)

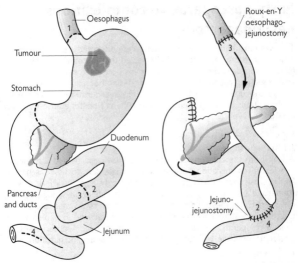

Fig. 7.3 Operative diagram of a total gastrectomy with a Roux-en-Y reconstruction.

Early postoperative complications: oesophagectomy

The two most common oesophagectomies performed are the Ivor Lewis oesophagectomy (laparotomy + right-sided thoracotomy) and the transhiatal oesophagectomy (laparotomy + cervical incision). After oesophageal resection, a conduit is created from another part of the GI tract (e.g. gastric tube, jejunum, transverse colon), in order to restore continuity. Complications can be present in up to 40%, and postoperative mortality is ~ 10%.

Operative site bleeding (📖 p.154)

Anastomotic leak

A leak from the anastomosis between the oesophagus and the conduit is a feared complication. Late leaks are usually due to tissue ischaemia and necrosis, due in part to poor blood supply. Signs of a leak may be subtle, and are usually manifest by a change in patient physiology, e.g. new onset AF. The suspected diagnosis can be proven by a water-soluble contrast swallow study. Early leaks (< 72h postoperatively) in stable patients require re-operation. Late leaks can often be managed conservatively by intercostal drainage, NG suction, IV antibiotic therapy, and nutrition.

Chylothorax

The thoracic duct crosses posteriorly from the right to the left of the lower oesophagus. A right-sided thoracic procedure or a transhiatal resection can damage the thoracic duct, leading to the leakage of chyle into the right thoracic cavity. This usually presents as the appearance of chylous (milky) fluid in the intercostal drains, or the development of a pleural effusion (if the drains have been removed). A senior surgeon should carefully place an intercostal drain, avoiding the oesophageal conduit. If the milky discharge continues after a period of observation and medium chain triglyceride nutrition, surgical re-exploration is indicated. At surgery, the injured thoracic duct should be identified and ligated.

Recurrent laryngeal nerve palsy

Mild unilateral recurrent laryngeal nerve damage presents with voice changes, and is usually reversible. Bilateral partial nerve injury is rare, but can cause airway obstruction. This is apparent on extubation in theatre and requires re-intubation. Tracheostomy may be required.

Early postoperative complications: laparoscopic Nissen's fundoplication

This is the most common form of surgical antireflux procedure. The gastro-oesophageal junction is defined, any hiatus hernia present reduced, and the hiatal defect repaired. The gastric fundus is then mobilized off the spleen, wrapped around the gastro-oesophageal junction, and sutured on to itself.

Severe dysphagia

Mild dysphagia is very common in the early postoperative phase, and regresses with dietary modification and time. Severe or complete dysphagia can present with bolus obstruction, retching, and severe retrosternal or epigastric pain on swallowing. An oral water-soluble contrast study demonstrates a hold-up proximal to the wrap. Patients who present in the early postoperative period usually require revision surgery.

Pneumothorax

This is most commonly due to injury of the left parietal pleura during dissection around the mediastinal oesophagus. The CO_2 used to create the pneumoperitoneum leaks into the pleural space. These are often detected intraoperatively, but may present immediately postoperatively. Clinical features, investigations, and management are discussed elsewhere (📖 p.460). Small pneumothoraces causing minimal symptoms often do not require intercostal chest drain insertion, as CO_2 within the pleural cavity is rapidly absorbed.

Operative site bleeding (📖 p.154)

Gastrointestinal perforation

Unrecognized perforation of the oesophagus, stomach, or the more distal tract may occur in up to 1% of cases. Presentation may be delayed up to 5 days postoperatively.

- Clinical features. The patient complains of fever and abdominal pain. On examination, tachycardia and abdominal tenderness with peritonism are present.
- Investigations. FBC shows ↑ WCC. Erect CXR may show a pneumoperitoneum, but this would be expected to be present for up to 5 days after laparoscopy anyway. CT of the abdomen may demonstrate peritoneal fluid collections, but these may be difficult to distinguish from normal postoperative changes.
- Management. As CT is often unhelpful, clinical suspicion of a GI perforation mandates a return to theatre for surgical repair of the perforated viscus and washout of the abdominal cavity. This can be performed either via a laparoscopic or open approach.

Gastric volvulus (📖 p.206)

Early postoperative complications: laparoscopic gastric banding

This is a bariatric procedure, designed to restrict the volume of food entering the gut by placing a band around the proximal stomach. The inner cuff of the band can be inflated/deflated by way of a subcutaneous port. Most major complications relate to the band and should be managed in consultation with a bariatric surgeon. These may present some weeks or months postoperatively, once the band has been inflated.

Severe dysphagia

Overinflation of the band causes retching with difficulties in swallowing or, occasionally, total obstruction. Irritation and distension of the gastric pouch may lead to mild haematemesis. Clinical examination is usually unremarkable, and bloods and plain X-rays are normal. These patients require urgent deflation of the band, usually under radiological guidance.

Band slippage

If a portion of the stomach slips above the band it can cause an acute gastric pouch obstruction. The obstructed stomach can undergo necrosis and perforate.
- Clinical features: upper abdominal pain and vomiting, with tachycardia and upper abdominal tenderness on examination.
- Investigations: FBC usually shows ↑ WCC, and a plain AXR may demonstrate the distended gastric pouch. Urgent upper GI contrast studies and/or CT scan are needed to confirm the diagnosis.
- Management. The immediate management after IV fluid resuscitation of the patient and analgesia is to deflate the gastric band via the percutaneous port. Exploratory laparoscopy may be required to exclude gastric necrosis, to reposition, or even to remove the band.

Band erosion

Erosion of the band through the stomach wall causes gastric necrosis and perforation. A port infection or an intraabdominal collection in a patient after gastric band placement should be considered to be associated with band erosion with or without underlying gastric perforation until proven otherwise. After resuscitation of the patient and IV antibiotic therapy, CT-guided percutaneous drainage of any collections should be performed. An upper GI endoscopy is needed to identify an eroding gastric band and, if shown, the patient should proceed to surgery for band removal, washout, and repair of the gastric defect.

Early postoperative complications: laparoscopic gastric bypass

Unlike laparoscopic gastric banding, this bariatric operation aims to induce both a restrictive and malabsorptive effect. A small gastric reservoir is created and a Roux-en-Y gastric bypass is performed, reducing the absorptive intestinal surface (Fig. 7.4).

Anastomotic leak

Leaks from the gastric staple line, or the two small bowel anastomoses may occur. This is the most worrying of all complications, and may present insidiously with a delayed recovery, or more overtly with tachycardia, pyrexia, and peritonitis. A low threshold for suspecting an anastomotic leak is essential. A contrast study and/or CT scan may prove the diagnosis, or the patient may proceed directly to laparoscopy.

Marginal (stomal) ulcers

These ulcers form at the gastro-jejunal anastomosis and can occur in up to 10–15% of patients postoperatively. Marginal ulcers can erode and cause upper GI haemorrhage or can perforate. The investigation and management are the same as for those of peptic ulcers (🕮 p.190, p.196).

Gastric remnant dilatation

The large volume gastric remnant can become blocked with blood clots and gastric secretions in the early postoperative phase, or develop an ileus. The patient complains of nausea, vomiting, and abdominal pain, and epigastric tenderness and fullness are found on examination. Abdominal X-ray may show a distended stomach, but CT is usually required to make the diagnosis. NG tube and endoscopic access to the remnant is impossible due to the surgically altered anatomy; decompression of the remnant can be achieved by CT-guided transgastric aspiration of the gastric remnant. Surgical decompression is indicated if this fails.

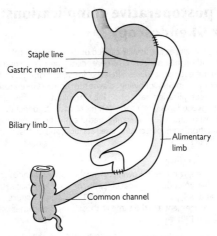

Fig. 7.4 Operative diagram of a gastric bypass.

Early postoperative complications: upper GI endoscopy

Diagnostic procedures are usually carried out with pharyngeal local anaesthesia only, although short-acting IV benzodiazepine (e.g. midazolam) may be used. Therapeutic procedures often require midazolam and an IV opioid.

Major complications following diagnostic upper GI endoscopy are rare, with a complication rate of < 1%. Complications after therapeutic endoscopic procedures are more common, and are dependent on the technique used and the underlying pathology. Therapeutic techniques include dilatation, stent placement, laser ablation, and endoscopic mucosal resection (EMR).

Upper GI bleeding

Significant bleeding is rare following diagnostic upper GI endoscopy unless the patient has an underlying coagulopathy, or is on anticoagulation. Rates after EMR and polypectomy are as high as 10%. Clinical features, investigations, and management are the same as those for other causes of upper GI bleeding (📖 p.190).

Oesophageal perforation (📖 p.200)

Gastric or duodenal perforation

Perforation of the stomach or duodenum is rare, except during therapeutic procedures such as gastric or duodenal dilatation, gastric EMR, and duodenal stent placement. Perforations are usually recognized or suspected during the procedure, but may present within 24h.

- Clinical features: abdominal pain, with tachycardia, abdominal distension, and signs of peritonitis.
- Investigations: FBC shows ↑ WCC; erect CXR shows free gas in > 90% of cases. When clinical features suggest perforation and the CXR is normal, abdominal CT can show small volumes of free gas.
- Management.
  - Patients with localized signs and minimal systemic upset are suitable for a trial of non-operative management, i.e. IV fluid resuscitation, NBM, NG suction, broad-spectrum IV antibiotics (e.g. cefuroxime 750mg tds + metronidazole 500mg tds) and an IV PPI (e.g. omeprazole 40mg od). Parenteral nutrition may be necessary.
  - Emergency laparotomy is indicated in those patients with large perforations, generalized peritonitis, and those who do not respond to non-operative therapy. Depending on the operative findings, simple repair or gastric resection may be necessary.

Oversedation

❶ If assistance is needed urgently, call for the resuscitation team.

This may manifest itself as a collapse, decreased level of consciousness, confusion, hypotension, hypoxia, or difficulty maintaining an airway. While naloxone and flumazenil are being drawn up, adopt an 'ABC' approach.

- Airway: maintain with head tilt, chin lift, and jaw thrust. Insert an oropharyngeal airway (Guedel) if required. Give high-flow O_2 via a non-rebreathing mask.

- Breathing: start bag-valve-mask ventilations if breathing is inadequate.
- Circulation: if hypotensive or tachycardic, insert 2 large-bore peripheral IV cannulae and give stat crystalloids.
- Naloxone: reverses the sedative and analgesic effects of opioids. Give IV in 100–200mcg boluses every 1–2min until the opioid effects are reversed. Patients with renal failure do not clear opioids normally, and need large doses of naloxone to reverse the effects, which are often cumulative—a naloxone infusion is usually required since the opioid half-life is very prolonged.
- Flumazenil: reverses the sedative effects of benzodiazepines. Give 200mcg IV, then 100mcg boluses every 1–2min until benzodiazepine effects are reversed.

❶ Both naloxone and flumazenil have shorter half-lives than the drugs that they antagonize, and may have to be given repeatedly.

❶ Don't forget to consider other diagnoses such as dehydration, TIA/CVA, MI, or PE.

Aspiration

This should be suspected if the patient vomits and becomes cyanosed with a decreased SaO_2. The patient's airway should be protected and maintained (chin lift, jaw thrust) and the pharynx suctioned. Supplemental O_2 should be given, and any sedation reversed. The patient should be encouraged to sit up, and cough. Admission is required for O_2 therapy, aggressive physiotherapy, and broad spectrum IV antibiotics (either cefotaxime 1g bd + metronidazole 500mg tds, or as per local protocol).

Liver and biliary tree

Introduction

The majority of acute hepatobiliary diseases are associated with gallstones. Gallstones are very common in the West, but < 30% of people with gallstones become symptomatic. Knowledge of biliary anatomy (Fig. 8.1) is essential to enable an understanding of the different clinical manifestations of gallstone disease. Almost all gallstones form in the gall bladder (cholecystolithiasis).

Common complications of gallstones

Gallstones within the gall bladder and cystic duct

- Biliary colic (📖 p.226). Transient obstruction of the gall bladder outflow (Hartmann's pouch or cystic duct) leads to gall bladder spasm and pain.
- Acute (calculous) cholecystitis (📖 p.228). The presence of stones in the gall bladder may lead to inflammation and infection.
- Mucocele. Obstruction of the gall bladder outflow with ongoing mucus secretion leads to gall bladder distension.
- Empyema of the gallbladder (📖 p.228). Infection of a mucocele leads to pus within the gall bladder.
- Gangrene of the gall bladder (gangrenous cholecystitis; 📖 p.230). Infection and distension can lead to thrombosis of the arterial supply of the gallbladder. Gall bladder perforation (📖 p.230) may ensue.

Gallstones within the biliary tree

Gallstones in the bile ducts (choledocholithiasis) usually originate from the gall bladder. Primary ductal stones are rare. Small gallstones (< 5mm diameter) commonly pass unnoticed into the duodenum, but larger stones impact in the CBD or ampulla of Vater, causing complications.

- Obstructive jaundice (📖 p.232). Obstruction to the biliary flow without infection.
- Acute cholangitis (📖 p.234). Obstruction to the biliary flow with infection.
- Acute pancreatitis (📖 p.244).

Very large gallstones are unable to pass into the cystic duct. Continued irritation and inflammation within the gall bladder leads to fistula formation.

Other complications of gallstones

- Mirizzi's syndrome: jaundice resulting from obstruction of the common hepatic duct due to compression from, or inflammation due to, a gallstone in Hartmann's pouch or the cystic duct.
- Gallstone ileus: gallstone obstruction of the distal small bowel after formation of a fistula between the gall bladder and duodenum (📖 p.239).

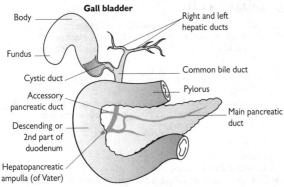

Fig. 8.1 The anatomy of the gall bladder and biliary tree. The long-term presence of gallstones in the gall bladder neck leads to dilatation of this region (Hartmann's pouch).

① Biliary colic

Biliary colic is the most common manifestation of gallstone disease and is generally straightforward to diagnose and manage. Most patients go on to have their gall bladder and gallstones removed (usually laparoscopically).

History

- Severe RUQ/epigastric pain, often radiates through to the angle of the right scapula.
- Pain is usually constant (biliary colic is a misnomer), develops rapidly, and usually resolves within 12h. Pain is triggered by fatty foods.
- Nausea is common; vomiting less so.

Examination

- Apyrexial.
- RUQ tenderness of variable severity.
- ❶ Fever, jaundice, Murphy's sign, and signs of peritonitis are absent. Their presence indicates an alternative diagnosis.

Initial investigations

- FBC, U&Es, LFTs and serum amylase: typically ↔. Abnormalities suggest other disorders (e.g. acute cholecystitis, acute pancreatitis). Mild obstructive changes to the LFTs (↑ ALP, ↑ GGT) can be seen if small stones are in the CBD.
- CRP: ↔ or mildly ↑.
- Erect CXR: request in all patients with RUQ/epigastric pain to exclude free subdiaphragmatic gas (☐ p.109). Supine AXR is not required; only 10% of gallstones are radio-opaque.
- ECG: if history of cardiac disease or age > 40 years to detect Myocardial ischaemia as a possible cause of the pain, and to assess fitness for anaesthesia.
- Urine dipstick: exclude right-sided renal colic.
- G&S: if surgery is likely.

Initial management

- Keep NBM.
- Start maintenance IV fluids.
- Give thromboprophylaxis (☐ p.26).
- Prescribe parenteral analgesia, usually IV morphine with an anti-emetic.

Further investigations

- USS RUQ: detects gall bladder stones and assesses the gall bladder and other upper abdominal organs. A dilated CBD (> 8mm) implies stones in the duct.
- Upper GI endoscopy: if USS doesn't show stones (ΔΔ PUD).

Further management

If USS confirms biliary colic, laparoscopic cholecystectomy should ideally be performed on the same admission.

① Acute cholecystitis

Acute cholecystitis is usually due to stones in the gall bladder (acute calculous cholecystitis). Mild cases of acute calculous cholecystitis may initially be difficult to distinguish from biliary colic. Inflammation of the gall bladder without the presence of stones or sludge (acute acalculous cholecystitis) is uncommon (Box 8.1).

> **Box 8.1 Acute acalculous cholecystitis**
>
> Patients with shock or sepsis of any cause can develop gall bladder ischaemia and infection without stones. Clinical diagnosis is often difficult due to coexistent pathology. USS shows a thickened, distended gall bladder, with pericholecystic fluid but no gallstones. CT scanning is useful to exclude other intraabdominal causes of pain or sepsis. Treatment is with broad spectrum IV antibiotics and emergency cholecystectomy if the patient is fit enough for a GA. If not, percutaneous transhepatic cholecystostomy can be performed under LA with USS-guidance.
>
> ❶ Acute acalculous cholecystitis has a mortality of up to 50%.

History
- Severe RUQ pain with radiation through to the right scapula.
- Previous history of biliary colic.
- Pain persists for longer than that of biliary colic.
- Vomiting is more of a feature than with biliary colic.
- Rigors suggest acute cholangitis (📖 p.234).

Examination
- Pyrexia and mild tachycardia without hypotension.
- Marked RUQ tenderness with signs of localized peritonitis.
  - ❶ Signs of peritonitis outside the RUQ suggest gall bladder rupture or perforated PU disease (📖 p.196).
- Usually Murphy's sign positive (inspiration with the examiner's hand placed low in the RUQ causes significant pain and prevents deeper inspiration).
- A palpable mass in the RUQ is present in ~ 25% and is due to an inflammatory phlegmon or gall bladder empyema (Box 8.2).
- ❶ Jaundice suggests acute cholangitis (📖 p.234).

> **Box 8.2 Gall bladder empyema**
>
> Abdominal signs are less marked than in gangrenous cholecystitis, and swinging pyrexia is seen. The gall bladder is palpable. Drainage can be performed surgically or radiologically. Percutaneous transhepatic cholecystostomy can be performed if multiple co-morbidities or cardiovascular instability make GA unsuitable.

Initial investigations
- FBC: ↑ WCC.
- U&Es: may show mild dehydration. CRP is ↑↑.

- LFTs: often normal, but mild obstructive changes to the LFTs (↑ ALP, ↑ GGT) can be seen if small stones are in the CBD.
- Serum amylase (📖 p.246): usually normal, but mild ↑ < 3 × the upper limit of normal can occur.
- G&S.
- Erect CXR: mandatory to exclude free intraabdominal gas (📖 p.109) or right basal pneumonia.
- Supine AXR: rarely helpful.
- ECG: if history of cardiac disease or age > 40, to detect Myocardial ischaemia as a possible cause of the pain, and to assess fitness for anaesthesia.
- Urine dipstick: exclude right-sided renal colic with an infected system.
- Blood cultures.

Initial management
- Keep NBM.
- Start appropriate IV fluids (📖 p.17).
- Give thromboprophylaxis (📖 p.26).
- Prescribe IV opioid for analgesia, with an anti-emetic.
- Start antibiotics according to local protocols (e.g. ciprofloxacin 500mg bd PO with metronidazole 500mg tds IV).

Further investigations
- USS RUQ is > 90% sensitive and specific. Sonographic features of acute calculous cholecystitis include:
  - gallstones (or sludge) within a thickened, sometimes distended gall bladder;
  - pericholecystic fluid.
- If USS is negative despite high clinical suspicion of acute cholecystitis, consider endoscopic USS.
- Abdominal CT and/or upper GI endoscopy is required if endoscopic USS is negative and the pain continues.

Further management
- Laparoscopic cholecystectomy may be performed within 72h of the onset of symptoms. After 72h the surgery is more difficult and has higher risks of conversion and major bile duct injury.
- If laparoscopic cholecystectomy is not performed, the majority of patients settle with antibiotics.
  - Once the pyrexia and pain settle, change to oral antibiotics (for a total course of 7–10 days); re-introduce oral fluids and a low-fat diet.
  - Arrange elective laparoscopic cholecystectomy at > 6 weeks to allow inflammation to resolve.

❶ Patients treated conservatively require regular clinical assessment and blood tests. Those with worsening peritonitis and/or inflammatory markers may be developing gang renous cholecystitis (Box 8.3). A sudden onset of generalized peritonitis in a patient with acute cholecystitis implies gall bladder perforation (Box 8.4).

Box 8.3 Gangrenous cholecystitis

Severe acute cholecystitis (both calculous and acalculous) can lead to gangrene of the gall bladder. Clinical features include septic shock, marked RUQ peritonitis, and deterioration despite resuscitation and appropriate IV antibiotics. Gas within the gall bladder wall may be seen on AXR or USS. Emergency cholecystectomy is needed and HDU/ITU care postoperatively is required. Discuss antibiotic treatment with a microbiologist.

Box 8.4 Perforated gall bladder

Rarely, acute cholecystitis can progress rapidly to perforation. Patients present with septic shock and widespread peritonitis due to bile and pus. Free gas will not be seen on erect CXR. The diagnosis may only be made at emergency laparotomy. Aggressive IV fluid resuscitation is needed beforehand and HDU/ITU care will be needed.

① Obstructive jaundice

Partial or complete obstruction to biliary flow leads to obstructive jaundice, characterized by jaundice, pruritus, dark urine, and pale stools. The most common causes are gallstones, tumours in or around the biliary tree, or blockage of biliary stents placed at ERCP.

History

- Jaundice, pruritus, dark urine, pale stools.
- RUQ pain, commonly due to gallstones.
- Pancreatic head malignancy often causes pain and weight loss as well as jaundice.
- Painless obstructive jaundice usually indicates periampullary carcinoma or cholangiocarcinoma.
- ❶ Rigors indicate acute cholangitis (📖 p.234).

Examination

- Jaundice, first seen in the sclera when bilirubin 30–40µmol/L.
- Palpable gall bladder in malignant obstruction (Courvoisier's law).
- Palpable left supraclavicular lymph node (Virchow's node) due to malignancy (Troisier's sign).

Initial investigations

- FBC: ↓ Hb may indicate malignancy; ↑ WCC indicates acute cholangitis.
- U&Es, serum amylase, and CRP: usually ↔.
- LFTs: ↑ conjugated bilirubin, ↑↑ ALP, ↑↑ GGT.
  - ❶ If ↑↑ ALT or AST, then check viral hepatitis serology.
- PT, APTT and INR: PT and INR ↑, due to failure to absorb fat-soluble vitamin K.
- Serum CA-19.9: marker of pancreatobiliary malignancy.
- Urinary conjugated bilirubin is present on dipstick.
- Erect CXR: exclude metastatic malignancy in the chest.

Initial management

- Allow clear fluids by mouth.
- Keep well-hydrated with maintenance IV fluids.
- Start antibiotics, e.g. ciprofloxacin 500mg bd PO.
- Give slow IV vitamin K 10mg for 3 days.
- Start thromboprophylaxis if there are no contraindications (📖 p.26).
- Re-check FBC, U&Es, LFTs, CRP, PT, APTT, and INR daily.

Further investigations and management

Definitive assessment and treatment depends on the underlying cause of the obstruction.

- USS RUQ: detects a dilated (obstructed) biliary tree and stones within the gall bladder. Often unable to visualize distal obstructing lesions, as gas in the duodenum obscures the distal CBD.
- If gall bladder stones are present and the CBD is dilated on USS, the obstruction is likely to be due to a stone, and ERCP is needed.
- If gall bladder stones are absent and the CBD is dilated on USS, then an obstructing lesion at the distal CBD is likely (e.g. adenocarcinoma

of the head of the pancreas), and CT pancreas should be performed before ERCP.

- If the intrahepatic ducts are dilated but the CBD is normal diameter on USS, hilar cholangiocarcinoma (Klatskin tumour) is likely. Request an MRCP. PTC may be necessary.
- If a biliary stent is present, ERCP will be needed to remove the blocked stent and insert a new stent.

❶ Patients with jaundice and a non-dilated biliary tree on USS should be referred to a gastroenterologist/hepatologist for consideration of intrahepatic causes of jaundice.

✪ Acute cholangitis

Acute cholangitis (also known as ascending cholangitis) is secondary infection of an obstructed biliary tree, commonly due to stones, tumour, or a blocked biliary stent. The presence of septic shock (📖 p.482) or persisting/intermittent fever despite appropriate antibiotic therapy indicates severe acute cholangitis.

❶ Severe acute cholangitis has a mortality of ~ 20% and requires emergency assessment, resuscitation, and biliary drainage.

History
- Rigors (50%).
- RUQ pain, can be mild.
- Jaundice with dark urine/pale stools.
- History of gallstones or biliary disease/interventions.

Examination
- Pyrexia, often high-grade.
- Tachycardia, hypotension.
- Confusion.
- Dehydration.
- Jaundice.
- Mild RUQ tenderness.

❶ Charcot's triad (pyrexia with rigors, jaundice, RUQ pain) is present in only 25%.

Initial investigations
- FBC: ↑↑ WCC; ↓ platelets in DIC.
- U&Es: ↑ urea and ↑ creatinine, electrolyte abnormalities.
- CRP: ↑↑.
- LFTs: obstructive changes (↑ bilirubin, ↑↑ ALP, ↑↑ GGT).
  - ❶ If ↑↑ ALT or AST, then check viral hepatitis serology.
- Serum amylase: usually normal, but mild ↑ < 3 × the upper limit of normal can occur.
- PT, APTT, and INR: ↑ PT and INR.
  - ❶ Beware of DIC (↑ PT, ↑ APTT, ↓ fibrinogen, ↑ FDPs).
- ABG and serum lactate: ↓ PaO_2 with ↓ pH, ↓ $PaCO_2$, and ↓ base excess is often seen. Lactate ↑.
- G&S.
- Blood cultures.
- Urine dipstick: to exclude UTI, and detect urinary conjugated bilirubin.
- ECG: if history of cardiac disease or age > 40 years, and to assess general fitness.
- Erect CXR: mandatory to exclude free intraabdominal gas, right basal pneumonia, and to assess general fitness.
- Supine AXR: rarely alters management, though gas in the biliary tree (aerobilia) or a biliary stent may be seen.

Initial management
- Keep NBM.
- Give O_2 15L/min via a non-rebreathing mask to keep SaO_2 > 94%.

- Insert a urinary catheter and aim for a urine output > 0.5mL/kg/h.
- Aggressive IV fluid resuscitation with 10–20mL/kg crystalloid boluses to correct hypotension (📖 p.17).
- ❶ Patients may require a central venous line if septic shock or a history of cardiac disease are present. Discuss with the on-call intensivist regarding HDU/ITU admission.
- Give low-dose IV opioid for analgesia, titrated to effect, with an anti-emetic.
- Correct deranged clotting: give FFP if invasive procedures are required, otherwise start vitamin K 10mg od IV.
  - ❶ Discuss with the on-call haematologist if DIC is a possibility.
- Start thromboprophylaxis (📖 p.26), unless contraindicated.
- Start antibiotics according to local protocol as soon blood cultures are taken (e.g. ciprofloxacin 500mg bd PO or cefuroxime 1.5g tds IV + metronidazole 500mg tds IV).

Further investigations

USS RUQ: detects a dilated (obstructed) biliary tree and stones within the gall bladder.

Further management

Cholangiography and drainage of the infected bile is required.
- This is usually achieved with ERCP; less commonly with PTC.
- PTC is preferred to ERCP if the obstructing lesion is near the liver hilum, or if ERCP is contraindicated, e.g. previous gastric surgery.
- Surgical drainage is required if ERCP/PTC fails, but mortality is high.

The urgency with which drainage is needed depends on the patient's response to resuscitation and IV antibiotics.
- Patients who respond rapidly to resuscitation and IV antibiotics can undergo semi-urgent cholangiography and decompression.
- Those who worsen or fail to improve require urgent cholangiography and biliary decompression.

Definitive treatment depends upon the underlying cause of the obstruction.

☼ Liver trauma

The liver is commonly damaged during blunt abdominal trauma due to its large size and relative immobility. Penetrating injuries are less common in the UK. Patients with significant liver trauma commonly have other intra-abdominal injuries. Morbidity and mortality are high in major liver trauma.

History

- Determine the mechanism of injury.

❶ Resuscitation and primary survey usually take precedence over history-taking (📖 p.42).

Examination

- RUQ tenderness and peritonism are invariably present in the responsive patient.
- Overlying bruising may be present in blunt trauma.
- Signs of shock vary with the volume of blood lost.

Initial investigations

- FBC: ↓ Hb in those with significant blood loss.
- U&Es, LFTs, and PT/INR and APTT: to assess baseline renal and hepatic function and determine the degree of coagulopathy. ↑ ALT/AST is due to hepatocyte damage.
- Cross-match 2–6 units of packed RBCs, depending on the degree of shock and other injuries.

❶ Blood loss can be **massive**. Contact the on-call haematologist early.

Initial management

- Give O_2 at 15L/min via a non-rebreathing mask.
- Insert 2 × large-bore peripheral cannulae.
- Start IV fluids, initially crystalloid, although severe or ongoing hypotension requires transfusion of packed RBCs.
- Insert a urinary catheter and maintain urine output > 0.5mL/kg/h.
- Correct any coagulopathy with FFP, platelets, etc., as needed.
  - ❶ Adequate warming is essential to counteract the effects of hypothermia on clotting.

Further investigations

- Abdominal CT (Fig. 8.2): is indicated in patients with suspected liver trauma who are haemodynamically stable after fluid resuscitation.
  - Liver injuries can be graded I (subcapsular haematoma < 10% of surface area or laceration < 1cm depth) to VI (complete liver avulsion) on CT.
- ❶ Patients with haemodynamic instability despite fluid resuscitation require emergency laparotomy. There may be other indications for laparotomy in polytrauma (📖 p.71).

Further management

Most blunt and some penetrating liver injuries can be managed non-operatively.

- Patients should be observed in HDU/ITU with regular FBC, U&Es, LFTs, PT/INR, and APTT.
- Repeat CT scanning in 4–7 days may be necessary to detect injury progression. Biliary leaks or abscesses can develop.
- Laparotomy is required in those failing non-operative management, i.e. ongoing requirement for packed RBCs and fluid resuscitation.
- At laparotomy, the best management of significant liver injuries is to pack several large gauze pads around the liver to slow haemorrhage and enable transfer to a specialist liver surgery centre.

❶ Correction of coagulopathy, hypothermia, and metabolic acidosis is essential.

❶ All significant liver injuries should be referred to a specialist liver centre.

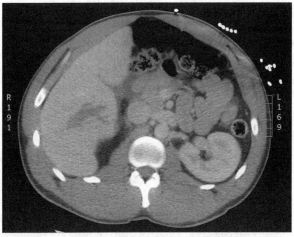

Fig. 8.2 Abdominal CT showing a deep liver laceration after high energy blunt trauma.

☼ Liver abscess

Causative organisms include bacteria, amoebae, and (rarely) fungi. Bacterial abscesses usually arise after biliary tract obstruction and ascending infection. Haematogenous spread can also occur (e.g. with appendicitis, diverticulitis, Crohn's colitis). Amoebic liver abscesses are more common in developing countries.

Clinical features

- Those with solitary abscesses often present with vague, poorly localized symptoms.
- Multiple abscesses present acutely with RUQ pain, rigors, and vomiting.
- Symptoms from the original focus of infection may predominate.
- A history of travel to developing countries suggests amoebic infection.
- On examination, the patient may have swinging pyrexia, with tachycardia, hypotension, and RUQ tenderness or a palpable mass.
- Signs from the original focus of infection are often present.

Investigations

- Initial investigations and findings are similar to those of acute cholangitis (📖 p.234).
- Send blood for *Entamoeba histolytica* serology to exclude amoebic abscesses.
- Erect CXR: may show a right pleural effusion, a raised right hemidiaphragm, right basal atelectasis, or (rarely) a gas–fluid level within the liver.
- Liver abscesses are diagnosed on RUQ USS or abdominal CT.

Management

- Initial management is supportive.
- Start broad spectrum IV antibiotics (e.g. gentamicin (dosage according to local protocols) + ampicillin 500mg qds + metronidazole 500mg tds).
- Give thromboprophylaxis (📖 p.26).
- If amoebic serology is negative, bacterial abscesses > 1–2cm diameter can be aspirated or drained under radiological guidance with fluid sent for culture.
- If biliary tree obstruction is found on USS/CT, drainage with ERCP or PTC is required.
- Laparotomy is rarely needed, but is indicated if percutaneous drainage fails or if surgery is required for the causative lesion.
- Amoebic abscesses generally do not need to be drained, as metronidazole often results in rapid clinical resolution.

☼ Gallstone ileus

Gallstone ileus is mechanical small bowel obstruction (📖 p.268) due to an intraluminal gallstone. A large gallstone can erode into the duodenum from the gall bladder, forming a cholecystoduodenal fistula, eventually impacting in the distal ileum. Gallstone ileus typically occurs in those > 65 years old.

Clinical features

- Patients present with symptoms and signs of small bowel obstruction, which may be subtle or intermittent due to repeated impaction and disimpaction of the stone.
- There may be no history of symptoms of gallstone disease.

Investigations

- Supine AXR: shows dilated small bowel loops. Occasionally, gas can be seen in the biliary tree (aerobilia) and a radio-opaque gallstone may be present.
- Abdominal CT confirms the diagnosis.

Management

As for any other cause of mechanical small bowel obstruction (📖 p.268).

- Emergency laparotomy/laparoscopy: simple enterolithotomy and small bowel closure alone is appropriate for the majority of patients. Cholecystectomy is not usually attempted.

Early postoperative complications: liver resection

Liver resections are most commonly performed for colorectal cancer metastases. Refinements to surgical and anaesthetic techniques have led to significant improvements in both mortality and morbidity rates, but liver resection is major, complex surgery. It is performed in tertiary hepatobiliary centres only.

Bile leaks

Bile leaks can occur from the cut surface of the liver or from biliary anastomoses.

- Clinical features. Leaks that are well-contained and drained fully by surgical drains may cause minimal systemic upset. Bile is seen in the drain fluid. Poorly contained leaks lead to biliary peritonitis and sepsis. Contained leaks away from operative drains develop into intraabdominal abscesses.
  - ❶ Suspect a bile leak in any liver resection patient with worsening abdominal pain or features of sepsis.
- Investigations. FBC shows ↑ WCC, and CRP is ↑. Abdominal CT detects intraabdominal collections, and radiologically guided drainage confirms the presence of bile and drains sepsis.
- Management. The mainstay of management is percutaneous drainage of the bile collection with decompression of the biliary system by ERCP + sphincterotomy or stenting. If sepsis is present, fluid resuscitate and start broad-spectrum IV antibiotics. Where surgical drains have failed to drain the bile collection, CT- or USS-guided percutaneous drainage is necessary. Laparotomy may be required if the above fail.

Operative site bleeding (📖 p.154)

Liver failure

Removal of an excessive liver volume results in failure of the remainder to cope with the body's physiological requirements. This is rare, but can occur in patients with unrecognized chronic liver disease.

- Clinical features. Patients have worsening jaundice, ascites, and confusion (hepatic encephalopathy).
- Investigations. LFTs and INR are progressively deranged. Sepsis and bleeding must be excluded as underlying causes, or contributing factors. Request a CXR and culture body fluids. A CT abdomen is necessary to exclude an intraabdominal collection and bleeding.
- Management. Septic foci must be drained and treated with IV antibiotics. Early involvement of a liver surgeon and a hepatologist is essential. Prognosis is poor. N-acetylcysteine may be given.

❶ Involve your senior early if progressive dysfunction of LFTs is seen in a patient post-hepatic resection.

Early postoperative complications: laparoscopic and open cholecystectomies

Laparoscopic cholecystectomy

By far the most common biliary operation is removal of the gall bladder, usually laparoscopically. Conversion to an open cholecystectomy is needed in ~ 5% of cases, but is dependent on the technical difficulty and the skill of the surgeon.

Biliary tree damage

Damage to the biliary tree occurs after ~ 0.25–0.5% of laparoscopic chole-cystectomies and usually manifests as a bile leak. Occasionally, complete occlusion of the CBD can occur. Bile leaks can occur from the gall bladder bed, the cystic duct stump, or occasionally from damage to the CBD or CHD.

- Clinical features. Patients present 0–5 days postoperatively with abdominal pain starting in the RUQ and signs of peritonitis.
- Investigations. FBC shows ↑ WCC, and CRP is ↑. LFTs may be non-specifically deranged due to sepsis. CXR to exclude bowel perforation is usually unhelpful as subdiaphragmatic gas can be seen for up to 5 days post-laparoscopy.
- Management. Resuscitate with IV fluids and give IV antibiotics. Patients with localized signs need an urgent USS to identify and drain the fluid collection. If the fluid is bile, ERCP is needed for placement of a biliary stent and to decompress the biliary tree. Those with widespread peri-tonitis require emergency laparotomy/laparoscopy. Complex biliary damage requires referral to a specialist centre for reconstructive biliary surgery.

❶ Complete occlusion of the CBD presents as progressive obstructive jaundice apparent from 24–48h post-operatively. USS shows a dilated biliary tree and ERCP confirms complete occlusion. This requires referral to a specialist hepatobiliary centre.

❶ Call your senior if biliary tree damage is suspected.

Operative site bleeding (📖 p.154)

Bowel perforation Small, unrecognized bowel injuries can present 1–5 days postoperatively with abdominal pain and sepsis. Examination reveals peritonitis. Emergency laparotomy/laparoscopy is required.

Open cholecystectomy

The majority of open cholecystectomies performed now are conversions from the laparoscopic procedure, indicating that the operation was diffi-cult or that complications occurred. Open surgery carries a higher rate of wound (📖 p.166) and cardiorespiratory complications, but lower rates of unrecognized bowel and biliary injuries.

Early postoperative complications: ERCP and PTC

ERCP

ERCP can be a complex procedure, with morbidity of ~ 10% and mortality of ~ 1%.

Acute pancreatitis (📖 p.244) The risk of acute pancreatitis post-ERCP is highest in females < 60 years old and in patients where the papilla has been difficult to cannulate. Clinical features, investigations, and the principles of management are the same as for any other cause of acute pancreatitis. Transient hyperamylasaemia without acute pancreatitis (i.e. without abdominal pain) occurs in ~ 50% of patients post-ERCP, but has no clinical importance.

Upper GI bleeding (📖 p.190) The risk of upper GI haemorrhage is higher if sphincterotomy has been performed. Clinical features, investigations, and the principles of management are the same as for any other cause of upper GI bleeding, except that repeat endoscopy is usually not necessary, as the bleeding should settle with supportive management.

Gastroduodenal perforation

This should be apparent during the ERCP, but can present late.
- Clinical features. Patients complain of lower chest or upper abdominal pain post-ERCP.
- Investigations. FBC shows ↑ WCC. Request an erect CXR and supine AXR to look for free gas and retroperitoneal gas. Abdominal CT may be required to confirm periduodenal retroperitoneal gas.
- Management. A contained perforation may be able to be managed non-operatively with percutaneous drainage of collections, NG drainage, IV antibiotics, and nutrition via a feeding jejunostomy or TPN. Free perforations require emergency laparotomy.

Acute cholangitis (📖 p.234)
Oversedation (📖 p.220)

PTC The widespread availability of ERCP means that PTCs are rarely performed. Indications for PTC include failed ERCP, intrahepatic biliary obstruction, or inability to perform ERCP due to difficulty accessing the CBD (e.g. choledochojejunostomy).

Bile leak (see 'Early postoperative complications: liver resection')

Bleeding (📖 p.154) May settle with supportive management and correction of anaemia and coagulopathy. Laparotomy is required if shock persists despite fluid resuscitation.

Bowel perforation This is rare post-PTC. Patients complain of severe upper abdominal pain and FBC shows ↑ WCC. Request an erect CXR to look for free subdiaphragmatic gas. Abdominal CT may be required. Free perforations require emergency laparotomy.

Acute cholangitis (📖 p.234)

Pancreas and spleen

⚙ **Acute pancreatitis**

Acute pancreatitis (AP) is acute inflammation of the pancreas. It can be a life-threatening condition, with an inpatient mortality of 10–15%. AP can be defined as either mild or severe.

- Mild AP (80% of cases) is associated with minimal extrapancreatic organ dysfunction and a rapid recovery. Severe AP may develop as the disease progresses.
- Severe AP (20% of cases) is defined as being associated with organ failure and/or local complications such as infected pancreatic necrosis, pancreatic abscess formation, or pancreatic pseudocyst formation.

❶ As 95% of deaths from AP occur in patients with severe AP, the **early** identification of patients who may go on to develop severe AP is essential.

Anatomy and physiology

- The pancreas is situated retroperitoneally in the upper abdomen, draped across the vertebral column. It is formed from dorsal and ventral pancreatic buds from the primitive foregut that come together to form the main and accessory pancreatic ducts.
- Two developmental anomalies may occur, both of which are associated with pancreatitis. Pancreas divisum occurs when the dorsal and ventral pancreatic ducts fail to fuse. Annular pancreas occurs where a band of pancreatic tissue of varying thickness surrounds the second part of the duodenum.
- The pancreas has two components: the endocrine pancreas, which principally produces insulin and glucagon, and the exocrine pancreas, which produces digestive enzymes such as amylase, lipase, and trypsin (responsible for the breakdown of carbohydrate, fat, and protein, respectively). The enzymes are stored in intracellular zymogen granules and secreted in response to vagal and hormonal stimuli (e.g. CCK and secretin). Trypsin is secreted as the pro-hormone trypsinogen which is activated by enterokinase in the duodenum.

Pathophysiology

AP occurs when the normal defence to local enzyme activation breaks down. Destruction of cellular integrity, due to alcohol, drugs, or hypothermia, results in local release of enzymes and autodigestion. Reflux of enterokinase up the pancreatic duct may follow passage of small gallstones and results in local activation of trypsinogen.

The ensuing inflammatory process initiates a positive feedback loop by causing further cellular destruction and enzyme release and activation.

Causes

- Obstruction of the pancreatic duct or papilla, e.g. gallstones (~ 40%), pancreatic/ampullary tumours, pancreas divisum/annular pancreas.
- Toxins, e.g. ethanol (~ 40%), methanol, scorpion venom.
- Drugs, e.g. prednisolone, azathioprine, ACE inhibitors.
- Infections, e.g. mumps, cytomegalovirus, HIV.
- Metabolic, e.g. hypercalcaemia, hypertriglyceridaemia, pregnancy.
- Trauma, e.g. blunt trauma, ERCP.
- Miscellaneous, e.g. hypothermia.

- Ischaemia, e.g. after cardiopulmonary bypass, vasculitis.
- Familial.
- Idiopathic (~ 10%), i.e. no identifiable cause found.

History

- Rapid onset of upper abdominal pain, that usually radiates through to the back.
- Relief may be gained by sitting forwards; more commonly patients lie still.
- The pain extends to the RIF when inflammatory material passes through the epiploic foramen (of Winslow) and tracks down the right paracolic gutter.
- Frequent vomiting and/or retching is common.
- There may be a history of a recent alcohol binge, or previous symptoms consistent with biliary colic.

❶ Take a full drug history and family history.

Examination

- Low-grade pyrexia.
- Tachycardia.
- Marked upper abdominal tenderness.
- Rarely, skin nodules (subcutaneous areas of fat necrosis) are present.
- In severe cases:
  - pale appearance, sweaty;
  - hypotension and shock;
  - generalized abdominal tenderness with involuntary guarding;
  - Cullen's sign or Grey Turner's sign (periumbilical or flank bruising, respectively, due to haemorrhagic pancreatitis).

Initial investigations

There are two priorities in the initial investigation phase. The first is to confirm the clinical diagnosis of AP (and exclude ΔΔ); the second is the determination of disease severity.

Investigations to confirm the clinical diagnosis of AP

❶ Finding the cause of the attack is not an immediate priority.

- FBC: ↑↑ WCC is common.
- U&Es: dehydration is reflected in ↑ urea and creatinine.
- LFTs: ↑ in bilirubin, ALP, ALT, or GGT suggest gallstone pancreatitis.
- Serum amylase: in the presence of appropriate symptoms and signs, serum amylase > 3 x the upper limit of normal is usually diagnostic of AP.
  - Many other conditions can cause a moderately raised amylase, but it is very rare for these to cause elevations > 5 x the upper limit of normal (see Box 9.1).
  - Rises early (4–6h), but can fall quickly, meaning that the diagnosis can be missed if the patient presents > 24h after the onset of pain. Interpret levels in the light of symptom duration.
- Serum lipase: preferable to amylase for the diagnosis of AP, due to its longer half-life and greater sensitivity and specificity. It is not yet widely available.
- ECG: to exclude myocardial ischaemia as a possible cause of epigastric pain, sweating, and tachycardia.

- Erect CXR: to exclude perforated PU. ALI/ARDS or pleural effusions may develop.
- Supine AXR: useful to exclude small bowel obstruction. In AP, the AXR is often normal, although it may show loss of the left psoas shadow, the 'colon cut-off' sign, or a sentinel loop (a dilated gas-filled duodenum).
- ❶ If the diagnosis remains in doubt despite these investigations, request an emergency abdominal CT (Fig. 9.1). The presence of an inflamed pancreas on CT confirms AP, and excludes ΔΔ, e.g. perforation, bowel infarction.

Box 9.1 Causes of raised serum amylase

1–4 × the upper limit of normal
- Abdominal causes: perforated PU, acute cholecystitis, ruptured AAA, ruptured ectopic pregnancy, bowel obstruction, mesenteric infarction, pancreatic trauma.
- Impaired renal excretion: renal failure (occasionally amylase is very high), macroamylasaemia.
- Salivary gland disease: salivary gland calculi, parotitis (e.g. mumps).
- Miscellaneous: alcohol binge, morphine.

> 5 × the upper limit of normal
- AP
- DKA

❶ Hypertriglyceridaemia can prevent some laboratories from measuring serum amylase. Request serum lipase or urinary amylase instead

---

Investigations for predicting disease severity
- Once a diagnosis of AP has been made, further investigations (e.g. ABG, LDH, Ca^{2+}) are necessary for predicting severity. A number of multifactorial scoring systems have been identified (e.g. Ranson, APACHE II, Glasgow (Box 9.2)).
- Serum CRP > 150mg/L within 48h of admission, and obesity are also independent predictors of severity.
❶ By definition, a patient with AP and organ failure (e.g. shock) has **severe** disease without the need for further scoring.

Box 9.2 The modified Glasgow (Imrie) criteria*

- Age > 55 years
- WCC > 15 × 10^9/L
- Blood glucose > 10mmol/L
- Serum urea > 16mmol/L
- PaO_2 < 8kPa (60mmHg)
- Serum albumin < 32g/L
- Serum calcium < 2mmol/L (uncorrected)
- LDH > 600U/L

The presence of > 2 of the above variables within 48h of admission predicts severe AP.

* Blamey, S.L. *et al.* (1984). *Gut* **25**, 1340–6.

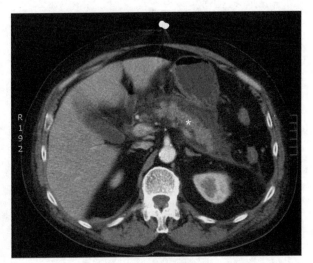

Fig. 9.1 Abdominal CT showing an enlarged, oedematous pancreas (*) with peri-pancreatic fat stranding, consistent with acute pancreatitis.

Initial management

Initial management is determined by disease severity (actual or predicted). Management is supportive, with specific treatment for complications.

Mild AP

- Admit all cases, even if the pain is minimal, as the disease may progress rapidly.
- Keep NBM.
- Start thromboprophylaxis (📖 p.26).
- Insert a urinary catheter, and give IV fluids to keep output > 0.5mL/kg/h.
- Start an insulin sliding scale if CBG > 12mmol/L (📖 p.24).
- Give O$_2$ to keep SaO$_2$ > 95%.
- Give parenteral analgesia, e.g. morphine 5–10mg IM/IV prn up to every 4h, with prn anti-emetics.
  - Pethidine is preferred to morphine in some units, as morphine may cause sphincter of Oddi spasm and exacerbate AP.
  - If pain is poorly controlled, start a PCA.
- Daily bloods, including CRP. Serial amylase is not required once a diagnosis of AP has been made, as it is not a prognostic indicator.
- An NG tube may be required for ongoing vomiting.

Severe AP is managed as for mild AP, except for the following.

- HDU/ITU care is required.
- Insert an NG tube.

- Insert a central venous line for CVP monitoring.
  - ❶ Extensive fluid sequestration can occur and it is not uncommon to require 5–6L in first 24h to maintain urine output.
- Bloods and ABGs may be needed twice-daily or more, initially.

Further investigations

- All patients require USS RUQ to detect gallstones and/or a dilated CBD. USS has no role in the diagnosis of AP.
- Those with severe AP, signs of sepsis, or deterioration in clinical status 6–10 days after admission require IV and oral contrast-enhanced abdominal CT using a pancreatic protocol.
  - The presence of pancreatic necrosis (non-enhancing areas post-contrast) or complications such as fluid collections indicates severity. Radiological severity assessments (e.g. the Balthazar score) are more accurate prognostic indicators than clinico-biochemical scores.
  - If extensive pancreatic necrosis (> 30%) is present on CT, start IV antibiotics to help prevent infected pancreatic necrosis (e.g. cefuroxime 1.5g tds, or imipenem 500mg qds).
  - ☞ This last point is contentious, as the evidence base is still evolving.[1]

Further management

- Reassess: review the patient regularly to detect deterioration (or failure to progress) and manage as severe AP. Request pancreatic CT to detect local complications.
- Patients with improving clinical and biochemical parameters whose pain has resolved can have oral fluids, and eventually food, re-introduced.
  - Where this does not occur within 5–10 days of admission, start naso-jejunal or nasogastric feeding. If these are not tolerated, start TPN.
- Patients with severe gallstone pancreatitis, cholangitis, jaundice, or a dilated CBD require early ERCP and sphincterotomy.
- The development of infected pancreatic necrosis carries a mortality of > 40%.
  - Patients developing sepsis require contrast-enhanced CT scanning to identify pancreatic necrosis/abscesses. CT-guided aspiration may be necessary to confirm infected pancreatic necrosis.
  - Consider multiple CT-guided or minimally invasive external drainage of infected pancreatic necrosis/abscesses.
  - Surgical pancreatic necrosectomy may be necessary and should only be performed in specialist units.
  - ❶ Consider transfer of patients with severe AP to a specialist unit, especially those with pancreatic necrosis.
- All patients with mild gallstone pancreatitis should undergo cholecystectomy before leaving hospital or electively within 2 weeks of discharge. Patients who are not fit for an operation should have an ERCP and sphincterotomy as a definitive procedure.

- Further outpatient investigations should be done following recovery if the aetiology is not clear.

Reference

1 UK Working Party on Acute Pancreatitis (2005). UK guidelines for the management of acute pancreatitis. *Gut* **54** (Suppl. 3), iii1–iii9.

:O: **Pancreatic trauma**

Pancreatic trauma is uncommon. It usually occurs intraoperatively, e.g. during splenectomy or left nephrectomy, but may result from penetrating or blunt abdominal trauma. Penetrating trauma is often associated with catastrophic injuries to neighbouring structures such as the IVC, abdominal aorta, and superior mesenteric vessels, so the majority of traumatic cases present after blunt trauma.

Pathophysiology of blunt trauma

A direct epigastric blow compresses the pancreas against the lumbar vertebrae, sometimes resulting in fracture of the pancreatic neck. It is more common in young children due to horse kicks, bicycle handlebar injuries, and ill-fitting seat belts. The injury may disrupt the main pancreatic duct leading to leakage of enzymes into the peritoneal cavity (pancreatic ascites). Other complications include AP, pancreatic pseudocyst, pancreatic abscess, and pancreatic fistula.

❶ Significant trauma is required to disrupt the pancreas and therefore multiple injuries are usually coexistent, e.g. liver, spleen, small bowel, lumbar vertebrae. These may obscure a pancreatic injury, so think of it specifically.

History

• History of blunt compression trauma or penetrating trauma to trunk.
• Abdominal pain. This may be minimal following isolated trauma, leading to delayed presentation.

❶ Resuscitation and primary survey often take precedence over history-taking (◻ p.42).

Examination

• Tachycardia, low-grade pyrexia.
• Abdominal distension.
• Epigastric bruising may be present with blunt trauma, or an entry site may be seen with penetrating trauma.
• Tenderness in the epigastrium.

Initial investigations

• FBC: ↓ Hb if coexistent large vessel injury.
• U&Es: often normal.
• LFTs: ↑ ALT/AST if significant liver trauma is also present.
• G&S: all patients. Cross-match 4–6 units of packed RBCs if shock is present (suggesting other associated injuries).
• Serum amylase: may be **normal** in the first 3h, but ↑ later. Seldom > 5 × the upper limit of normal.
• Erect CXR or supine AXR: no specific signs of pancreatic trauma are seen, although retroperitoneal gas may be due to a ruptured duodenum, making pancreatic trauma likely.

❶ Because pancreatic trauma may present with non-specific symptoms or signs, and the serum amylase is often normal initially, a high index of suspicion is required. Diagnosis is often delayed.

In **haemodynamically stable** patients where the mechanism of injury raises the possibility of pancreatic trauma, request abdominal CT.

- CT abdomen: pancreatic injury may be manifested by pancreatic oedema or retroperitoneal haematoma. Parenchymal fracture of pancreas ± free fluid in the lesser sac suggests pancreatic ductal injury.
  - Other solid organ trauma is often seen.
  - CT within 8h of the injury may be falsely negative; repeat later if pancreatic injury is likely.

❶ In haemodynamically unstable patients or those with peritonitis or evisceration, laparotomy is required. Pancreatic injury is often diagnosed at laparotomy.

Initial management

❶ Death following pancreatic trauma is commonly from other associated injuries. Seek and treat immediately life-threatening injuries first.
- Transfer to HDU/ITU is usually required.
- Keep NBM.
- Give parenteral opioid analgesia.
- Give O_2 to keep SaO_2 > 95%.
- Insert a urinary catheter and resuscitate with IV fluids, aiming for a urine output > 0.5mL/kg/h.
- Start thromboprophylaxis (📖 p.26) if active bleeding is not present.
- Consider IV antibiotic prophylaxis to prevent peripancreatic infections.

Further investigations
- ERCP: to assess whether main duct injury has occurred, but only where this is not clear from CT and the patient is stable.
- MRCP: increasingly used in the assessment of possible ductal injuries.

Further management
- Begin feeding via TPN or feeding jejunostomy.
- Patients with blunt trauma who are haemodynamically stable and with no parenchymal fracture on CT may be able to be treated non-operatively. Repeat CT scanning is necessary to detect evolving injuries.
- Surgery is required if injury to the main pancreatic duct is suspected.
  - Intraoperative pancreatography may be necessary.
  - If the main pancreatic duct is fractured, the ruptured distal duct can be drained into a Roux loop. If the distal pancreas is not viable, distal pancreatectomy and splenectomy are required.
  - Major injuries to the head of the pancreas require a Whipple's pancreaticoduodenectomy if the patient is stable.

❶ The management of pancreatic trauma is complex. Consider early referral to a specialist unit.

✸ Splenic trauma

The spleen is the 2nd most commonly injured abdominal organ following blunt trauma. This usually leads to significant haemorrhage, although a contained splenic haematoma may form, avoiding shock. Late rupture of a splenic haematoma can occur. A pathologically enlarged spleen can rupture with seemingly trivial trauma. The spleen is infrequently injured in penetrating trauma due to its relatively small size and protection from overlying ribs 9–11.

Iatrogenic splenic trauma is common, especially with surgery involving the left kidney, left colon, stomach, or distal pancreas.

Anatomy and physiology
- The spleen lies in the LUQ, lateral to the greater curve of the stomach and immediately beneath the diaphragm. The tail of the pancreas is intimately associated with the hilum of the spleen. It has peritoneal attachments to the parietal peritoneum laterally, as well as to the stomach, left kidney, and splenic flexure of the colon. It is a highly vascular organ.
- Splenomegaly due to glandular fever (infectious mononucleosis) is associated with an increased tendency to rupture. Other causes of splenomegaly (e.g. portal hypertension) do not have a significantly increased risk of rupture.
- The spleen is important for protection against encapsulated bacteria (e.g. *Streptococcus pneumoniae*, *Neisseria meningitidis*, *Haemophilus influenzae*).

History
- Blunt LUQ or left-sided chest trauma; this may be trivial (e.g. coughing, sneezing) with splenic rupture after glandular fever.
- Left shoulder tip pain due to diaphragmatic irritation by blood (Kehr's sign).

❶ Resuscitation and primary survey may take precedence over history-taking (📖 p.42).

Examination
- Tachycardia, hypotension, pallor.
- Bruising over the LUQ.
- Tenderness ± crepitus over the left chest wall due to fractured ribs.
- Abdominal tenderness ± guarding may be localized to the LUQ, or may be generalized.
- Tipping the bed head down may precipitate Kehr's sign.

❶ Significant blunt trauma is associated with multiple other injuries.

Investigations
- FBC: may show ↓ Hb, but a ↔ Hb does not exclude a significant splenic injury.
- U&Es, LFTs, and serum amylase are ↔ in isolated splenic trauma.
- G&S: in all patients with suspected splenic trauma. Cross-match 4–6 units of packed RBCs if the patient is haemodynamically unstable.
- Erect CXR and supine AXR: usually normal, although large splenic haematomas can lead to an elevated left hemidiaphragm, left pleural effusion/haemothorax, left basal atelectasis, medial displacement of the stomach, or inferior displacement of the splenic flexure.
- FAST scan: free fluid is seen in the LUQ.

❶ Have a low threshold for investigation if splenic injury is suspected, even in the haemodynamically normal patient.

Management
The haemodynamically unstable patient
- Keep NBM.
- Give high-flow O_2 via a non-rebreathing mask.
- Establish 2 × large-bore peripheral venous cannulae and resuscitate with IV fluids ± blood products as required.
- Insert a urinary catheter (📖 p.504), if time permits.
- Unless the patient responds rapidly to fluid resuscitation, transfer to theatre immediately. While splenic conservation is often spoken about, the priority is to save the patient, the urgency of which may preclude preservation.

❶ All patients undergoing emergency splenectomy require postoperative immunization and antibiotic prophylaxis to prevent overwhelming post-splenectomy infection (📖 p.259).

The haemodynamically stable patient where splenic injury is suspected
- Keep NBM.
- Insert a urinary catheter (📖 p.504).
- Give maintenance IV fluids.
- Request emergency abdominal CT (Fig. 9.2) with the facility for immediate transfer to theatre should deterioration occur suddenly.
  - Splenic injury can be graded I–V (Box 9.3).
  - Coexistent haemoperitoneum is common.

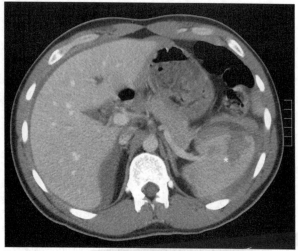

Fig. 9.2 CT showing a deep splenic laceration (*) after LUQ blunt trauma. Intraperitoneal blood is seen around the liver.

Box 9.3 AAST splenic injury grading

- Grade I: subcapsular haematoma < 10% of surface area, or capsular tear < 1cm deep.
- Grade II: subcapsular haematoma 10–50% of surface area, intraparenchymal haematoma < 5cm diameter, or laceration 1–3cm deep.
- Grade III: subcapsular haematoma > 50% of surface area, ruptured parenchymal or subcapsular haematoma, intraparenchymal haematoma > 5cm diameter, or laceration > 3cm deep.
- Grade IV: laceration involving hilar vessels with devascularization > 25%.
- Grade V: shattered spleen or hilar vascular injury.

- A contained splenic haematoma in an otherwise stable patient can be treated non-surgically.
  - Close monitoring may require HDU admission.
  - Twice-daily FBC may be necessary initially.
  - Radiological embolization of bleeding sites may be useful in haemodynamically stable patients with ongoing transfusion requirements.

❶ Haemodynamic instability or peritonitis mandate immediate laparotomy.

Early postoperative complications: Whipple's procedure (pancreaticoduodenectomy)

The pancreas is a difficult organ upon which to operate and has a high frequency of postoperative complications. The most common pancreatic operation is Whipple's pancreaticoduodenectomy, where the head of pancreas, duodenum, CBD, and gall bladder are resected. Three anastomoses are fashioned: between the cut duct in the body of pancreas with a Roux-en-Y loop of jejunum, between the cut end of the common hepatic duct and the Roux loop, and between the stomach remnant and proximal jejunum. Expect to come across one or all of these complications at some time.

Pancreatic anastomotic leak/pancreatic fistula

An anastomotic leak from the remnant pancreas is the most feared complication, associated with the greatest mortality

❶ This should be considered in all patients who become unwell following a Whipple's.

- Clinical features. A leak may present with increased abdominal pain, tachycardia, pyrexia, oliguria, and an increasing respiratory rate (often the first sign that something is wrong). Abdominal tenderness is often difficult to distinguish from wound pain. Wound discharge may be present.
- Investigations. Send drain and wound fluid for measurement of amylase (> 1000U/L is suggestive of a leak). Abdominal CT shows an abnormal fluid collection in the region of the pancreatic anastomosis.
- Management. Is initially non-operative. Leave the abdominal drains in until the leak has settled and arrange CT-guided percutaneous drainage of any residual collections. Start subcutaneous octreotide to reduce pancreatic secretion, and feed via feeding jejunostomy or nasojejunal tube (or TPN if enteral feed is not tolerated). If sepsis develops despite non-operative treatment, further laparotomy with washout and extensive drainage, or a completion pancreatectomy, may be needed.

Delayed gastric emptying

This is common after a Whipple's, and may be secondary to a subclinical pancreatic leak or neurapraxia of the retroperitoneal nerves. The presentation is similar to GOO (i.e. high volume vomiting every 1–2 days). Management is non-operative.

- Keep NBM and drain the stomach via an NG tube.
- Arrange abdominal CT to rule out mechanical obstruction or peripancreatic collections.
- Start feeding via TPN or through a feeding jejunostomy/nasojejunal tube.
- Begin prokinetic agents such as IV erythromycin or metoclopramide.

It may take several weeks to settle.

Operative site bleeding (📖 p.154)

Upper GI bleeding

Bleeding may occur from the gastroenterostomy or the entero-enterostomy. The clinical features, investigations, and management are the same as for other causes of upper GI bleeding (📖 p.190). Gastroenterostomy bleeding can be halted endoscopically with adrenaline injections. Entero-enterostomy bleeding is usually self-limiting, and requires supportive therapy. If bleeding is heavy a return to theatre and revision of anastomosis is indicated.

Bile leak/biliary fistula

Breakdown of the hepatico-jejunostomy biliary anastomosis is uncommon, and bile leaks are more common from accessory bile ducts. Patients present with worsening RUQ pain, becoming generalized. The RUQ is tender with guarding, and bile may be seen in the drains. Serum bilirubin is raised, and CT scan reveals a RUQ collection. Percutaneous drainage reveals bile. Check fluid amylase to exclude a pancreatic leak. Bile leaks usually resolve with external biliary drainage and drainage of collections. Large leaks from the anastomosis may require laparotomy and revision of the biliary anastomosis.

Early postoperative complications: splenectomy

Pancreatic leak/pancreatic fistula

The tail of pancreas is close to the splenic hilum and may be damaged during a splenectomy. For this reason a silicone drain should be placed in the LUQ. Postoperatively drain fluid amylase can be measured, and > 1000U/L suggests a significant injury. Abdominal CT may demonstrate a fluid collection associated with the pancreas and separate from the drain, which may warrant percutaneous drainage. The amount of pancreatic secretion can be reduced using octreotide. The fistula usually heals spontaneously within a few weeks.

Acute gastric dilatation (📖 p.205) ± short gastric artery bleeding

Acute gastric dilatation is avoided by placement of an NG tube at surgery, with frequent aspiration postoperatively. Patients with vomiting or LUQ pain post-splenectomy should have CXR and AXR to assess stomach size. Insert an NG tube if the stomach is dilated, and keep the patient NBM. Dilatation of the stomach post-splenectomy carries the risk of initiating bleeding from the short gastric vessels that were ligated on the greater curve of the stomach. If shock is present, resuscitate with IV fluids and packed RBCs, correct any coagulopathy, give high-flow O_2, and discuss with your seniors immediately. A return to theatre may be needed.

Thrombocytosis

The platelet count typically rises following splenectomy and can be associated with thromboembolic events. When platelet counts are > 750 × 10^9/L, aspirin 75mg od PO should be started, albeit with little evidence as to its efficacy in this setting. Platelet counts eventually return to normal.

Overwhelming post-splenectomy infection (OPSI)

Splenectomy leaves a patient susceptible to infection, particularly from encapsulated organisms. While most infections occur in the first 2 years following splenectomy, there is an increased lifetime risk. Post-splenectomy infection with these organisms is rapidly progressive and has a high mortality. Reducing the risk of OPSI can be achieved through immunization, oral antibiotic prophylaxis, and patient education (Box 9.4). Re-immunize according to current guidelines.

❶ It is the surgeon's responsibility to ensure that immunization and antibiotic prophylaxis are given before discharge.

Box 9.4 Prevention of OPSI*

- Give meningococcal group C vaccine 2 weeks post-splenectomy.
- Give pneumococcal vaccine 2 weeks post-splenectomy.
- Give *H. influenzae* type B vaccine 2 weeks post-splenectomy.
- Give influenza vaccine as soon as possible post-splenectomy.
- Start lifelong prophylactic oral antibiotics (phenoxymethylpenicillin or erythromycin).
- Patient education is essential. Inform the patient of the risk of OPSI and give written information. Those who develop symptoms of infection require urgent admission for IV antibiotics. Encourage the patient to carry a card documenting asplenism. When travelling, anti-malarial prophylaxis must be strictly adhered to.
- Inform the GP of splenectomy and vaccinations/prophylaxis given.
- Hospital records must clearly document splenectomy.

* Davies, J.M. *et al.* (2002). *Clin. Med.* **2**, 440–3.

Small and large bowel

⦸ **Appendicitis**

The appendix is a vestigial blind-ending tube of variable length (2–12cm) with its base at the pole of the caecum. In 60% of the population it lies retrocaecally; in the rest the intraperitoneal position probably varies with time, although often the tip lies in the pelvis.

Acute appendicitis is the most common abdominal surgical emergency, affecting ~ 10% of the UK population. It may occur at any age, but is most common between the ages of 10 and 30, and uncommon in the very young (< 2 years old). The incidence of appendicitis declines progressively with age.

Accurate diagnosis can be challenging but should be made predominantly on **clinical** evaluation rather than overreliance on investigations. Close and repeated clinical examination is the key to reaching an appropriate decision on the need for surgery, especially in marginal cases. Unnecessary delays in diagnosis may allow perforation to occur but, conversely, removal of a normal 'lily-white' appendix occurs in up to 20% of cases. While removal of a normal appendix is undesirable, it is in some cases inevitable if genuine appendicitis is not to be overlooked.

- ❶ Because of its frequency, appendicitis should always be borne in mind as a possible cause of an acute abdomen.
- ❶ The seriousness of appendicitis should never be underestimated; it has a mortality of 1%.

Pathophysiology

- Appendicitis may occur in an unobstructed appendix but in the majority of cases it is due to obstruction of the lumen by a faecolith or enlargement of lymphoid tissue within the appendix wall. Occasionally, a caecal or appendiceal tumour may obstruct the lumen.
- Inflammation in the mucosa extends to involve the full thickness of the appendix wall and overlying serosa with eventual formation of intraluminal pus and local fibropurulent exudate.
- Mild inflammation may resolve spontaneously, particularly if the appendix is unobstructed. In most cases it progresses, leading to ischaemia of the wall (from increased intraluminal pressure and thrombosis of the branches of the appendicular artery), gangrene, and eventually perforation.
- Perforation usually results in localized peritonitis (and an appendix abscess) due to walling off by the omentum and small bowel, but may also produce generalized peritonitis (▢ p.108).

History

❶ The clinical findings are variable (Box 10.1) and depend partly on the patient's age and the anatomical position of the appendix.

- Acute abdominal pain, usually 1–3 days duration. Classically, colicky periumbilical pain shifting after several hours to become a constant RIF pain. Pain is worse with movement and coughing.
- Nausea and vomiting.
- Anorexia.
- There may be history of similar, less severe episodes.

Box 10.1 Common variations in clinical presentation

- Children < 10 years old: vomiting and malaise may predominate. Tenderness in the RIF can be variable. May also present with pain in the right hip and RIF on walking.
- The elderly: as with young children, RIF tenderness can be variable. May present with vomiting, confusion, and sepsis.
- During pregnancy: upwards displacement of the appendix by the enlarging uterus may lead to RUQ pain and tenderness.
- Retrocaecal appendicitis: poorly localized right flank or RUQ pain and tenderness, positive psoas stretch test.
- Pelvic appendicitis: diarrhoea or urinary frequency with RIF tenderness. Urine dipstick often shows mild pyuria or haematuria due to bladder irritation.
- Generalized peritonitis and septic shock: more common in young children and the elderly and those with a delayed presentation.
- ❶ Never forget to exclude testicular torsion as a cause of RIF pain in young males.

Examination
- Flushed facies.
- Pyrexia (37.5–38°C) in uncomplicated appendicitis; it may be higher if perforation has occurred.
- Mild tachycardia.
- Coated tongue with foetor.
- Tenderness in the RIF with signs of localized peritonitis (📖 p.102).
- A RIF mass may occasionally be palpable (Box 10.2).

Box 10.2 Tender RIF mass

An appendix mass may occur if acute appendicitis is present for several days because of delayed presentation or intervention.
- The inflammatory mass is localized to the RIF and is made up of loops of small bowel and/or omentum surrounding the inflamed appendix. It may progress to an appendix abscess resulting from localized perforation.
- Typically, presentation is with RIF pain of several days duration, pyrexia, and a tender, palpable mass in the RIF, without peritonitis.
- Exclude other causes of a RIF mass (appendix abscess, Crohn's disease, caecal carcinoma, torted ovarian cyst, gall bladder mucocele, psoas abscess, pelvic kidney) by urgent abdominal CT or USS.
- If an appendix mass is confirmed, treat non-surgically initially, with IV fluids, analgesia, and IV antibiotics (see 'Initial management'). If, as is most likely, the appendix mass resolves spontaneously, interval appendicectomy after 3 months is scheduled. If there is no clinical improvement on non-surgical treatment, surgery is indicated.
- Appendix abscesses can be drained radiologically or surgically.

- Rovsing's sign (pain in RIF on palpation of LIF) is often present.
- Extension of the right hip may provoke pain (psoas stretch test) in retrocaecal appendicitis.
- DRE may reveal pelvic tenderness in pelvic appendicitis.

Differential diagnoses

Although acute appendicitis is common, watch out for pitfalls (Box 10.3) and don't neglect other possible diagnoses.

- Mesenteric adenitis: in young children, associated with sore throat, cervical lymphadenopathy, and upper respiratory symptoms.
- Meckel's diverticulitis: very difficult to distinguish, clinically (Box 10.4).
- Acute Crohn's ileitis: there may be a past history of colicky abdominal pain, diarrhoea, and weight loss.
- Pelvic inflammatory disease: in sexually active females, usually with vaginal discharge. Pain is often in the LIF also, and cervical excitation is present on vaginal examination.
- Torted ovarian cyst: pain is of sudden onset and a mass is not always palpable.
- Testicular torsion: may present with minimal scrotal pain but with vomiting and RIF pain. An abnormal testis is found on examination.
- Urinary tract infection: dysuria is present, and urine dipstick is abnormal.
    - **❶** Pelvic appendicitis may cause very similar symptoms with similar dipstick abnormalities, but with tenderness on DRE.
- Ureteric calculi: spasms of pain shooting to the groin, usually with dipstick haematuria.
- Gastroenteritis: diarrhoea and vomiting are major features. Pain is crampy and associated with passing loose stools.
    - **❶** Beware of diagnosing gastroenteritis in a child with abdominal pain and vomiting, but without diarrhoea. Appendicitis is more likely.
- Acute cholecystitis: pain more in the RUQ, but on occasion it can be difficult to distinguish from a retrocaecal appendicitis.
- Caecal diverticulitis: usually in older patients and very difficult to distinguish from appendicitis. Sigmoid diverticulitis from a long sigmoid colon lying in the RIF can cause similar diagnostic difficulties.
- Perforated PU: gastric contents can run down the right paracolic gutter to cause RIF pain. The onset of pain is sudden and located in the epigastrium. Check an erect CXR for free gas.
- Perforated caecal or ascending colon cancer: the patient is almost always > 40 years old and a mass may be palpable. Microcytic anaemia is usually present and there may be free gas on an erect CXR.
- Rectus sheath haematoma (📖 p.128): the patient is often on warfarin and the pain and tenderness are slightly more medial than McBurney's point.

Initial investigation

- FBC: ↑ WCC is common.
- CRP: commonly ↑.
- MSU: dipstick urinalysis to exclude renal colic and UTI, and βhCG pregnancy test in women of child-bearing age.
- Erect CXR: usually not required. Request if peritonitis suggests a perforated hollow viscus.

- Supine AXR: usually not required. If vomiting is a major feature, or the abdomen is distended, request AXR to exclude bowel obstruction.

Box 10.3 Pitfalls in diagnosis

- In males, **always** examine the testes to exclude torsion.
- In females of child-bearing age, **always** check βhCG to exclude an ectopic pregnancy.
- Patients recently prescribed oral antibiotics for presumed UTI may present with partially treated appendicitis. Their presentation is often delayed, and signs are atypical. Have a low threshold for admission and observation.
- In patients > 40 years old, consider colonic pathology, e.g. carcinoma, diverticulitis.

Box 10.4 Meckel's diverticulitis

Meckel's diverticulum is a remnant of the embryological vitello-intestinal duct. The rule of 2s states that they:
- occur in 2% of the population;
- are usually 2 inches long;
- are located on the anti-mesenteric border of the ileum approximately 2 feet from the caecum.

They can have 3 types of heterotopic mucosa within them (gastric, pancreatic, and colonic), and are 3–5 times more common in males. Most never cause a problem but occasionally they may present acutely with inflammation. The diagnosis usually only becomes apparent during surgery undertaken for suspected acute appendicitis. If a Meckel's diverticulum is found to be the cause of an acute abdomen then surgical treatment comprises local resection of the diverticulum or of the segment of bowel containing it. A normal Meckel's discovered incidentally should be left alone. Other possible symptoms from a Meckel's diverticulum include:
- bleeding;
- perforation;
- chronic peptic ulceration;
- intussusception;
- small bowel volvulus (if the Meckel's is still attached to the umbilicus);
- umbilico-ileal fistula.

Initial management

Where appendicitis is being queried, and there are no other features of significant disease, patients can be broadly classified into four groups.
- Appendicitis is very unlikely: discuss discharge with the patient. If discharge agreed, tell them to return if symptoms worsen or if they have other concerns.

- Appendicitis possible, but unlikely.
  - Admit for observation, review in 6h.
  - Keep NBM, start IV fluids, analgesia, anti-emetics, and thromboprophylaxis (📖 p.26).
  - ❶ Do **not** give antibiotics, as this will confuse further assessment.
- Appendicitis probable.
  - Admit, keep NBM, start IV fluids, analgesia, anti-emetics, and thromboprophylaxis (📖 p.26).
  - Book and consent for theatre, either open appendicectomy or diagnostic laparoscopy ± appendicectomy (Box 10.5).
  - If imminent perforation is a concern or if theatre is likely to be delayed, consider IV antibiotics (e.g. cefuroxime 750mg tds + metronidazole 500mg tds) after discussion with your senior.
- Appendicitis probable, features of severe sepsis (📖 p.482).
  - Admit, keep NBM, start analgesia, anti-emetics, and thromboprophylaxis (📖 p.26).
  - Check for metabolic acidosis on ABG and serum lactate.
  - Insert a urinary catheter, and aggressively IV fluid resuscitate.
  - Give O_2 as required to keep $SaO_2 > 95\%$.
  - Start IV antibiotics (see previous bullet point for 'Appendicitis probable') after taking blood cultures.
  - Book and consent for emergency theatre.
  - Discuss with ITU/anaesthetic team.

Further investigations

Patients admitted for observation or diagnostic uncertainty often require further investigations.

- In females of child-bearing age with ongoing RIF pain that does not reach the threshold for surgery, consider transvaginal pelvic USS to exclude gynaecological pathologies, e.g. ruptured or torted ovarian cyst, ectopic pregnancy, tubo-ovarian abscess.
- USS of the appendix: accuracy is highly dependent on the expertise of the ultrasonographer.
- USS RUQ: may be useful to differentiate between biliary pathology and retrocaecal appendicitis.
- CT abdomen and pelvis: use selectively because of the relatively high dose of ionizing radiation exposure it involves. CT should generally be reserved for cases of particular diagnostic doubt. It is especially helpful in elderly patients with an atypical presentation where there is a higher chance of alternative pathology, and in whom the lifetime risk from radiation exposure is less.

Box 10.5 Appendicectomy

The choice between open and laparoscopic appendicectomy depends on the skills of the surgeon, the availability of laparoscopic equipment, and patient preference. Laparoscopy is particularly useful in females of child-bearing age due to far superior visualization of the gynaecological organs.

At open or laparoscopic surgery, if the appendix is not inflamed a careful search should be made for other causes of RIF pain, including a Meckel's diverticulitis, Crohn's ileitis, and gynaecological causes of abdominal pain in the female.

❶ If during appendicectomy the appendix is found to be normal but there is acute inflammation in the terminal ileum consistent with Crohn's disease, appendicectomy should be performed as this will avoid any future diagnostic confusion. There is little risk that it will lead to development of an enterocutaneous fistula.

Open appendicectomy
- Usually performed through a Lanz, muscle-splitting incision. Even if the appendix is not inflamed it should always be removed; otherwise subsequent appendicitis might be wrongly diagnosed in the presence of a RIF scar.
- Consider midline laparotomy in the elderly because of the likelihood of other causes for abdominal pain.

Diagnostic laparoscopy ± appendicectomy
- Might best be avoided if clinical suspicion of perforated appendicitis exists, so as not to risk further dissemination of intraabdominal infection.
- If the appendix looks normal and there are no other causes for RIF pain found, some surgeons would advocate appendicectomy anyway.
- Where appendicitis is seen, and the appendix is removed laparoscopically, the incidence of wound infection and postoperative pain and hospital stay may be reduced. Laparoscopic appendicectomy may increase the incidence of intraabdominal abscess formation.
- Difficulty in removing the appendix laparoscopically mandates conversion to open appendicectomy.

Further management
Repeated clinical assessment every 6–12h is essential.
- If symptoms and signs resolve, and normal diet is tolerated, the patient can be discharged.
- Where alternative pathologies have been excluded, and symptoms and signs have not improved significantly with observation over 24–48h, open appendicectomy or diagnostic laparoscopy should be considered.

☼ Mechanical bowel obstruction

Intestinal obstruction is a common surgical emergency accounting for up to 20% of emergency general surgical admissions. Obstruction is usually due to mechanical causes but functional intestinal obstruction (ileus (📖 p.295) or pseudo-obstruction of the colon (📖 p.276)) may occur as a result of disordered neural activity in the bowel. Mechanical obstruction of the small bowel is 3 x more common than that of the large bowel.

A combination of history and examination aided by plain abdominal X-rays is usually sufficient to:
- confirm the diagnosis of mechanical rather than functional bowel obstruction;
- determine whether it is small or large bowel obstruction;
- indicate the likely cause;
- reveal whether or not strangulation is present.

❶ These distinctions are essential since they influence management and the need for urgent surgery.

Classification
Mechanical intestinal obstruction can be classified according to:
- cause: luminal, intramural, or extrinsic;
- location: small or large bowel, proximal or distal;
- extent: partial or complete;
- time course: acute, subacute, or chronic;
- nature: open-ended or closed loop (occluded proximally and distally);
- simple or complicated (i.e. accompanied by ischaemia or perforation).

Causes
There is a wide variety of potential causes and these are often classified according to whether the obstruction is:
- extrinsic, e.g. adhesions, hernia (abdominal wall or internal), volvulus, malignant or inflammatory masses;
- intramural, e.g. intussusception, inflammatory stricture (diverticular and Crohn's disease), malignant stricture, polypoid tumour, benign tumour, ischaemic stricture (radiotherapy, ischaemic colitis), congenital atresia;
- luminal e.g. gallstone, foreign bodies, meconium, parasites, bezoars.

In adults, the most common causes of mechanical small bowel obstruction are adhesions (60%), strangulated hernias (20%), and malignancy (10%). Adhesions may result from previous abdominal surgery or from previous intraperitoneal inflammation.

The most common causes of large bowel obstruction are colorectal carcinoma (70%), diverticular disease (10%), and sigmoid volvulus (5%). Caecal malignancies may cause a clinical picture of small rather than large bowel obstruction.

Pathophysiology
Intestinal obstruction leads to a combination of bacterial overgrowth, increased luminal pressure, disordered motility, and intestinal distension. These disrupt the normal flux of fluid and electrolytes across the bowel wall proximal to the obstruction and large volumes of fluid accumulate

within the proximal bowel. The extensive loss of extracellular fluid into the bowel lumen, combined with loss of fluid and electrolytes from vomiting, causes severe hypovolaemia and electrolyte disturbances.

Increased intraluminal pressure reduces perfusion of the bowel wall and this may lead to ischaemia and eventually intestinal perforation. This is particularly likely in a closed loop obstruction. The caecum is at particular risk of perforation in distal large bowel obstruction because of its greater diameter: Laplace's law states that the intraluminal pressure needed to cause distension is inversely proportional to its diameter.

History

The cardinal features of mechanical intestinal obstruction are:

- colicky central abdominal pain, the exact location of which depends on whether the midgut or hindgut is involved (📖 p.98);
- abdominal distension;
- vomiting;
- often constipation of faeces alone.

Mechanical small bowel obstruction

- Abdominal pain is typically colicky and occurs early.
- Vomiting occurs early especially in high obstruction.
- Vomitus is bilious in high obstruction.
- Vomitus may be become 'faeculent' due to bacterial overgrowth.
- Abdominal distension may be mild if the obstruction is very proximal.
- Constipation occurs late and may be absent.
- There may be a history of previous abdominal surgery, adhesive obstruction, pelvic radiotherapy, or of a painful swelling consistent with a strangulated hernia.

Mechanical large bowel obstruction

- Pain may not be colicky in nature.
- Abdominal distension occurs early and is often marked.
- Constipation occurs earlier.
- Vomiting appears late.
- Partial obstruction may allow passage of liquid stool (spurious diarrhoea).
- There may be a history of altered bowel habit, weight loss, or rectal bleeding consistent with colorectal cancer, or a history of previous sigmoid volvulus. Recurrent LIF pain suggests diverticular disease.

Examination

- Dehydration is often severe.
- Pyrexia is not usually present in uncomplicated obstruction.
- Abdominal distension.
- A palpable mass may be due to colonic carcinoma, severe diverticular disease, or a strangulated internal hernia containing small bowel.
- ❶ Features of strangulation may be present (Box 10.6). A strangulated hernia may be palpable, and abdominal wall hernial orifices must be checked thoroughly (📖 p.175).
- ❶ In possible large bowel obstruction, check specifically for caecal tenderness indicating imminent caecal perforation.
- Check for hepatomegaly, RUQ mass, or jaundice, suggesting metastatic colorectal carcinoma.

- Increased resonance to abdominal percussion.
- Auscultation reveals the presence of bowel sounds that in small bowel obstruction are classically high-pitched ('tinkling') and occur coincidentally with peaks in abdominal pain.
- DRE may be normal or reveal blood and mucus suggesting colorectal cancer.

Box 10.6 Clinical features of bowel strangulation

- Continuous rather than colicky abdominal pain, worse with movement.
- Severe abdominal pain.
- Pyrexia.
- Tachycardia.
- Abdominal tenderness with guarding.
- Palpable abdominal mass.

❶ Some of these features may be present in the absence of strangulation and strangulation can occur in the absence any of these signs in 10% of patients.

Initial investigations

- FBC: Hb may be ↑ due to haemoconcentration, while ↓ Hb may indicate colorectal carcinoma, especially of the caecum and ascending colon. ↑↑ WCC suggests strangulation.
- U&Es: ↓ K^+ is due to loss of K^+-rich vomitus. Urea and creatinine are ↑ due to dehydration.
- LFTs: ↑ ALP if hepatic colorectal metastases.
- G&S: for all patients.
- ABG: check for metabolic acidosis if severe dehydration is present or strangulation is suspected.
- Supine AXR.
  - Small bowel can be identified by the presence of valvulae coniventes, which extend across the entire diameter of the bowel, and the central position within the abdomen (Fig. 10.1). Small bowel should be < 3.5cm diameter. Obstructed, fluid-filled small bowel may not be visible on AXR.
  - Large bowel usually lies peripherally and has haustra that do not cross the entire bowel (Fig. 10.2). The transverse colon should be < 10cm diameter. A caecal diameter > 12cm identifies impending perforation.
  - If perforation has occurred, free gas may be visible.
  - Distension of both the large and small bowel implies either mechanical large bowel obstruction with an incompetent ileocaecal valve or non-mechanical bowel obstruction (ileus). Gas in the rectum is consistent with ileus.
  - Look specifically for signs of sigmoid or caecal volvulus (Box 10.7).
  - Gas in the biliary tree or a large calcification in the pelvis consistent with a gallstone suggests gallstone ileus (📖 p.239).
- Erect CXR: to identify free gas under the diaphragm. Metastatic colorectal carcinoma may be present.

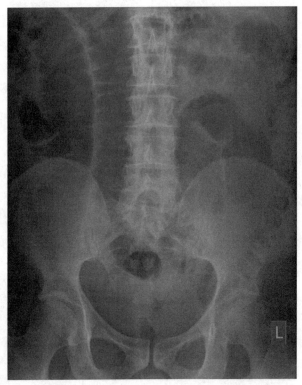

Fig. 10.1 Supine AXR of small bowel obstruction due to a band adhesion. Valvulae conniventes are clearly seen.

Initial management
- Keep NBM.
- 'Drip and suck'.
  - Begin aggressive IV fluid resuscitation. Severe dehydration is often present and commonly undertreated: > 5L of crystalloid in the first 24h may be needed. Those with significant cardiorespiratory co-morbidities may require a central venous line.
  - Insert a urinary catheter and keep urine output > 0.5mL/kg/h.
  - Insert an NG tube, aspirate, and place on free drainage.
- Start thromboprophylaxis (📖 p.26), as long as this will not interfere with any planned epidural anaesthesia.

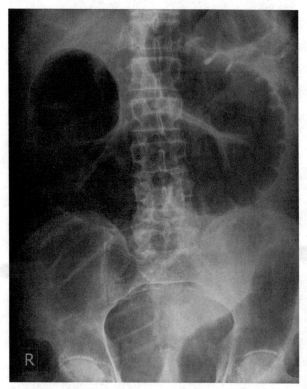

Fig. 10.2 Supine AXR showing an obstructing rectosigmoid carcinoma. The ileocaecal valve is competent, so only large bowel distension is seen.

- If strangulation or perforation are suspected, emergency surgery is indicated following resuscitation. Start broad spectrum IV antibiotics (e.g. cefuroxime 750mg tds + metronidazole 500mg tds).
- If strangulation or perforation are not suspected, continue 'drip and suck', observe, and investigate as appropriate.

Box 10.7 Colonic volvulus

A volvulus is a rotation of the intestine on its mesenteric axis causing bowel obstruction and compromising the blood supply (especially the venous drainage) of the involved segment of bowel. Eventually this may lead to venous infarction and perforation. Most cases of colonic volvulus involve the sigmoid colon although caecal volvulus may also occur

Sigmoid volvulus is common in Africa and Asia where diets are very high in fibre. In the West it occurs most often in the elderly and the institutionalized.
- Clinical features: are those of large bowel obstruction. Pain and vomiting usually occur late. There is minimal abdominal tenderness initially, but persistence of volvulus with venous gangrene leads to signs of peritonitis.
- Investigations: as for intestinal obstruction. Supine AXR is usually diagnostic and shows a grossly dilated loop of sigmoid arising from the LIF. Where AXR features are not clear and in the absence of signs of strangulation, water-soluble contrast enema or CT abdomen and pelvis are diagnostic.
- Non-operative management. Dehydration should be corrected. Uncomplicated sigmoid volvulus in the absence of suspected colonic ischaemia is treated by rigid sigmoidoscopy and gentle insertion of a flatus tube (📖 p.514) beyond the neck of the obstruction. Successful decompression results in the dramatic passage of flatus and faeces. The flatus tube is left in situ for 24–48h. Decompression can also be achieved colonoscopically. Recurrence is likely, so elective surgery should be considered.
- Operative management. Clinical suspicion of ischaemia/strangulation or failure of non-operative decompression requires emergency laparotomy and sigmoid colectomy ± end colostomy.

Caecal volvulus occurs when there has been abnormal rotation of the midgut and a lack of caecal fixation posteriorly.
- Clinical features are of distal small bowel obstruction.
- Supine AXR may show a grossly distended loop of large bowel originating from the RIF, although abnormal caecal fixation means that this sign is highly variable. As above, when AXR features are not clear, and in the absence of signs of strangulation, water-soluble contrast enema or CT abdomen and pelvis are diagnostic.
- Caecal volvulus is best treated by right hemicolectomy.

Further investigations
- CT abdomen and pelvis: confirms dilated bowel, may identify the site of obstruction (Fig. 10.3), and can reveal metastatic cancer.
- Water-soluble contrast studies (e.g. gastrograffin).
  - Some surgeons favour a water-soluble contrast enema over CT in order to more accurately define the site, completeness, and likely cause of a large bowel obstruction.
  - Contrast given via an NG tube may help to distinguish mechanical small bowel obstruction from ileus. The appearance of contrast in the large bowel within 24h on AXR identifies those patients with adhesive small bowel obstruction who may not require surgery.

Further management

Small bowel obstruction

- Non-strangulated small bowel obstruction thought to be due to adhesions is treated non-operatively initially and resolves spontaneously in ~ 50% of cases.
- Resolution of obstruction is indicated by decreasing NG tube output, the passage of flatus, and improving appearance on serial supine AXRs.
- If after 24–48h there is no improvement on non-operative therapy, surgical intervention is indicated. Surgery may vary from simple division of a single band adhesion to time-consuming and extensive division of multiple adhesions.
- Malignancy causing small bowel obstruction normally requires surgical intervention but non-operative treatment may be preferred if widespread intraabdominal malignancy is present.
- A palpable mass is usually an indication for early surgery.

Large bowel obstruction

- Mechanical large bowel obstruction rarely resolves without surgery. An exception is sigmoid volvulus (Box 10.7).
- A complete colonic obstruction with a competent ileocaecal valve is a closed loop obstruction and requires urgent surgery to avoid caecal perforation.
- Large bowel obstruction due to colorectal cancer is best treated with colonic resection but, in those with metastatic disease or significant co-morbidities, a defunctioning stoma may be more appropriate. In selected patients with advanced or metastatic colorectal cancer, palliation of an obstructing colon cancer may be achieved by endoscopic insertion of an expandable stent.
- ❶ In the absence of metastatic disease, it can be very difficult to distinguish between malignant and diverticular large bowel obstruction on CT appearances and at surgery.

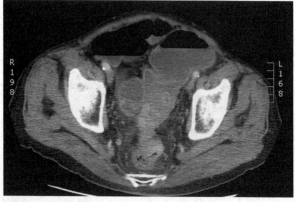

Fig. 10.3 CT abdomen and pelvis showing a rectosigmoid carcinoma with proximal large bowel distension.

ⓘ **Non-mechanical large bowel obstruction**

Failure of propulsive peristalsis of any part of the GI tract leads to a non-mechanical obstruction. This is most commonly seen after GI surgery, where it is known as an ileus and is part of the postoperative recovery period (📖 p.295). Non-mechanical obstruction can occur in the absence of abdominal surgery, particularly in the large bowel, and occasionally in the stomach (📖 p.205).

Reversible non-mechanical large bowel obstruction is also known as colonic pseudo-obstruction or Ogilvie's syndrome. It occurs almost exclusively in hospitalized patients and there is nearly always an identifiable precipitating cause. If not adequately treated it may lead to caecal ischaemia and perforation.

Colonic pseudo-obstruction is thought to be due to an imbalance in the autonomic control of the colon. The nature of the dysregulation is not completely clear but reduced sacral parasympathetic stimulation may result in an adynamic distal segment of colon leading to a functional obstruction and dilatation of the proximal colon.

Causes

These are numerous, and multiple causes may contribute.
- Metabolic and endocrine, e.g. ↓ K^+, ↓ Na^+, uraemia, DKA, ↓/↑ Ca^{2+}, ↓ Mg^{2+}, hypothyroidism.
- Recent surgery.
- Cardiac, e.g. MI, CCF.
- Drugs, e.g. opioids, anticholinergics, calcium channel antagonists, phenothiazines.
- Trauma, especially to the pelvis or retroperitoneum.
- Systemic infection.
- Miscellaneous, e.g. stroke, burns.

History

Suspect in any hospitalized patient who develops symptoms of large bowel obstruction. The clinical picture is broadly similar to that of mechanical large bowel obstruction:
- history of constipation, abdominal pain (tends to be less severe than in mechanical large bowel obstruction), distension, and vomiting.

Examination

- Abdominal distension.
- Marked resonance to percussion.
- Tenderness is often minimal, and bowel sounds may or may not be present.
- DRE usually reveals a grossly distended, empty rectum.
- ❶ Check for caecal tenderness indicating imminent caecal perforation.

Initial investigations

- Investigate as for mechanical large bowel obstruction. AXR shows dilated colon with no distal cut-off of gas. Serial AXR can be used for monitoring.

- • ❶ Caecal diameter of > 12cm on AXR implies imminent perforation.
- In addition, check serum Ca^{2+}, Mg^{2+}, glucose, and thyroid function.

Initial management

Non-operative management is the rule, as pseudo-obstruction usually resolves with supportive measures.

- 'Drip and suck' and keep NBM, as for mechanical bowel obstruction (see 'Mechanical bowel obstruction', 'Initial management').
- Correct the underlying cause, where possible, including correction of any metabolic and endocrine abnormalities.
- Stop all non-essential opioid and anticholinergic medications.

Further investigations

- Water-soluble contrast enema is diagnostic, excluding mechanical large bowel obstruction, and can be therapeutic, stimulating bowel motility.
- CT abdomen and pelvis can exclude mechanical obstruction.

Further management

In patients with significant distension and discomfort where mechanical obstruction has been excluded, consider the following.

- Decompression via colonoscopy. Successful deflation occurs in 80% of cases, though 40% have recurrence. Many patients with non-mechanical large bowel obstruction are not fit enough to undergo this procedure.
- Neostigmine (1–2mg IV) has been shown to be effective at stimulating gut motility. Relative contraindications include recent MI, asthma, bradycardia, peptic ulcer disease, and β-blockers.
- Insertion of a flatus tube (📖 p.514) may help, but they often become blocked.
- ❶ Neostigmine should only be given under cardiac monitoring in an HDU/ITU setting after review by senior clinicians. Treat bradycardia with atropine 0.6–1.2mg IV.

If impending perforation remains a risk despite non-operative treatment (i.e. caecal diameter remains > 12cm) surgical decompression is indicated, but has a high mortality.

① Colonic diverticulitis

Acquired colonic diverticulae are mucosal out-pouchings of the large bowel wall. They occur predominantly in the sigmoid colon as a result of a low-fibre diet. The presence of colonic diverticulae is widespread in the West, where its incidence increases dramatically with age. Up to half the elderly population may have the condition, although the majority are asymptomatic (diverticulosis). When symptoms occur, this is known as diverticular disease. Emergency presentations of diverticular disease include:

- colonic perforation and generalized peritonitis (📖 p.108);
- lower GI bleeding (📖 p.280);
- large bowel obstruction due to diverticular strictures, inflammation, or pressure from local abscesses (📖 p.268).

The most common acute presentation of diverticular disease is diverticulitis. It should be considered as a diagnosis in patients > 40 years old with lower abdominal pain, especially if it is predominantly left-sided.

The severity of the condition varies considerably, from mild symptoms associated with limited inflammation of the pericolic tissues and parietal peritoneum to severe disease with associated pericolic abscesses and sepsis resulting from localized perforation.

History
- Progressive lower abdominal and LIF pain, worse with movement.
- Anorexia.
- Rigors may occur if a pericolic abscess is present.
- Vomiting may occasionally be present due to an associated ileus.
- A history of previous episodes of LIF pain, altered bowel habit, or rectal bleeding may be present.
- ❶ Ask specifically for symptoms of recurrent UTI, pneumaturia, or vaginal discharge suggestive of colovesical or, in the latter, colovaginal fistulae.

Examination
- Pyrexia.
- Tachycardia.
- LIF and suprapubic tenderness, often with guarding.
- A vague LIF mass may be palpable, due to either a thickened sigmoid colon or a pericolic abscess.
- Abdominal distension may be present as a result of colonic obstruction or an ileus in response to a pericolic abscess.

Initial investigations
- FBC: ↑ WCC is common.
- U&Es: may show mild to moderate dehydration.
- Take blood cultures if pyrexial.
- Urine dipstick: to exclude UTI and pyelonephritis. Debris in the urine may suggest a colovesical fistula.
- Erect CXR: mandatory to exclude free intraabdominal gas due to perforation.
- Supine AXR: usually unremarkable, but may show colonic or small bowel dilatation.

Initial management

This is essentially non-operative and comprises antibiotics and management of fluid balance with careful monitoring of clinical progress. Most patients (> 80%), including those with marked peritoneal signs, show a good clinical response with resolution of symptoms over 24–48h.

- Depending on severity, keep NBM or limit to clear fluids.
- IV broad-spectrum antibiotics, e.g. cefuroxime 750mg tds + metronidazole 500mg tds.
- Give IV fluid resuscitation.
- Insert a urinary catheter (depending on severity).
- Start thromboprophylaxis (📖 p.26).
- Parenteral opioid analgesia.

Further investigations

- Patients with known diverticular disease whose symptoms settle rapidly with non-operative management do not require further inpatient imaging.
- When the diagnosis is uncertain, or clinical features fail to settle within 48–72h, CT abdomen and pelvis (Fig. 10.4) is indicated to confirm the diagnosis and identify pericolic abscesses.

Further management

- Large (> 3–5cm) pericolic abscesses identified on CT may be treated by radiologically-guided percutaneous drainage.
- Severe cases that fail to settle with non-operative management may require emergency surgery to drain intraabdominal collections and carry out sigmoid colectomy. Hartmann's procedure (sigmoid colectomy with LIF end colostomy) is often performed in preference to resection and primary anastomosis.

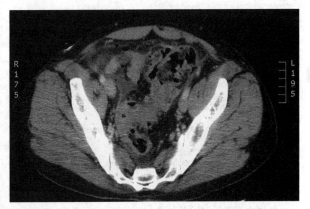

Fig. 10.4 CT abdomen showing multiple rectosigmoid diverticulae with fat stranding, indicating diverticulitis.

:✪: **Acute lower GI bleeding**

Acute lower GI haemorrhage is a common emergency surgical presentation. Acute upper GI bleeding is discussed in Chapter 7 (📖 p.190). The colour of the blood can sometimes give a vague indication to the site of bleeding, as bleeding from the left colon and rectum is usually bright red, while more proximal bleeding usually results in the passage of dark red blood. This is highly dependent on the rate of blood loss, however. Heavy upper GI bleeding may present with bright red or dark red PR bleeding.

In the elderly patient, significant acute lower GI bleeding is most often due to diverticular disease. The management of PR bleeding in children is covered in Chapter 14 (📖 p.368). Other causes of lower GI bleeding include:

- haemorrhoids;
- colonic polyps;
- colorectal carcinoma;
- ischaemic colitis (📖 p.285);
- inflammatory bowel disease (IBD; 📖 p.288);
- infective colitis;
- radiation proctitis;
- diversion proctitis;
- aorto-enteric fistula after a previous AAA repair.

History

- Usually sudden onset, painless PR bleeding.
- Bleeding with abdominal pain and diarrhoea suggests ischaemic colitis, infective colitis, or IBD.
- Recent change of bowel habit, weight loss, or tenesmus suggests colorectal cancer.
- There may be a history of collapse, or symptoms of anaemia.
- Ask specifically for a history of IBD, pelvic radiotherapy, previous AAA repair, anticoagulants, bleeding diatheses, and stomas.
- ❶ Check for a history of PUD; NSAID, oral steroid, or alcohol use; and epigastric pain that may indicate a possible upper GI bleed.

Examination

- Often pale and clammy, occasionally confused or obtunded.
- Tachycardic, hypotensive.
  - ❶ The physiological response to blood loss may be altered by cardiac medications.
- Look for stigmata of chronic liver disease that may indicate a variceal upper GI bleed.
- Look for scars and stomas suggesting an aorto-enteric fistula or diversion proctitis, respectively.
- Significant abdominal tenderness is rare.
- Colonic angiodysplasia is associated with aortic stenosis.
- Perform a DRE to identify low rectal cancers and confirm the colour of the blood.
  - ❶ Proctoscopy should be performed to exclude haemorrhoids as the source of the blood loss. Rigid sigmoidoscopy in the acutely

bleeding patient is difficult to perform and rarely adds any useful information.

Initial investigations

❶ Shocked patients require emergency resuscitation. This should not be delayed while awaiting the results of investigations.

- FBC: ↓ Hb is frequent, and may be severe.
- U&Es: usually ↔, but ↑ urea may indicate an upper GI or small bowel bleed.
- LFTs: usually ↔, but check for evidence of chronic liver disease.
- PT, APTT: in all patients with lower GI bleeding.
- G&S: In all patients with lower GI bleeding. Cross-match 2–4 units of packed RBCs if Hb is ↓ or bleeding is severe.
- ECG and CXR: request in the elderly and in those with cardiorespiratory co-morbidities, as baseline investigations.
- Supine AXR: if diarrhoea or abdominal pain are present, look for the mucosal 'thumbprinting' of ischaemic colitis.

Initial management

❶ Consider the diagnosis of aorto-enteric fistula in any patient who has had previous AAA repair or untreated AAA with a significant lower GI bleed. Discuss with your senior **immediately**.

The early goals of management are to resuscitate and monitor the patient and correct abnormal clotting.

- Keep NBM.
- Fluid resuscitation.
  - Insert at least 2 large-bore peripheral IV cannulae.
  - Start aggressive IV fluid resuscitation with either crystalloids or colloids, appropriate to the degree of shock.
  - If shock is present, or Hb < 10g/dL with ongoing bleeding, packed RBCs will be needed. Give high-flow O_2 via a non-rebreathing mask.
- Correction of abnormal clotting.
  - Stop warfarin and anti-platelet agents. **Do not** give LMWH.
  - If INR > 1.5 give 10–15mL/kg FFP and consider vitamin K 1mg IV. Patients with severe bleeding with abnormal PT or APTT should be discussed with the on-call haematologist.
- Monitoring.
  - Insert a urinary catheter, and aim for hourly urine output of > 0.5mL/kg/h.
  - Twice-daily FBC, at least initially.
  - Ask the nurses to start a stool chart.
  - In those with significant cardiorespiratory co-morbidities and heavy bleeding, consider inserting a central venous line to guide resuscitation and HDU admission for monitoring.

Further management

Bleeding stops spontaneously in the majority of patients. Once the Hb is normal and stable, and the bowels have opened with no sign of blood, the patient can be discharged. Arrange urgent outpatient colonoscopy.

- Profusely bleeding haemorrhoids can be treated according to local preference, e.g. banding.

Invasive inpatient investigations are reserved for those with ongoing heavy bleeding requiring repeat transfusions.

- Consider upper GI endoscopy to exclude an upper GI source if profuse bleeding is present.
- Colonoscopy is often unable to identify the site of bleeding, as vision is obscured. Intubation of the terminal ileum can be useful to exclude the small bowel as the source of blood loss. When sites of bleeding can be identified:
  - angiodysplasia can be diathermied;
  - bleeding diverticulae can be injected with adrenaline;
  - polyps can be removed.
- If colonoscopy fails to identify the bleeding site and blood loss is ongoing, consider either a nuclear medicine labelled RBC scan, or selective mesenteric angiogram, depending on local availability and expertise.
- Once the bleeding site is identified, emergency surgery and bowel resection are required for ongoing bleeding.

❶ The management of patients with heavy GI bleeding requires close co-operation between senior surgeons, gastroenterologists, intensivists, and radiologists.

:**⚙**: Ischaemic bowel

Ischaemic bowel may occur when arteries or veins are blocked by thrombi or emboli. Secondary causes include external compression of the bowel or its mesentery, impairing capillary flow or venous return.

Small bowel ischaemia

Small bowel ischaemia is a very serious condition that is usually recognized late and carries a high mortality. Occlusion of the SMA by a thrombus or an embolus occurs most commonly in the elderly and those with severe cardiovascular disease. Emboli usually arise from the left atrium (AF) or LV (mural thrombus or LV aneurysm). SMA or SMV thrombosis occurs in those with reduced cardiac output or hypercoagulable states. Aortic dissection (📖 p.468) can cause small bowel ischaemia, and it may occur as a complication of angiography due to the catheter or guidewire dislodging debris.

Clinical features
- Severe central abdominal pain, poorly responsive to parenteral opioids.
- Vomiting; may contain altered blood.
- There may be a history of AF or recent MI.
- On examination, the patient may be shocked, tachycardia and hypotension are common, and AF may be present.
- Abdominal tenderness may be mild initially, but signs of peritonitis are present later.
- Bowel sounds are usually absent.

❶ The reported severity of the pain may be disproportionate to the initial abdominal findings.

Investigations
- FBC: usually ↑↑ WCC (> 20 x 10⁹/L).
- U&Es: usually reflect dehydration.
- Serum amylase (📖 p.246): mild–moderately raised, usually < 5 x the upper limit of normal.
- ABG and serum lactate: metabolic acidosis is usually present late in the disease process.
  - **❶** Normal ABG and serum lactate do **not** exclude ischaemic bowel.
- ECG: may show cardiac dysrhythmias or signs of LV aneurysm.
- Supine AXR: can be normal, but usually shows a few mildly dilated small bowel loops.
- Erect CXR: usually normal, but may show a thoracic aortic aneurysm or LV aneurysm.
- Emergency CT abdomen and pelvis: may show thickened, poorly enhancing small bowel loops, but can be normal.
- Emergency mesenteric angiography: can confirm the diagnosis and indicate the nature of the occlusion.

❶ When signs of peritonitis are present, surgery should not be delayed for unnecessary investigations.

Management
Management is dependent on the overall clinical picture.
- Patients with severe multiple co-morbidities with advanced signs of peritonitis are unlikely to survive surgery, and palliative care should be considered.

- ❶ This decision should only be made after discussion with a senior surgeon.

Otherwise, if small bowel ischaemia is suspected, emergency surgery is indicated. In addition, do the following.
- Give high-flow O_2 via a non-rebreathing mask.
- Insert an NG tube.
- Start thromboprophylaxis (📖 p.26).
- Begin broad-spectrum IV antibiotics (e.g. cefuroxime 750mg tds + metronidazole 500mg tds).
- At laparotomy, the cause and extent of the small bowel ischaemia should be assessed.
  - Non-viable small bowel should be resected.
  - When the bowel appears to be viable, mesenteric embolectomy or aorto-mesenteric bypass may be possible.
  - Second look laparotomy after 24–48h may be necessary to detect further bowel ischaemia.
  - Elderly patients with gangrene of most or all of the small bowel are unlikely to survive extensive resection, and continuation of surgery may not be appropriate.
  - An aggressive approach should be taken in younger patients, with resection of all the ischaemic bowel and early discussion with a specialist intestinal failure unit. These patients can survive with home TPN and may be candidates for intestinal transplantation.
- Consider postoperative anticoagulation.

Large bowel ischaemia

This typically occurs in patients > 50 years old with atherosclerosis. It results from impaired blood supply to the colon causing mucosal ischaemia and inflammation. This may arise from large vessel disease (thrombus or embolus), small vessel disease (e.g. radiation damage or diabetes), or a low flow state (e.g. cardiogenic shock). The splenic flexure is particularly vulnerable because it is a watershed area between the SMA and IMA. The resulting mucosal inflammation may resolve without complication. In a minority of cases it may progress to gangrene of the colonic wall, colonic perforation, or necrotizing colitis. In the longer term, ischaemic colitis may heal with fibrosis and form a chronic colonic stricture.

Clinical features
- Acute abdominal pain, often left-sided.
- Diarrhoea with dark blood and clots.
- Symptoms of cardiovascular disease may be present.
- On examination, mild pyrexia and tachycardia are present with mild left-sided abdominal tenderness.
- DRE may confirm blood-stained diarrhoea.
- Signs of atherosclerosis may be present, e.g. decreased peripheral pulses.

Investigations
- FBC: usually ↑↑ WCC.
- U&Es: may be ↔ or reflect dehydration.
- Serum amylase: usually ↔.

- ABG and serum lactate: mild metabolic acidosis may be present.
- ECG: may show cardiac dysrhythmias or signs of old ischaemic events.
- Supine AXR: often normal, but may show thickened large bowel with 'thumbprinting' due to mucosal oedema and ulceration.
- Erect CXR: mandatory to exclude perforation.
- CT abdomen and pelvis: shows thickened large bowel.
- In patients without peritonism, lower GI endoscopy can be used to confirm diagnosis and exclude IBD and colonic carcinoma.

Management

Most cases settle with non-operative treatment.

- Keep NBM initially.
- Resuscitate with IV fluids and insert a urinary catheter. Aim for urine output > 0.5mL/kg/h.
- Start thromboprophylaxis (📖 p.26).
- Parenteral opioid analgesia.
- Give broad spectrum IV antibiotics, e.g. cefuroxime 750mg tds + metronidazole 500mg tds.

❶ If colonic gangrene or perforation are suspected either clinically or on CT, laparotomy with colonic resection is required.

① **Inflammatory bowel disease**

Ulcerative colitis and Crohn's disease may present as an emergency with a similar clinical picture of abdominal pain and bloody diarrhoea.

Crohn's disease

This is a chronic inflammatory disorder of the GI tract. It is most common between the ages of 15 and 45 but may present at any age. The cause is unknown.

In ~ 50% of cases the disease is confined to the small bowel, usually the terminal ileum (ileocaecal disease or 'terminal ileitis'). It may affect both the small and large bowel or the colon alone (Crohn's colitis). Perianal disease is common. Intestinal inflammation is full thickness (transmural) and typically involves discrete segments of bowel with intervening segments of uninvolved intestine (skip lesions). Non-caseating granulomas may be present. Chronic inflammation leads to fibrosis and stricturing. There is associated thickening of the mesentery and enlargement of the mesenteric lymph nodes.

Acute presentations are variable, but include:

- Acute exacerbation of chronic Crohn's is the most common acute presentation. The clinical features, investigations, and management are outlined in the following sections.
- Acute inflammation of the ileum (terminal ileitis). This may be the first presentation of Crohn's and mimics acute appendicitis (📖 p.262) although the history is often more protracted and may include diarrhoea and weight loss.
- Intestinal perforation: often localized and contained.
- Intestinal obstruction: due to acute inflammation or chronic strictures.
- Fistula formation, e.g. ano-rectal, enterocutaneous, enteroenteric, enterovesical.

Clinical features

An acute exacerbation of Crohn's presents with the following.

- Abdominal pain, often in the RIF, vomiting, and diarrhoea (bloody if colonic involvement).
- Anorexia with general malaise and weight loss is common.
- On examination, a mild pyrexia and tachycardia are found, and the patient is usually pale.
- Dehydration is present, especially if diarrhoea or vomiting have occurred.
- Abdominal tenderness is often worse in RIF, and a RIF mass may be palpable.

Investigations

- FBC: may reveal ↓ Hb and ↑ WCC.
- U&Es: may show ↑ urea from dehydration.
- LFTs: may show ↓ serum albumin.
- Stool culture: to exclude infective colitis.
- ESR and CRP: usually ↑↑.
- Supine AXR: loops of mildly dilated small bowel are common.
- Erect CXR: perforation with free gas is rare.

- CT abdomen and pelvis: thickened loops of SI are common. Free gas and intraabdominal collections can be detected.
- Small bowel enemas and radiolabelled white cell scans help confirm the diagnosis and assess the extent of disease.

Management
If the diagnosis is clear, treatment is predominantly non-operative.
- Resuscitate with IV fluids, and correct electrolyte abnormalities.
- Insert a urinary catheter if the disease is severe.
- Give packed RBCs if Hb < 8g/dL is present.
- Start thromboprophylaxis if bleeding is not marked (🕮 p.26).
- Start high-dose aminosalicylates and steroids (either IV hydrocortisone or oral prednisolone).
- Azathioprine is sometimes used.
- ❶ Patients with acute exacerbations of Crohn's are best managed by gastroenterologists working closely with colorectal surgeons.
- Surgery is reserved for complications such as intestinal perforation, obstruction, and fulminant colitis.

❶ Acute inflammation of the ileum discovered at laparotomy should be left alone unless there is associated perforation or obstruction, in which case resection of the affected segment should be undertaken.

Ulcerative colitis (UC)
This most commonly affects young adults. It has a relapsing/remitting clinical course. UC is an inflammatory disease of the mucosa and submucosa of the large bowel characterized by the formation of crypt abscesses, superficial ulceration, and pseudopolyps. Eventually, dysplastic changes occur that may progress to carcinoma after several years. UC always involves the rectum and may extend proximally in continuity towards the caecum for a variable distance. So-called 'backwash ileitis' may also be present.

The acute presentations of UC and Crohn's colitis are often indistinguishable. Disease severity may range from a mild bowel disturbance and minimal systemic upset with distal proctitis to a life-threatening illness with major systemic upset in the presence of severe pancolitis. Pancolitis may progress to toxic megacolon, a serious condition requiring urgent total colectomy and end ileostomy to avoid colonic perforation and generalized faecal peritonitis.

In patients presenting with severe bloody diarrhoea in the absence of a known history of UC, the differential diagnosis includes Crohn's colitis, infective colitis, and ischaemic colitis.

Clinical features
- Symptoms include profuse bloodstained diarrhoea with urgency of defecation and tenesmus.
- Colicky lower abdominal pain is common, as are anorexia, general malaise, and weight loss.
- On examination, there is usually a pyrexia, with signs of dehydration (profound in severe disease) and anaemia.
- Abdominal tenderness is generalized.

Investigations
- FBC: may reveal ↓ Hb and ↑ WCC.
- U&Es: may show ↑ urea, ↓ K⁺, and ↓Na⁺.
- LFTs: may show ↓serum albumin.
- Stool culture: to exclude infective colitis.
- Supine AXR: to detect toxic megacolon (colon > 5.5cm or caecum > 9cm in diameter).
- Rigid sigmoidoscopy and biopsy of posterior rectal wall for histology.

Management
First-line management is medical rather than surgical.
- Resuscitate with IV fluids, and correct electrolyte abnormalities.
- Insert a urinary catheter if the disease is severe.
- Give packed RBCs if marked Hb < 8g/dL) is present.
- Start thromboprophylaxis if bleeding is not marked (📖 p.26).
- Medical therapy with aminosalicylates and corticosteroids. Prednisolone enemas are given for mild disease, but for more severe disease additional high dose systemic steroids are required.
- Daily supine AXR to detect toxic megacolon.
- Total colectomy and end ileostomy is indicated for fulminant disease that fails to respond adequately to medical therapy and toxic megacolon.

❶ Patients with acute exacerbations of UC are best managed by gastro-enterologists working closely with colorectal surgeons.

① **Rectal foreign bodies**

Patients occasionally present with irretrievable rectal foreign bodies. Most commonly, these have been inserted by the patient or their partner. The variety of foreign bodies inserted PR is surprising, as is the difficulty they may cause in removal.

❶ Foreign bodies inserted PR can cause rectal or sigmoid perforation.

Clinical features

- Get an accurate description of the foreign body, as this may facilitate extraction.
- A history of significant abdominal or pelvic pain raises the possibility of rectal or sigmoid perforation, as does PR bleeding.
- On abdominal examination, look for signs of peritonitis.
- On DRE, check if the foreign body is palpable, although it often isn't, as the patient's attempts at removal may have pushed it proximally.

Investigations

- The object may be visible on rigid sigmoidoscopy, although this examination is best performed under GA.
  - ❶ Be careful not to push the object proximally.
- Supine AXR: to confirm the presence of the foreign body and its position. Look for retroperitoneal air, indicating rectal perforation. A lateral pelvic view may also be of use (Fig. 10.5).

If abdominal signs or PR bleeding are present request:
- FBC: check for ↓ Hb or ↑ WCC.
- U&Es: usually ↔.
- G&S: in case laparotomy is required.
- Erect CXR: to check for free gas under the diaphragm.

Management

If the object is readily palpable on DRE and there are no signs of rectal or sigmoid injury (bleeding, abdominal/pelvic pain, signs of peritonitis), then attempts at removal may be fruitful.

- Biopsy forceps inserted under direct vision via a rigid sigmoidoscope may be used to grasp the object.
  - ❶ Be **very** careful not to push the object proximally or to damage the rectum.

Removal under GA may be required. If there are signs of bowel injury, or the object cannot be removed rectally under GA, laparotomy ± end colostomy is required.

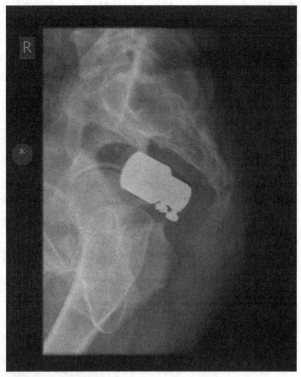

Fig. 10.5 The end of a gardening tool is seen in the rectum.

Early postoperative complications: small or large bowel resection

Anastomotic or suture/staple line leak

This is the most common serious complication after bowel surgery when an anastomosis has been formed or a suture or staple line is present. It may occur after small bowel resection but is less common. Clinically apparent leaks are most common after low rectal anastomoses. Anastomotic leaks may still occur in the presence of a proximal defunctioning stoma, although the consequences of the leak are less marked.

The presentation is highly variable ranging from the very dramatic (sudden generalized peritonitis and circulatory collapse from septic shock) to the insidious (e.g. new onset AF, prolonged ileus), with most cases falling somewhere in between.

❶ A high index of suspicion is needed **whenever** a patient becomes unwell or fails to progress as expected.

- Clinical features. May include: fever, increasing tachycardia or hypotension, oliguria/anuria, abdominal pain resulting from localized/generalized peritonitis, and abdominal distension from an associated ileus.
- Investigations. FBC may show ↑ WCC, and U&Es show ↑ creatinine. Erect CXR may show free gas (Fig. 10.6), although its presence is a normal finding within the first 3–7 days after laparotomy. CT of the abdomen and pelvis shows free gas and increased intraabdominal fluid. In the case of colonic surgery a water-soluble contrast enema is possibly the most useful investigation as it can demonstrate a leak directly.
- Management. Depends on the mode of presentation. In all patients start broad-spectrum IV antibiotics (e.g. cefuroxime 750mg tds + metronidazole 500mg tds), and resuscitate with IV fluids. If generalized peritonitis is present then resuscitate and arrange emergency laparotomy. For patients with localized peritonitis who are systemically well, non-operative treatment may be considered. If systemic symptoms ensue or fail to progress satisfactorily, surgical intervention is necessary.

❶ Anastomotic leaks that are not recognized early may present later as a wound infection and enterocutaneous fistula.

Wound problems (📖 p.166) Wound infection is common and bleeding may occur. Wound dehiscence is uncommon.

Operative site bleeding (📖 p.154)

Intraabdominal abscesses

These are localized collections of intraabdominal pus. They may occur after any type of elective or emergency abdominal surgery but are more common in patients who have had resections of the GI tract or treatment for perforated GI disease. They also arise commonly from intraabdominal inflammatory conditions (e.g. diverticular disease, acute appendicitis, and pancreatitis) and GI perforations. An abscess may form after a well-localized anastomotic or suture/staple line leak. The anatomical location may be subphrenic, subhepatic, pelvic, paracolic, lesser sac, interloop (between loops of small bowel), or localized to an area of pathology, e.g. an anastomosis or perforation (Fig. 10.7).

• Clinical features. Intermittent fever and rigors, local abdominal discomfort, local symptoms (e.g. urinary or rectal symptoms with pelvic abscesses), symptoms from an associated ileus, weight loss, swinging pyrexia, tachycardia, palpable abdominal mass, tenderness, abdominal distension. A pelvic abscess may be palpable on DRE.

❶ The presentation is variable and a high index of suspicion is required.

• Investigations. FBC shows ↑ WCC. If severe, ↓ WCC may be present. U&Es and LFTs may be mildly deranged from sepsis. Blood cultures may reveal bacteraemia. Erect CXR may show pleural effusion and basal collapse if a subphrenic abscess is present. Supine AXR may show an ileus, but is often normal. CT of the abdomen and pelvis confirms the diagnosis.

• Management. Depends on the size and location of the collection and the degree of systemic upset. In all patients start broad-spectrum IV antibiotics (e.g. cefuroxime 750mg tds + metronidazole 500mg tds) and resuscitate with IV fluids. If systemic upset is mild, or in children post-appendicectomy, IV antibiotics alone may be sufficient. If symptoms are more significant, drainage is required, preferably percutaneously via radiological guidance. When this fails or is not possible, laparotomy is required. Large pelvic abscesses palpable on DRE may be drained surgically through the rectum.

Prolonged ileus

Laparotomy and manipulation of the intestine invariably cause impaired peristalsis. It typically lasts for 72h. An ileus lasting for > 5 days may be due to electrolyte abnormalities, retroperitoneal injury, or drugs (e.g. anticholinergics, opioids). However, other diagnoses should also be considered, e.g. mechanical obstruction (📖 p.268), acute gastric dilatation (📖 p.205), anastomotic leak, and intraabdominal abscesses.

• Clinical features. Vomiting, constipation, and abdominal distension. Bowel sounds are usually reduced. Abdominal pain is related to the laparotomy wound.

• Investigations. FBC and U&Es show normal postoperative changes. Supine AXR shows distended small and large bowel. Free gas may normally be present on erect CXR for up to 5–7 days post-laparotomy.

• Management. Keep NBM, and 'drip and suck' (📖 p.271). Correct any electrolyte abnormalities and reduce or stop all non-essential opioids and anticholinergics. Encourage mobilization. When gut function fails to return within 7 days postoperatively or if an anastomotic leak or intraabdominal abscess is suggested clinically, consider starting parenteral nutrition and excluding other diagnoses with an abdominal CT scan or water-soluble contrast enema or follow-through.

Lower GI bleeding (📖 p.280)

PR bleeding may occur after small or large bowel surgery and often arises from a stapled anastomosis. It usually settles spontaneously. Check FBC and PT, APTT. Resuscitate with IV fluids, correct any coagulopathy, and give packed RBCs if anaemic. If the patient is haemodynamically unstable, aggressively resuscitate, give high-flow O_2, and discuss with your seniors immediately. If bleeding is heavy a return to theatre and revision of the anastomosis may be necessary.

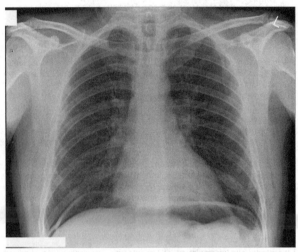

Fig. 10.6 Free gas under both hemidiaphragms on erect CXR.

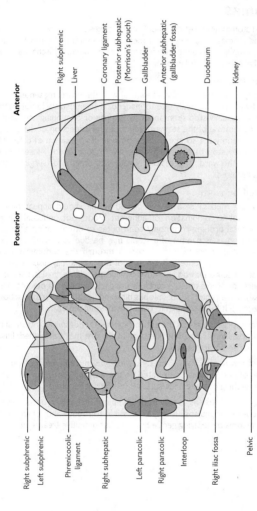

Fig. 10.7 Common sites of intraabdominal abscesses. (Adapted, with permission, from Leaper, D.J. and Peel, A.L.G. (2003) *Oxford Handbook of Postoperative Complications*, Chapter 11, p. 201. Oxford University Press.)

Early postoperative complications: stomas

Bowel stomas are most commonly colostomies or ileostomies. These may be end stomas or looped, permanent or temporary. The most common early complications after stoma formation are bleeding, ischaemia, parastomal abscess, and prolapse.

Stomal bleeding

Bleeding may arise from the abdominal wall, the bowel mesentery, or the bowel wall. This is usually due to inadequate haemostasis. Minor haemorrhage will usually stop spontaneously. Profuse or continuing haemorrhage requires removal of the stoma bag and careful inspection of the stoma to try and identify the source of haemorrhage. If application of direct pressure fails to stop the bleeding, discuss with your senior—insertion of a suture on the ward or, occasionally, return to theatre for surgical correction is required.

Stomal ischaemia

Ideally, the mucosa of a newly formed stoma should appear pink and healthy, but a combination of adherent blood clot, mucosal oedema, and mucosal bruising commonly contributes to discoloration of recently formed stomas. Ischaemia of a stoma may be due to constriction of the bowel and its mesentery as it passes through the abdominal wall or tension on the mesentery. Retraction of the stoma may also be present. Stomal ischaemia may be indicative of widespread intestinal ischaemia.

- Check the stoma mucosa carefully using a bright light (a pen torch is ideal). If the central mucosa looks pink and healthy, no further action is needed. If it looks ischaemic, discuss with your senior.

❶ Don't forget to assess the entire patient—is widespread intestinal ischaemia possible (📖 p.284)? A return to theatre may be needed. Discuss with your senior immediately.

Parastomal abscesses present with swelling, inflammation, and discharge of pus. They can be treated on the ward by gently opening up the cavity, washing out, and packing. LA is usually not required.

Stomal prolapse is usually a late complication but may occur early. For an acute major prolapse it may be possible to reduce and retain the prolapsed stoma by applying gentle pressure but definitive treatment requires surgery.

Early postoperative complications: lower GI endoscopy

Colonoscopy requires IV pre-medication with an opioid (e.g. pethidine) and a short-acting benzodiazepine (e.g. midazolam), while flexible sigmoidoscopy is typically performed without either. Complications of the endoscopy itself are perforation and haemorrhage. A transmural diathermy injury after polypectomy can mimic the abdominal symptoms of a perforation, but the absence of free gas on abdominal CT confirms the diagnosis of 'post-polypectomy syndrome'.

Side-effects from the pre-medications are common. Elderly patients may occasionally develop cardiac events arising either from electrolyte disturbances associated with bowel preparation, or as a result of sedation combined with visceral stimulation during the procedure.

Colonic perforation

The incidence of perforation is approximately 0.1% for diagnostic endoscopy and 0.2% for therapeutic endoscopy. Perforation may result from pneumatic pressure, mechanical trauma from the colonoscope or associated instruments, or from thermal injury during diathermy polypectomy. The presence of perforation may be recognized during the procedure or it may only become apparent afterwards.

- Clinical features. Abdominal pain that persists, worsens, or becomes generalized. Tachycardia, pyrexia, abdominal distension with signs of peritonitis may be present.
- Investigations. FBC shows ↑ WCC, erect CXR shows free gas in ~ 90% of cases. When clinical features suggest perforation and the CXR is normal, abdominal CT can show small volumes of free gas.
- Management. Some patients with contained perforations after polypectomy (and those with post-polypectomy syndrome) are suitable for a trial of non-operative management that includes IV fluids, NG drainage, and broad-spectrum IV antibiotics (e.g. cefuroxime 750mg tds + metronidazole 500mg tds). Emergency laparotomy is indicated in those patients with traumatic perforations, those with peritonitis, and those who do not respond satisfactorily to non-operative therapy. Depending on the operative findings simple surgical repair, colonic resection and anastomosis, or the creation of a temporary stoma may be necessary.

Lower GI bleeding

Clinically relevant bleeding occurs in up to 0.2% of patients undergoing lower GI endoscopy and is usually confined to those undergoing polypectomy. It may present immediately, or after a delay of up to several days. Manage as for any other acute lower GI bleed (📖 p.280). Bleeding nearly always stops spontaneously. Occasionally, repeat therapeutic colonoscopy is required. Interventional radiology or surgery is rarely needed.

Oversedation (📖 p.220)

The anus and anal canal

Introduction

Patients with perianal disorders commonly present acutely, although many can be discharged home the same day with outpatient follow-up. There is significant variation between surgeons in their preferred management of many perianal conditions; be sure that you are aware of the preferences of your seniors.

Perianal anatomy

A sound grasp of perianal anatomy (Fig. 11.1) is essential to avoid misdiagnosis and ensure correct management. In the adult, the anal canal is ~ 4cm long. The dentate line marks the boundary between insensate ano-rectal mucosa superiorly, and sensate anal canal skin inferiorly. Anal glands open into the base of the anal columns, which end at the dentate line. Vascular anal cushions above the dentate line assist in maintaining continence, although continence is primarily due to the presence of two anal sphincters.

- Internal anal sphincter:
  - a continuation of the inner circular muscle of the rectum;
  - an involuntary muscle, under autonomic control.
- External anal sphincter:
  - a continuation of the pelvic floor musculature (levator ani);
  - a skeletal muscle, under somatic control.

Between the internal and external anal sphincters lies the intersphincteric groove. The ischioanal fossa (sometimes called the ischiorectal fossa) is a fat-filled space outside the external anal sphincter bounded laterally by the ischial tuberosities. Posteriorly, the perianal skin merges with that of the natal cleft. The management of natal cleft pilonidal abscesses is covered elsewhere (📖 p.476).

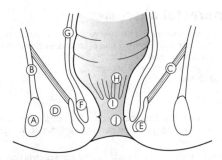

Fig. 11.1 Perianal anatomy in the coronal plane. (A) Ischial tuberosity; (B) obturator internus; (C) levator ani; (D) ischioanal fossa; (E) external anal sphincter; (F) internal anal sphincter; (G) circular muscle of the rectum; (H) anal columns; (I) dentate line; (J) intersphincteric groove.

① **Anorectal abscesses**

These vary in site, severity, and hence clinical presentation. They are most common in the third and fourth decades of life and are classified according to their anatomical location (Fig. 11.2):

- perianal (most common—60% of cases);
- ischioanal (20% of cases);
- intersphincteric;
- submucosal.

❶ Occasionally, an intraabdominal infection (e.g. appendicitis, diverticulitis) may present with deep pelvic or perianal pain due to a supralevator (pelvirectal) abscess.

Most anorectal abscesses are thought to arise from obstruction and infection within an anal gland and subsequent spread of infection into the intersphincteric space and adjacent tissue spaces. The organisms responsible are variable but *E. coli* and enterococci are common. Spontaneous discharge or failed surgical drainage of anorectal abscesses may also lead to a fistula. Many anorectal abscesses coexist with anal fistulae (Box 11.1).

Box 11.1 Fistula-in-ano

Most anal fistulae present initially as anorectal abscesses. After spontaneous or surgical drainage, ongoing discharge suggests that a fistula track is present. Although associated anorectal abscesses require emergency treatment, definitive treatment of fistulae should be undertaken on an elective or semi-elective basis.

❶ Inappropriate fistula surgery risks damaging the anal sphincters, resulting in faecal incontinence. Only specialist surgeons should undertake fistula surgery.

History

- Severe, dull perianal pain, exacerbated by sitting, lying supine, or bowel motions.
- Occasionally, spontaneous discharge of perianal pus occurs.
- Previous failed treatment with oral antibiotics in the community is common.
- ❶ A history of recurrent anorectal abscesses and fistulae raises the possibility of Crohn's disease.
- ❶ Check for a history of diabetes or immunosuppressive diseases.

Examination

- Tachycardia may be present; pyrexia is uncommon.
- Examination of the anus reveals an exquisitely tender, fluctuant swelling in the perianal region with redness of the overlying skin.
- Ischioanal abscesses may not be apparent on external examination.
- DRE is usually not possible due to pain. Where possible, a 'boggy' mass may be palpated.
- ❶ Skin necrosis indicates Fournier's gangrene (📖 p.376).

Investigations

The majority of cases in systemically well young people do not require investigation, but the CBG should be checked to exclude diabetes.

- Radiological imaging (MRI, CT, or anal ultrasound) is rarely necessary but may be helpful to delineate suspected intersphincteric or supralevator abscesses.

If symptoms or signs of sepsis are present:
- FBC: ↑ WCC, with ↑ CRP;
- U&Es: ↑ urea and creatinine, reflecting dehydration;
- ABG: metabolic acidosis with ↑ serum lactate;
- blood, urine, and sputum cultures;
- CXR to exclude pneumonia.

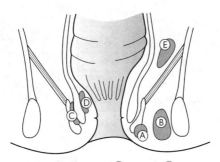

Fig. 11.2 Anorectal abscesses. Ⓐ Perianal; Ⓑ ischioanal; Ⓒ intersphincteric; Ⓓ submucosal; Ⓔ supralevator.

Management

The treatment of an anorectal abscess is surgical drainage. Primary treatment with antibiotics is ineffective.

- The standard treatment for most anorectal abscesses is drainage under GA via a cruciate incision, followed by digital disruption of loculations, washout, and loose packing of the wound.
- Adjuvant treatment with antibiotics is unnecessary in straightforward anorectal abscesses in otherwise healthy individuals, except in the presence of widespread cellulitis.
- Small perianal abscesses may be suitable for drainage and packing under LA.
- Some surgeons advocate aspiration of small perianal abscesses using a green (21G) needle and a 10mL syringe under topical anaesthetic (ethyl chloride spray). If successful, prescribe a course of oral antibiotics (e.g. co-amoxiclav 625mg tds) for 7 days.
- Postoperative analgesia and stool softeners should be given.
- Arrange outpatient follow-up to enable identification of any fistulae.

- ❶ Aggressive probing to identify associated fistulous tracts should not be performed in the acute setting as false tracks are easily created.
- ❶ Patients with sepsis require **emergency** surgery and perioperative broad spectrum IV antibiotics (e.g. cefuroxime 750mg tds + metronidazole 500mg tds).

① Prolapsed internal haemorrhoids

Straining and passing small volume stools leads to enlargement of the anal cushions (internal haemorrhoids). Progressive enlargement eventually leads to prolapse (Fig. 11.3). Prolapsing internal haemorrhoids that fail to reduce can become strangulated, eventually leading to thrombosis. In time, thrombosed internal haemorrhoids fibrose, resulting in spontaneous cure.

Clinical features
- Acute, severe perianal pain, usually present for 1–2 days.
- On examination, large, fleshy, tender haemorrhoids are seen protruding through the anal canal.

Management
Thrombosed internal haemorrhoids may be treated non-operatively or operatively. Non-operative treatment is commonly practised as it avoids the risks of surgery.

Non-operative treatment
- Regular oral analgesia (e.g. paracetamol 1g qds + diclofenac 50mg tds + codeine phosphate 60mg qds).
- Regular stool laxatives/bulkers.
- Bed rest with elevation of the foot of the bed.
- Application of perianal cold compress (e.g. an ice pack or a bag of frozen peas).
- Arrange outpatient follow-up to ensure that symptoms have fully resolved.
- ❶ Gentle, firm, consistent pressure on the haemorrhoids can cause reduction, but this can very painful. LA gel (e.g. Instillagel™) should be applied for at least 30min prior to attempted reduction.
- ❶ Admission to hospital is occasionally required to adequately control symptoms.

Operative treatment Urgent haemorrhoidectomy under GA.

❶ This risks injury to the internal sphincter or anal stenosis due to inadequate skin bridges. This surgery should only be done by a colorectal surgeon.

① **Perianal haematomas**

Perianal haematomas (also known as thrombosed external haemorrhoids) lie below the dentate line of the anal canal and are covered by squamous epithelium with a rich sensory innervation (Fig. 11.3). Left untreated, perianal haematomas resolve spontaneously after several days.

Clinical features
- Acute, severe perianal pain, usually after straining.
- On examination, a blue/red cherry-sized, exquisitely tender bulge is seen adjacent to the anal verge.

❶ These should not be confused with prolapsed internal haemorrhoids, as the treatment is often very different. Perianal haematomas are unable to be 'reduced back' into the anal canal.

Management
Although resolution will eventually occur, perianal haematomas are often best treated in the acute phase by evacuation of the haematoma, as this relieves the pain immediately. This can be achieved through a small incision made under LA.

❶ Incision of a prolapsed internal haemorrhoid misdiagnosed as a perianal haematoma will result in profuse bleeding, which may require a procedure under GA to control. If you are unsure of the diagnosis, treat as a prolapsed internal haemorrhoid.

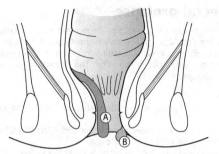

Fig. 11.3 Haemorrhoids. Ⓐ A prolapsed internal haemorrhoid; Ⓑ a perianal haematoma.

⏻ **Rectal prolapse**

Full-thickness prolapse of the rectum through the anus most often occurs in elderly females. Although the anus is usually patulous, large prolapses can occasionally impair venous return from the distal mucosa, leading to swelling and difficulties in reduction. The dramatic appearance often results in emergency referral.

Clinical features

- Recurrent rectal prolapse on straining that this time fails to reduce spontaneously.
- On examination, non-tender, oedematous circumferential full thickness rectal tissue protrudes through the anal canal.
- Unlike prolapsed piles, a rectal prolapse looks like a complete ring with a central orifice.
- Irritation of the rectal mucosa may lead to minor bleeding.

Management

With simple measures, these prolapses can often be easily reduced.

- Lie the patient in the left lateral position and tilt the bed head-down.
- An assistant is useful to retract the right buttock.
- Apply gentle, firm pressure to the distal rectum, squeezing the mucosa centrally to expel tissue oedema. Two (or three!) hands may be needed to control the prolapse.
- Continue to push the rectum back into the anal canal. Be patient!
- Once reduced, keep the patient in that position for at least an hour.

The patient can be discharged home with stool softeners (e.g. lactulose 10mL bd PO). Tell them to avoid straining and warn them that recurrence of the prolapse is likely. Arrange outpatient follow-up with a colorectal surgeon to discuss operative repair.

⑦ **Anal fissure**

This is a longitudinal tear in the skin and mucosa of the anal canal, usually in the posterior midline. Anal fissures are common, especially in 20–40 year olds, and may occasionally present acutely.

Clinical features

- Acute persisting perianal pain, often with a small amount of bright red blood, after passage of a large, hard stool.
- On examination, traction on the perianal skin may reveal an anal mucosal tear, usually in the posterior midline, although anal spasm may prevent exposure.

❶ DRE and instrumentation cause severe pain and should not be attempted unless the diagnosis is in doubt.

Management

Management is initially non-operative. Prescribe:
- GTN 0.4% ointment bd, to be placed around the anus, for 6 weeks.
  - ❶ Warn the patient that GTN ointment may cause throbbing headaches and may drop their blood pressure.
- Regular stool softners/bulkers to continue whilst on GTN.
- Oral analgesia, e.g. paracetamol 1g qds + ibuprofen 400mg tds.
  - ❶ Avoid opioids due to their constipating action.

Arrange outpatient follow-up with a colorectal surgeon to ensure healing and for full examination. If fissures do not heal, they can become chronic, and may need other treatments.

Early postoperative complications

The majority of perianal procedures are performed as day-case surgery and significant early postoperative complications are uncommon.

Open haemorrhoidectomy

Operative site bleeding (📖 p.154)

Bleeding from the highly vascular haemorrhoid pedicle results in profuse bleeding. Secondary haemorrhage due to infection may occur 5–10 days postoperatively, and can also be life-threatening. A return to theatre is essential.

Less dramatic bleeding can occur from the wound edges. Place a pressure dressing over the perianal area. Re-assess within 30min—ongoing bleeding may require a return to theatre.

Urinary retention This is common, especially in elderly men. Insert a urinary catheter (📖 p.504), and give adequate oral or parenteral analgesia. Admit overnight. Trial-without-catheter may be attempted the next morning, once pain is controlled. Failure requires re-catheterization, training in the use of a leg bag, and referral to the urology team.

Infection

Rarely, patients can develop a perianal infection. This usually occurs 5–10 days postoperatively and presents with pyrexia, malaise, increasing perianal pain, and pus-like discharge PR. Examination findings are limited by pain. Start IV metronidazole 500mg tds and admit. Examination under anaesthesia (EUA) or MRI may be necessary to exclude a collection.

❶ If sepsis is present (📖 p.482), fluid resuscitate and discuss with your senior immediately. Emergency EUA and drainage may be necessary.

❶ Very rarely, Fournier's gangrene (📖 p.376) can develop after open haemorrhoidectomy.

Stapled haemorrhoidopexy

Stapled haemorrhoidopexy (sometimes known as PPH—procedure for prolapse and haemorrhoids) lifts haemorrhoids by excising and stapling redundant proximal rectal mucosa.

Operative site bleeding (📖 p.154) Any significant bleeding after stapled haemorrhoidopexy is likely to arise from the staple-line and requires a return to theatre after resuscitation.

Rectal perforation

- Clinical features. Patients usually present 2–10 days postoperatively with low abdominal and perianal pain and features of sepsis. Pus may be visible on perianal inspection. DRE is often not possible due to pain.
- Investigations. FBC shows ↑ WCC. Supine AXR may reveal retroperitoneal gas. Definitive diagnosis often requires an abdominal and pelvic CT to identify the pelvic collection and retroperitoneal gas.
- Management. Resuscitate with IV fluids, insert a urinary catheter, and discuss with your seniors immediately. Start broad spectrum IV antibiotics (e.g. cefuroxime 750mg tds + metronidazole 500mg tds).

Drainage of the pelvic collection and a proximal defunctioning stoma is often required.

❶ Thankfully this complication is rare, but should be considered whenever patients present with perianal pain or pyrexia after stapled haemorrhoidopexy.

Breast and endocrine surgery

① **Breast abscesses**

Breast abscesses are common, particularly in breastfeeding women. *Staphylococcus aureus* is the most common causative organism. After breast surgery, haematomas may become infected, leading to a breast abscess (📖 p.317).

Clinical features

- The history includes breast pain and swelling.
- Systemic symptoms such as fever and vomiting may occur.
- Neglected abscesses can discharge spontaneously.
- On examination, overt signs of sepsis (📖 p.482) are rare, but mild tachycardia and low-grade pyrexia are common.
- An erythematous breast swelling is seen. Mature abscesses may show fluctuance.

❶ The differential diagnosis of inflammatory breast lesions includes inflammatory carcinoma.

Investigations

Systemically well, young, fit women do not require emergency investigations. If symptoms or signs of sepsis (📖 p.482) are present, the following are required:

- FBC: ↑ WCC, with ↑ CRP;
- U&Es: ↑ urea and creatinine, reflecting dehydration;
- ABG: metabolic acidosis with ↑ serum lactate;
- blood cultures;
- erect CXR: to exclude pneumonia.

Management

- The majority of breast abscesses are treated with needle aspiration, analgesia, and antibiotics as outpatients.
    - Unless systemic signs of sepsis are present, patients can be discharged home on oral antibiotics (e.g. flucloxacillin 500mg qds PO + phenoxymethylpenicillin 500mg qds PO).
    - Arrange for USS-guided aspiration of the abscess within 24h. Pus should be sent for microbiological analysis. Core biopsy of any suspicious lesions should be performed.
    - Follow-up must be arranged with a specialist breast team. Aspiration may need to be repeated.
- Patients with significant systemic symptoms or signs require admission for IV rehydration and IV antibiotics (e.g. flucloxacillin 1g qds IV + benzylpenicillin 1.2g qds IV) while USS-guided aspiration is arranged.
- Patients with sepsis require IV fluid resuscitation, IV antibiotics (e.g. flucloxacillin 1g qds IV + benzylpenicillin 1.2g qds IV) and emergency surgical drainage and washout.
- Abscesses that are pointing and about to discharge and those that have discharged spontaneously require surgical drainage and washout.
- In breastfeeding women, the infected breast should regularly be emptied of milk using a breast pump, and the milk discarded. Check the BNF for information on the safety of antibiotics excreted in breast milk.

Early postoperative complications: breast surgery

There are few early complications of breast surgery. Seromas and lymphoedema do not present acutely and can be managed in the outpatient clinic.

Operative site bleeding (see also 📖 p.154)

Wide local excision of breast lumps may result in a breast haematoma, despite wound drains. Large haematomas causing discomfort and breast distortion usually present within 24h of surgery and require urgent return to theatre for washout and haemostasis. Small haematomas may discharge spontaneously through the wound 1–7 days postoperatively, causing significant concern for the patient. Reassure the patient and arrange follow-up with their surgeon in the next available clinic.

Postoperative bleeding causing shock is rare after breast or axillary surgery.

Infection

Infection is uncommon after breast surgery. Extensive cellulitis or systemic signs of infection requires admission for IV antibiotics (e.g. flucloxacillin 1g qds + benzylpenicillin 1.2g qds). Patients with mild cellulitis can be given oral flucloxacillin 500mg qds. Arrange follow-up with their surgeon in the next available clinic.

Breast haematomas may become infected leading to deep abscesses. Admission for surgical drainage and washout through the original wound is required. Start IV flucloxacillin 1g qds if there are systemic signs of infection or significant overlying cellulitis.

Flap ischaemia

This may occur after reconstructive breast surgery or, rarely, after mastectomy. All flaps, especially free flaps requiring microvascular anastomoses (e.g. transverse rectus abdominis myocutaneous), require close monitoring. Signs of ischaemia include pale, mottled, dusky, or cyanotic skin. Capillary refill is slow in arterial ischaemia, but accelerated in venous congestion.

❶ Discuss with a senior surgeon immediately. Flap ischaemia may require emergency surgery.

Early postoperative complications: thyroid and parathyroid surgery

Airway compromise is the most feared early complication of thyroid and parathyroid surgery and may be due to many different causes. Other early complications may also occur.

Operative site bleeding (see also 📖 p.154)

Even small postoperative bleeds can rapidly compress the airway. Stridor may be present. Airway obstruction due to haematoma requires immediate re-opening of the wound on the ward, with removal of the strap muscle sutures and evacuation of the deep haematoma.

▶▶ Call for immediate anaesthetic support and arrange for emergency return to theatre.

❶ Failure to act rapidly may have fatal consequences.

Hypocalcaemia

This can occur after parathyroidectomy or total thyroidectomy with inadvertent parathyroid gland damage or removal. Check serum corrected Ca^{2+} on the night of surgery and daily thereafter until discharge.

Mild hypocalcaemia (> 2mmol/L) rarely causes symptoms but should be treated with oral calcium and vitamin D supplements. Severe hypocalcaemia (< 2mmol/L) may cause twitching progressing to tetany, laryngospasm, and airway obstruction. Chvostek's and Trousseau's signs may be present. Treat any symptoms **immediately** with 10mL of 10% calcium gluconate IV, followed by continuous infusion and regular serum calcium monitoring.

❶ IV calcium causes severe burns if extravasation occurs, so use a central venous line; otherwise use a freshly placed cannula in a large peripheral vein.

▶▶ If the airway is compromised, call for immediate anaesthetic assistance.

Laryngeal nerve damage

The recurrent laryngeal nerve supplies all intrinsic laryngeal muscles except for cricothyroid. Bilateral partial nerve injury may cause airway obstruction. This is apparent on extubation in theatre and requires re-intubation. Unilateral transection results in a weak, hoarse voice, while bilateral transection causes aphonia.

Superior laryngeal nerve damage results in subtle voice changes due to cricothyroid paralysis. Loss of supraglottic sensation can lead to aspiration. Airway obstruction does not occur.

Tracheomalacia

Rarely, airway obstruction post-extubation may be due to tracheal ring softening from a large multinodular goitre. This requires re-intubation.

Thyrotoxic crisis ('thyroid storm') can occur if the preoperative control of thyrotoxicosis in patients with Graves's disease is inadequate. This is now extremely rare after thyroidectomy. Clinical features include tachycardia, hyperpyrexia, and irritability. Treat promptly with rehydration and high-flow O_2. Involve the on-call intensivists early. Definitive treatment requires cooling, propylthiouracil, anti-dysrhythmics, and dexamethasone.

Vascular surgery

① **Deep venous thrombosis**

Deep venous thrombosis (DVT) is a common disease, occurring in up to 10% of general surgical patients, with potentially grave consequences:
- post-thrombotic syndrome (30%): chronic venous insufficiency with limb oedema, pain, and occasional venous ulceration;
- PE (📖 p.149), leading to death or pulmonary hypertension;
- extension of the thrombus with venous gangrene (phlegmasia caerulea dolens).

Risk factors for DVT follow Virchow's triad for thrombus formation.
- Alteration in the vessel wall (endothelial damage), e.g. venous surgery, long bone fracture, cannulation, phlebitis.
- Alteration in the flow:
  - stasis, e.g. long operation, plaster cast, bed rest, immobility, obesity;
  - turbulence, e.g. venous surgery, indwelling central venous lines.
- Abnormalities in the blood (hypercoagulable states):
  - inherited, e.g. factor V Leiden, factor II G20210A mutation, protein C or S deficiency, antithrombin III deficiency, lupus anticoagulant;
  - acquired, e.g. malignancy; oestrogens (oral contraceptive pill, hormone replacement therapy, pregnancy) thrombocytosis; poly-cythaemia; dehydration.

DVT/PE prophylaxis is essential, and all surgical patients should undergo a preoperative risk assessment (📖 p.27). Lower limb DVT is much more common than upper limb DVT (Box 13.1).

Box 13.1 Upper limb DVT

This is becoming more common due to the widespread use of intravas-cular catheters, cardiac pacemakers, and automated internal cardiac defi-brillators. Risk factors are the same as for lower limb DVT, as well as:
- thoracic outlet compression;
- effort thrombosis, i.e. where repeated, unaccustomed exercise of the arm results in venous impingement in the narrow thoracic outlet.

Patients present with a swollen, warm, painful arm. Duplex USS con-firms the presence of thrombus; more proximal thrombus may require contrast venography, or contrast-enhanced CT/MRI. Since the complica-tions of upper limb venous thrombosis mimic those of lower limb DVTs, treatment should be the same.

History

DVTs are often asymptomatic, but when symptoms occur, the following are typical features:
- aching calf pain;
- calf swelling.

Examination
- Low-grade pyrexia (< 37.5°C).
  - ❶ All surgical patients with pyrexia should be examined for DVT.

- Unilateral calf swelling with prominent superficial veins.
  - **❶** Bilateral swelling may occur if the DVT is bilateral, or has extended to occlude the IVC.
- Warmth and erythema (may be mistaken for cellulitis).
- Calf tenderness.
- **❶** Check for symptoms and signs of PE in all patients with DVT, and investigate appropriately (📖 p.146).

Severe pain, cyanosis, skin necrosis, and limb swelling extending to the groin are features of phlegmasia caerulea dolens (Box 13.2).

Box 13.2 Phlegmasia cerulea dolens (PCD)

This is a rare disease that is much more common in the lower limb and is associated with malignancies. Extensive proximal DVT with thrombosis of venous collaterals leads to complete venous outflow obstruction, and eventually venous gangrene. Patients present with limb oedema, severe limb pain, and distal cyanosis. Distal pulses are intact initially but are difficult to identify due to limb oedema. Duplex USS or MR venography show proximal thrombus. Mild cases can be treated with anticoagulation and limb elevation. Progressive PCD can be treated with thrombolysis or surgical thrombectomy. An IVC filter may be necessary. Amputation is needed if the limb is non-viable. Mortality is ~ 25%.

Initial investigations
- FBC: look for ↑ Hb and ↑ platelets; WCC can ↑ or ↓ with DVT.
- U&Es, LFTs, PT, APTT: as baseline investigations.
- D-dimers: a normal value excludes a DVT when the clinical probability is low.
  - **❶** D-dimers are usually raised postoperatively and are therefore of little use in surgical patients.

Initial management
- Anticoagulation: none of the above investigations can exclude a DVT, so start treatment dose LMWH (e.g. enoxaparin 1.5mg/kg od SC) or IV unfractionated heparin while awaiting the results of imaging.
  - **❶** LMWH are difficult to reverse, so avoid if the risk of bleeding is high. In the immediate postoperative phase unfractionated heparin is preferable.
  - **❶** Always discuss anticoagulation with your senior before starting.
  - **❶** Operative site haematoma due to anticoagulation is a particular concern in orthopaedics (📖 p.424), and where haemorrhage would have severe consequences, e.g. neurosurgery, ophthalmology.

Further investigations
- Duplex USS:
  - looks for lack of venous compressibility (due to solid intraluminal thrombus) and absence of flow;
  - highly sensitive (> 90% at detecting femoral DVT) and non-invasive;
  - widely available.

- Intravenous venography: more sensitive for calf DVTs, but invasive, expensive, and rarely used.
- MR venography: best for detection of pelvic venous thrombi.

Further management

If DVT is confirmed on duplex USS, start warfarin once bleeding is unlikely and aim for INR of 2.5. Stop LMWH once INR > 2 for 2 consecutive days.

- Warfarin duration: 6 weeks for calf DVT, 3 months if thigh DVT with temporary risk factors and a low risk of recurrence (6 months if idiopathic DVT or permanent risk factors).[1]
- Consider IVC filter insertion to prevent PEs if anticoagulation is contraindicated or if PEs recur despite therapeutic anticoagulation.[2] Free-floating thrombus is not an indication for an IVC filter.
- Thrombolysis: not recommended except in phlegmasia caerulea dolens.

References

1 Baglin, T.P. *et al.* (2005). Guidelines on oral anticoagulation (warfarin): third edition—2005 update. *Br. J. Haematol.* **132**, 277–85.

2 Baglin, T.P. *et al.* (2006). Guidelines on use of vena cava filters. *Br. J. Haematol.* **134**, 590–5.

☣ **Ruptured AAA**

An aneurysm is an abnormal permanent localized arterial dilatation. Aneurysms usually occur in the thoracic and abdominal aortas, the common and internal iliac arteries, and the popliteal and femoral arteries. AAAs are present in 5% of men over 65 years old, and are most commonly associated with atherosclerosis. They usually arise below the level of the renal arteries (infrarenal AAA). Complications of AAAs include the following.

- Rupture.
  - The risk of rupture is proportional to the diameter, and increases significantly once the AAA is > 5.5cm diameter.
- Distal embolization.
- Fistula formation, e.g. aorto-caval, aorto-enteric.
  - Aorto-enteric fistulae are uncommon in AAAs, but are more common following repair.
- Thrombosis (uncommon).

Surgical repair (either open or endovascular) is the only treatment for AAAs. Indications for AAA repair include:
- rupture: requires emergency repair;
- symptomatic: requires urgent repair, as new back pain or tenderness implies recent acute expansion and imminent rupture;
- diameter > 5.5cm: requires elective repair when the risk of rupture is greater than the expected mortality of the repair.

Rupture of an AAA is a much feared but relatively uncommon surgical emergency. Rupture into the peritoneal cavity results in exsanguination and death within minutes. If the rupture is contained within the retro-peritoneum, a large haematoma develops, blood pressure falls, and the rupture may be contained for some time, enabling transfer to hospital. Without repair, mortality is 100%.

❶ Maintain a high index of suspicion, especially in men over 60 years old, and in those with risk factors for atherosclerosis

History

The mode of presentation is variable.
- Collapse (📖 p.136).
- Sudden onset, severe abdominal, back, or left loin pain.
  - This may radiate to the groin or scrotum as the expanding haematoma strips the peritoneum away from the posterior abdominal wall.
- Symptoms of hypotension: SOB, chest pain, postural hypotension.
- History of known AAA undergoing USS surveillance.
- Risk factors for atherosclerosis: smoking, ↑ BP, diabetes, hyperlipidaemia, family history.

❶ In order to determine if AAA repair is suitable, an assessment of co-morbidities and pre-morbid functioning is essential (📖 p.12). The use of warfarin or aspirin increases the requirement for blood products if repair is required.

Examination

- Pale and clammy, cold peripheries, occasionally confused.
- Tachycardia, hypotension, tachypnoea, postural fall in BP.
- Epigastric and/or loin tenderness.
  - ❶ A palpable AAA is only present in ~ 50% due to obesity, hypotension, or extensive retroperitoneal haematoma.
  - ❶ The abdominal aorta bifurcates at the level of the umbilicus, so palpate it in the epigastrium.
- An aortic bruit may be audible.
  - A machinery murmur suggests an aorto-caval fistula; such patients may also have lower limb cyanosis with a high central venous pressure in the presence of hypotension.
- Exclude severe GI bleeding as a cause for ↓ BP by performing a DRE.
- Document the presence or absence of peripheral pulses in order to help interpret postoperative findings. An acutely lost pulse may be an indication for post-repair embolectomy.
- ❶ Ruptured AAAs are often mistaken for ureteric colic. Ureteric colic is uncommon in patients over 60 years old; AAAs are not.
- ❶ Ruptured AAAs should never be confused with an acute disc prolapse. By the age of 60 the intervertebral discs are desiccated and do not prolapse.

Initial investigations

❶ If a ruptured AAA is suspected, inform your senior and the theatre co-ordinator **immediately**.

Emergency investigations may be necessary to assist in excluding other causes of collapse/shock/epigastric and back pain and determine whether repair is appropriate (Box 13.3).

❶ Unnecessary investigations delay life-saving surgery.
- FBC: Hb often ↓, but normal Hb may be present acutely.
- U&Es: may show evidence of pre-existing renal impairment.
- PT, APTT: may be prolonged due to haemorrhage or anticoagulants.

Box 13.3 Determining suitability for emergency repair

Emergency repair of ruptured AAA has a mortality of ~ 20–30%. Patients with severe shock, multiple co-morbidities, and poor pre-morbid functioning have an operative mortality of 100%. Factors that are often taken into account to decide which patients are appropriate for emergency AAA repair include:
- age (repair is rare in those > 80 years old);
- co-morbidities and pre-morbid functioning;
- presence and degree of renal impairment and anaemia;
- ECG findings;
- level of consciousness following hospital admission.

❶ The decision on whether or not to offer repair should only be made by a consultant vascular surgeon.

❶ A patient suffering cardiac arrest prior to surgery will not survive surgery.

- Cross-match 6 units of packed RBCs.
- Serum amylase (📖 p.246): may be mildly raised in ruptured AAA, but acute pancreatitis is more likely if > 5 × the upper limit of normal.
- ECG. Exclude STEMI as a cause of shock and epigastric pain (📖 p.143). Other ischaemic changes may be due to hypotension and often improve with fluid resuscitation.

❶ These investigations must only be performed as an **emergency**. Bloods must be taken to the lab **immediately** and the labs must be aware that they need to be analysed and phoned through **immediately**.

❶ If there is clinical suspicion of peritonitis, and the patient's clinical state permits, an erect CXR is useful to look for free gas.

❶ USS in resus can detect an AAA, but **cannot** accurately identify if it is ruptured. An AXR (AP or dorsal decubitus) may show a calcified AAA sac or an absent psoas shadow on the left (Fig. 13.1), but is often unhelpful in ruptured AAA. Do not delay surgery by requesting these investigations in unstable patients.

Initial management
- Give high-flow O_2 via a non-rebreathing mask.
- Insert 2 × large-bore peripheral cannulae and give IV fluids (crystalloid or colloid) to restore systolic BP to ~ 90mmHg.
- ❶ Do not over-resuscitate, for fear of precipitating further haemorrhage.
- Give IV opioid analgesia.
- If time permits, insert a urinary catheter (📖 p.504).

Further investigations and management
Once co-morbidities and pre-morbid functioning are known, patients with suspected ruptured AAA must be discussed with the on-call consultant vascular surgeon.
- ❶ The decision to proceed to further investigations (i.e. CT) should only be made by a consultant. Delay can be fatal.
- ❶ Inform the patient and family of the suspected diagnosis and the possible outcomes. Occasionally, patients may decline emergency repair.

When the diagnosis is uncertain CT abdomen and pelvis (Fig. 13.2) is the investigation of choice, but only where the diagnosis is uncertain.

If ruptured AAA is likely and repair is appropriate
- Alert the on-call anaesthetist and theatre co-ordinator.
- Tell blood bank, as further packed RBCs, FFP, and platelets are often needed.
- Transfer the patient to theatre immediately.
- If transfer to another hospital is necessary:
  • arrange for an ambulance and make sure that they know exactly where the patient needs to go and that the receiving team are aware that the patient is on their way;
  • gather all notes, results, and imaging together;
  • make sure that the packed RBCs go with the patient;
  • where possible, a doctor trained in resuscitation (often the on-call anaesthetist) and a nurse should go with the patient.

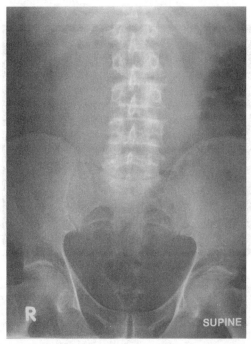

Fig. 13.1 AXR showing loss of the right psoas shadow due to a retroperitoneal haematoma from a ruptured AAA. (Reproduced, with permission, from Reynard, J. et al. (2006). *Oxford handbook of urology*, Chapter 3, p. 49. Oxford University Press, Oxford.)

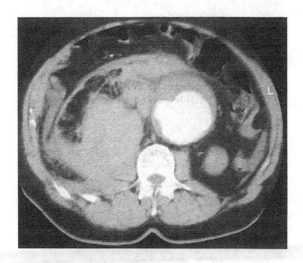

Fig. 13.2 A large AAA with intraluminal thrombus is seen on contrast-enhanced CT. The right retroperitoneal haemorrhage indicates rupture. (Reproduced, with permission, from Reynard, J. et al. (2006). *Oxford handbook of urology*, Chapter 9, p. 385. Oxford University Press, Oxford.)

❶ In some centres, emergency endovascular AAA repair is available and emergency CT scanning will be necessary.

If ruptured AAA is likely and repair is inappropriate or declined by the patient

- Admit to a ward side-room, and prescribe parenteral analgesia to keep the patient comfortable. A syringe-driver is often necessary.
- Ensure that a 'do not resuscitate' order is completed and documented in the notes.
- Keep the patient and family fully informed. Death is expected within 24h.

☠ Acute limb ischaemia

Acute limb ischaemia is much more common in the lower limb than the upper limb (Box 13.4). While acute limb-threatening ischaemia may manifest with the classical history of a painful, pale, pulseless leg, if it occurs on the background of chronic ischaemia the diagnosis may not be so clear. There are three key elements in the assessment of the acutely ischaemic limb:

- confirming the diagnosis;
- defining the aetiology;
- deciding whether the limb is salvageable.

Box 13.4 Acute upper limb ischaemia

Upper limb ischaemia presents with a painful, cold, numb hand. The causes and principles of treatment are similar to those of lower limb ischaemia. Most cases are secondary to embolization from a cardiac source, with emboli usually impacting at the brachial artery bifurcation. Brachial artery embolectomy via a transverse antecubital fossa incision is indicated.

Confirming the diagnosis

An ischaemic limb is defined by the presence of at least some of the '6 Ps': painful, perishingly cold, pallor, pulselessness, paraesthesia, and paralysis.

❶ Paralysis is a late sign and limb viability is dubious.

Causes

It is necessary to differentiate between thrombotic, embolic, and other causes, as the treatments are different.

- Embolism, e.g.:
  - left atrium (AF);
  - proximal bypass grafts;
  - left ventricle (LV aneurysm or post-MI mural thrombus);
  - left-sided heart valves;
  - aneurysm sac, e.g. AAA, popliteal aneurysm;
  - ruptured proximal atherosclerotic plaque;
  - patent foramen ovale (paradoxical embolus from a venous thrombosis);
  - iatrogenic, e.g. after angiography, angioplasty, or stenting.
- ❶ Proximal embolic sources may result in ischaemia of both lower limbs, and may embolize to other arteries, e.g. cerebral, mesenteric, renal.
- Thrombosis:
  - in an area of atherosclerosis;
  - of an aneurysm, e.g. AAA, popliteal aneurysm;
  - of a pre-existing vascular bypass graft;
  - because of septicaemia, e.g. pneumococcal or meningococcal.
- Aortic dissection (📖 p.468), as the false lumen excludes the arterial supply to the limb.
- Trauma (📖 p.337).
- ❶ Malignancies predispose to thromboembolic disease.

Assessing viability Muscle can survive 4–6h of ischaemia. Revascularization of ischaemic muscle results in reperfusion syndrome (📖 p.346), which can be life-threatening. It is therefore essential to accurately assess whether revascularization or amputation is the most appropriate treatment (Box 13.5).

Box 13.5 Indicators of reduced limb viability

Impending loss of viability
- Blotchy purpura that do not blanch on pressure (fixed staining) confined distally, e.g. to toes/forefoot.
- Pallor persisting when hanging dependent.
- Tender muscles.
- Reduced sensation to light touch.
- Partial paralysis.

Non-viable
- Fixed staining extending proximally, e.g. to forefoot/calf.
- Complete sensory loss.
- Muscles feel stiff on palpation.
- Total paralysis.

History
- Of acute limb ischaemia:
  - pain begins distally and progresses proximally;
  - paraesthesiae;
  - paralysis;
  - ❶ Elderly patients may also present with confusion.
- Of the underlying cause:
  - AF, recent MI, recent DVT, AAA;
  - aortic dissection (📖 p.468);
  - symptoms consistent with PVD;
  - hypercoagulable states, thrombophilia;
  - recent angiography, angioplasty, or stenting;
  - previous vascular graft (suspect thrombosis until proven otherwise).
- History favouring an embolic cause:
  - rapid onset pain (over minutes);
  - AF, recent MI, proximal aneurysm.
- History favouring a thrombotic cause:
  - delayed onset pain (over hours);
  - PVD, vascular graft.

Examination
- An irregularly irregular pulse suggests AF and an embolic cause.
- Colour of the limb:
  - pallor, reduced capillary refill, blotchy purpura;
  - failure of a pale limb to turn pink when hung dependent is suggestive of severe ischaemia.
- Cool to touch (compare the opposite limb and upper limb).
- Check for aneurysmal disease, e.g. AAA, popliteal aneurysm.
- Peripheral pulses (Fig. 13.3):
  - absent pulses in the non-ischaemic limb suggest underlying PVD and a thrombotic cause;
  - ABPI in both limbs. Use a handheld Doppler.

- Check carefully for sensory and motor loss.
- Tender muscles suggest muscle necrosis and compartment syndrome (📖 p.412).
- Assess the contralateral limb: look for evidence of embolic disease or PVD, e.g. trophic changes; ulceration, absent pulses.
- ❶ A thorough cardiovascular examination is necessary to identify other acute or chronic manifestations of vascular disease.

Initial investigations

❶ The investigation and management of aortic dissection is discussed in Chapter 18 (📖 p.468).
- FBC: ↑ Hb increases risk of thrombosis.
- U&Es: ↑ K^+ common in presence of ischaemia; ↑ creatinine and urea suggest pre-existing renal disease.
- PT, APTT: as baseline. Request INR if the patient is on warfarin.
- LFTs: usually normal, but ↑↑ AST/ALT suggests ischaemic hepatitis.
- CBG: may diagnose previously unknown diabetes.
- G&S: In most circumstances, as the patient will usually need surgery.
- ECG: Look for AF, Q waves (old MI), and ST elevation (LV aneurysm).
- CXR: May show a widened thoracic aorta (aneurysm or dissection), bronchial carcinoma, or metastatic malignancy.

Initial management

❶ If acute limb ischaemia is suspected, discuss with your senior immediately.
- Keep NBM.
- Give O_2 to keep SaO_2 > 95%.
- Insert a large IV cannula and give IV fluids to maintain systolic BP > 100mmHg.
  - ❶ Avoid unnecessary venepuncture as bleeding will occur if thrombolysis is required.
- Give IV opioid analgesia in small boluses.
- Treat ↑ K^+ (📖 p.18).
- Insert a urinary catheter (📖 p.504).
- If CBG > 11mmol/L start an IV insulin infusion regimen (📖 p.24).
- Anticoagulate: give an IV bolus of 5000 units of unfractionated heparin followed by an infusion to keep the APTT ratio at 1.5–2.5 to prevent clot propagation.
  - ❶ Contraindications to anticoagulation include dissection, trauma, and the expected need for spinal or epidural anaesthesia.

Further investigations and management

These depend on the likely underlying cause, the viability of the limb, and the fitness of the patient. If the cause of the ischaemia is an embolus, a search should be made for the source (e.g. echocardiogram, 24h ECG monitoring) once the patient has recovered from surgery.

❶ Postoperative complications are common, and revascularized limbs must be monitored carefully (📖 p.346).

Likely embolic cause in a viable limb
~ ~ergency surgery.

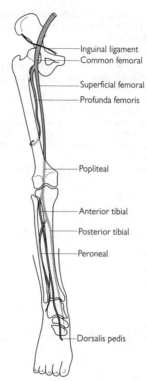

Fig. 13.3 Anatomy of the lower limb arteries. (Reproduced, with permission, from Longmore, M. *et al.* (2007). *Oxford handbook of clinical medicine*, 7th edn, Chapter 14, p. 597. Oxford University Press, Oxford.)

- Embolectomy via the common femoral artery is required to remove proximal or distal clots. This can be performed under LA, GA, or regional anaesthesia.
- On-table angiography confirms distal clearance of emboli.
- On-table thrombolysis may be indicated if there is persistent distal occlusion.
- A fasciotomy should be performed if compartment syndrome (□ p.412) may occur due to ischaemia reperfusion injury.

Likely thrombotic cause in a viable limb

- Emergency angiography: usually percutaneous angiography with digital subtraction angiography, but CT and MRI angiograms are also possible.

- Depending on the severity of the underlying PVD and the length of the occlusion, either emergency bypass surgery or percutaneous transfemoral thrombolysis may be used.

Non-viable limb or patient not fit for revascularization surgery

- Patients with non-viable limbs, or those not fit enough for complex revascularization surgery should undergo emergency amputation after adequate resuscitation.
- Patients with non-viable limbs who are unfit for either revascularization surgery or amputation should be given palliative care.
  - Admit to a ward side-room, and prescribe parenteral analgesia to keep the patient comfortable. A syringe-driver is often necessary.
  - Ensure that a 'do not resuscitate' order is completed and documented in the notes.
  - Keep the patient and family fully informed. Death is expected within 24h.

☼ Vascular trauma

Vascular trauma may be blunt or penetrating. Blunt trauma often occurs as a result of fractures around the knee, or supracondylar humeral fractures in children. Blunt trauma presents with ischaemia of the distal circulation. Penetrating arterial trauma is increasingly common (e.g. knife, gunshot, or shrapnel wounds) and usually presents with haemorrhage. Iatrogenic injury is also common (Box 13.6). Examples of traumatic arterial injury are shown in Box 13.7. Substance abuse can also lead to vascular injury (Box 13.8).

History
- Mechanism and timing of injury.
- Associated injuries to bones, nerves, organs, soft tissues, etc.
- Estimation of blood loss.
- Features of distal limb ischaemia (📖 p.333).
- Significant medical history:
  - pre-existing vascular disease: IHD, TIA/CVA, PVD;
  - risk factors for atherosclerosis: smoking, ↑ BP, diabetes, hyperlipidaemia, family history;
  - history of varicose veins: in case a vein graft is necessary;
  - anticoagulation or aspirin therapy.

❶ Resuscitation and primary survey may take precedence over history-taking (📖 p.42).

Examination
- General appearance: pale, clammy, poorly perfused peripheries; tachypnoea suggests significant blood loss.
- Tachycardia, hypotension if haemorrhage.
- Injury site.
  - Pulsatile haemorrhage or expanding/pulsatile haematoma.
  - Listen for a bruit.
  - ❶ Apply firm pressure directly over the site of bleeding.
- Distal limb:
  - colour (pale/cyanotic/fixed staining), temperature, movement, sensation;
  - pulses, particularly those distal to injury;
  - measure ABPI in the distal pulse if possible using a hand-held Doppler.
- ❶ Compare with the uninjured limb.
- ❶ Look for evidence of a compartment syndrome (📖 p.412).
- ❶ Repeated examination is essential to detect evolving ischaemia.

Initial investigations
- FBC: ↓ Hb due to haemorrhage.
- U&Es, PT, APTT: as baseline investigations.
- G&S for all vascular trauma, and cross-match 4–8 units of packed RBCs if severe haemorrhage has occurred.
- Limb X-ray: if fracture or foreign body (e.g. glass, bullet) is suspected.

Box 13.6 Iatrogenic vascular trauma

- Penetrating intraoperative injuries: usually detected intraoperatively, e.g. trocar injuries in laparoscopic surgery.
- Blunt intraoperative injuries: usually due to prolonged positioning of the patient with flexed joints (e.g. Lloyd–Davies position) or joint dislocation (e.g. total knee replacement).
- Intravascular procedures: false aneurysms, arteriovenous fistulae, and dissections may occur after percutaneous angiography, angioplasty, stenting, or intravascular catheter insertion.

Box 13.7 Types of traumatic arterial injury

- Traumatic spasm: reactive vasospasm without a gross injury.
- Intimal injury: the intima is less elastic than either the media or adventitia, and fractures first when an artery is stretched. This can lead to an intimal flap and arterial dissection.
- External compression, e.g. from a haematoma or bone fragment.
- False aneurysm: contained bleeding from artery into adjacent tissues.
- Arteriovenous fistula: occurs after penetration through an adjacent artery and vein.
- Laceration: a partial tear in an artery.
- Transection: a complete division of an artery.

Box 13.8 Substance abuse and vascular injury

Illicit substances can cause vascular injury because of vessel puncture (e.g. heroin) or as a result of the drug itself.

Injection-related vascular complications
- Arterial puncture: embolization, thrombosis, arterial spasm, false aneurysm, mycotic aneurysm.
- Venous puncture: thrombophlebitis, venous thrombosis, infective endocarditis.
- Simultaneous venous and arterial puncture leads to an arteriovenous fistula.

❶ Never examine a needle site wound with your fingers due to the risk of a retained needle and the possibility of hepatitis B, C, and HIV infection in the patient.

Drug-related complications Some recreational drugs have direct effects on the vascular tree that may result in acute presentation. Cocaine is both sympathomimetic and thrombogenic, and can lead to stroke, MI, aortic dissection, or arterial thrombosis. Management involves control of hypertension, anticoagulation (if thrombosis) has occurred), and treatment of the underlying vascular defect.

Initial management
- ❶ A bleeding penetrating injury should have direct pressure applied to it immediately while IV fluid resuscitation is begun (📖 p.52).
- Give high-flow O_2 via a non-rebreathing mask.
- Insert 2 × large-bore cannulae, preferably on uninjured limbs.
  - ❶ If possible, avoid using the long saphenous vein as it may be required to reconstruct an artery.
- Give IV fluid resuscitation, aiming for a systolic BP of 100mmHg to avoid further bleeding.
- Reduce and splint any long bone fractures/dislocations, and check the pulses afterwards.

Further investigations
In blunt trauma, further investigations may be necessary.
- Angiography is the gold standard investigation. If the patient is unstable, it can be performed on-table in theatre.
- Duplex USS may identify the injury site, thrombosis, false aneurysm, or fistula, but is very observer-dependent.

Further management
- Emergency surgical exploration is required for vascular injuries with distal ischaemia and for penetrating vascular injuries that do not stop after a period of direct pressure.
- Vascular trauma associated with orthopaedic injuries generally requires immediate reduction and fracture fixation, followed by vascular reconstruction.
- False aneurysms can usually be successfully treated by thrombin injection under duplex ultrasound guidance.
- Arteriovenous fistulas can be stented or embolized with coils.
- Large vessel trauma may be amenable to endovascular stenting.

⊙ **Varicose vein haemorrhage**

Varicose veins are abnormally dilated superficial veins. They usually arise in the legs as a result of incompetent valves within the deep and superficial venous systems as well as within the perforating veins which allow the superficial system to drain into the deep system. They are usually idiopathic, but may arise secondary to DVTs, proximal compression such as from a pelvic mass (or pregnancy), or as a result of an arteriovenous fistula. The only emergency associated with varicose veins is venous haemorrhage.

Clinical features

- There is a history of varicose veins.
- Bleeding may occur with or without trauma, and may be profuse.
- On examination the patient may be shocked, with a tachycardia and hypotension.
- The bleeding is from a small ulcer overlying a varix, usually around the ankle.

Investigations

- FBC: ↓ Hb due to blood loss. Repeat after IV fluid resuscitation to reveal true Hb.
- PT, APTT: to detect coagulopathy. Check the INR if the patient is on warfarin.
- G&S: in all patients. If severe haemorrhage has occurred, cross-match 2–4 units of packed RBCs.

Management

- ❶ Immediately elevate the affected limb above the level of the heart and apply pressure to the bleeding point. Bleeding stops immediately unless there is an underlying arteriovenous fistula (e.g. haemodialysis fistula).
- Give high-flow O_2 via a non-rebreathing mask.
- Insert 2 × large-bore cannulae and begin IV fluid resuscitation with crystalloid or colloid. Severe blood loss requires packed RBCs.
- Correct INR with FFP if on the patient is on warfarin.
- Continue limb elevation and pressure. If bleeding is ongoing, infiltrate with LA and suture across the bleeding point (📖 p.510).

In most cases the bleeding stops spontaneously and no further immediate treatment is required. Elective attention to the underlying varicose veins is necessary when the patient is fit.

Early postoperative complications: introduction

The most common complications after major vascular surgery are bleeding, and ischaemia of distal organs. Bleeding is dealt with elsewhere (📖 p.154). Ischaemia may occur because of thrombosis or embolism. ACS (📖 p.142) and AF (📖 p.158) can also occur, as generalized atherosclerotic vascular disease is present in nearly all patients undergoing major vascular surgery.

Early postoperative complications: open AAA repair

Many of the complications following repair of AAA are similar whether the repair is open or endovascular. Specific complications after endovascular aneurysm repair (EVAR) are discussed in the following section. Graft infection and aorto-duodenal fistulae (📖 p.190) tend to present late.

Emboli

Distal emboli originate within the aneurysm sac, within the prosthetic graft, or from the distal and proximal clamp sites. Distal embolization is particularly common after ruptured AAA repair, where anticoagulation is not given before the aorta is clamped. Distal emboli manifest with an acutely ischaemic foot or leg, depending on the extent. Embolectomy should be considered, combined with fasciotomy if the diagnosis was delayed.

Distal embolization into the small vessels of the foot produces pain and a rash (livedo reticularis) in the presence of palpable pedal pulses. This is known as trash foot, and is often due to cholesterol emboli from atherosclerotic plaques. It may progress to ulceration and gangrene. Treatment is with anticoagulation and supportive measures.

Ileus

As with any intraperitoneal operation, AAA repair is associated with ileus. Management follows standard principles (📖 p.295). Exclude pancreatitis by checking the serum amylase. Ileus may also occur in the presence of ischaemia and, if there was intraoperative concern with the appearance of the small bowel, exploration may be advisable.

Renal impairment

Renal impairment is common following AAA repair, especially after a rupture. If multiple renal arteries were present the more distal vessels arising from the aneurysm sac are sacrificed. Juxtarenal and suprarenal AAAs require suprarenal clamping and the kidneys suffer a prolonged period of ischaemia. Distal emboli and angiography exacerbate any renal injury.

The operation note will indicate the clamp position and likelihood of renal compromise. A fall in urine output postoperatively is the first sign of renal impairment. Assess the patient to ensure this is not due to postoperative haemorrhage. Investigations should include U&Es, with particular attention to the serum K^+ which may rise dangerously high.

Treat ↑ K^+ (📖 p.18), adequately rehydrate, and stop all nephrotoxic medications. Check ABG and serum lactate to assess the presence of metabolic acidosis. ITU referral for renal replacement therapy is needed for progressive metabolic acidosis, ↑ K^+ refractory to standard treatment, fluid overload with oliguria, or symptomatic uraemia.

Colonic ischaemia

The IMA arises from the abdominal aorta midway between the renal arteries and the bifurcation. In most patients with a large AAA the origin of the IMA is occluded. Where the IMA is patent it is oversewn during open repair, or excluded from the circulation in an endovascular repair.

Blood supply to the descending and sigmoid colon is then dependent on collaterals from the marginal artery (of Drummond) supplied by the middle colic artery above, and branches of the internal iliac artery below. Where the collateral supply is inadequate the colon becomes ischaemic. Other contributing factors include intraoperative use of vasopressors such as epinephrine and norepinephrine, operative exclusion of the internal iliac arteries (e.g. aorto-bifemoral graft), embolization to the internal iliac arteries, and prolonged aortic cross-clamping.

The incidence of symptomatic colonic ischaemia is 5–10%. Ischaemia may be mucosal, mucosal and muscular (heals with stricturing), or transmural (results in perforation).

- Clinical features. The classic triad is present in ~ 50% of cases (diarrhoea, blood in the stools, peritonitis—a late sign of impending or actual perforation).

❶ Other features include unexplained oliguria, sepsis, and shock.

- Investigation. FBC shows ↑↑ WCC early, but later ↓ and ↓ platelets. U&Es show ↑ urea and creatinine, and serum lactate is ↑. A coagulopathy may be present on PT and APTT. Check stool cultures to exclude infective colitis, and request CXR to exclude perforation. AXR shows left-sided mucosal oedema (thumb-printing). The diagnosis is confirmed by colonoscopy ± biopsies.
- Management. IV fluid resuscitation to treat ↓ BP. When transmural gangrene is suspected clinically or endoscopically, emergency colectomy is necessary.

Pancreatitis

Postoperative pancreatitis is a recognized complication of AAA repair, and is particularly common where the AAA has ruptured preoperatively. It is investigated and managed as for any case of pancreatitis (📖 p.244).

Graft thrombosis

An uncommon complication of AAA repair, thrombosis of the graft is usually related to a technical problem at one of the anastomoses. It presents with bilateral lower limb ischaemia. Diagnosis can be confirmed by angiography or contrast-enhanced CT; urgent thrombectomy is indicated.

Early postoperative complications: endovascular aneurysm repair (EVAR)

Early complications relate to accessing the femoral arteries to deploy the endovascular grafts, and include distal embolization (📖 p.332), thrombosis (📖 p.332), and bleeding (📖 p.154). Endoleaks (presence of blood flow outside the lumen of the endoluminal graft but within the aneurysm sac) usually occur late, are generally asymptomatic, and are usually only detected by radiological surveillance.

Early postoperative complications: limb revascularization

Limb revascularization is performed for the acutely ischaemic limb, e.g. embolectomy, or bypass surgery for thrombosis. Revascularized limbs must be monitored carefully for bleeding and other complications.

Graft thrombosis may present as an acutely ischaemic limb or a worsening of the pre-surgery ischaemic symptoms. There is typically no palpable distal pulse and no pulse (or Doppler signal) in the conduit. Check the operation note to see if pulses were present at the end of surgery. Duplex USS confirms thrombus in the graft. Early thrombosis (within 48h) merits re-exploration, thrombectomy, and on-table angiography. If there is a technical problem, revision surgery is necessary. If persistent thrombus is visible on-table, thrombolysis may be appropriate.

Reperfusion syndrome

Reperfusion of limbs of borderline viability leads to ischaemia reperfusion injury, and rhabdomyolysis. Lactic acid is flushed out of the limb, leading to a severe metabolic acidosis. Compartment syndrome can occur due to muscle swelling, as can ALI/ARDS. Rhabdomyolysis leads to $\uparrow K^+$, $\downarrow Ca^{2+}$, and CK > 5 × normal, and can cause acute renal failure. Check for myoglobinuria (dusky brown urine, positive for blood on dipstick) and monitor U&Es, urine output, and ABGs carefully.

Maintain good hydration and, if features of rhabdomyolysis occur, request urgent review by the on-call intensivist. HDU/ITU admission is often required for aggressive IV fluid resuscitation (e.g. with mannitol), alkalinization of urine with $NaHCO_3$, and correction of deranged electrolytes. Haemofiltration may be required if acute renal failure develops.

Compartment syndrome (📖 p.412)

Emboli

Emboli may arise from the arteries at the time of clamping, as a consequence of inadequate heparinization allowing thrombus to form adjacent to the clamps, and as a result of material from the vessel wall becoming dislodged as the circulation is restored. Symptoms may vary from those of an acutely ischaemic limb, to minor embolic changes in the skin of a digit or coolness of the limb. Large emboli merit re-exploration; small emboli (trash foot) cannot be retrieved and are best left alone. Consider anticoagulation.

Venous thrombi are common in ischaemic limbs, and may dislodge and cause PEs following revascularization.

Graft infection

This occurs with prosthetic grafts, and is more common where the groin has been explored or a postoperative wound infection occurs. Infection is inevitable when wound breakdown has occurred and has exposed the prosthetic material. If this occurs at an anastomosis, it will fail and catastrophic secondary haemorrhage will occur. Infected grafts should be removed before disaster strikes.

❶ Do not explore wounds overlying vascular grafts. If you suspect a wound infection over a vascular graft, discuss it with your senior.

Lymphocele

This is a collection of lymphatic fluid, common after exposure of the femoral artery via a groin incision. Lymphocele presents as a fluctuant swelling, occasionally with a lymphatic leak. Most resolve spontaneously. Where a leak is present infection must be assumed and antimicrobial therapy commenced to protect any underlying graft from infection. Discuss with your senior.

Early postoperative complications: carotid endarterectomy

Removal of an atherosclerotic plaque from the bifurcation of the common carotid artery has been shown to reduce the risk of stroke in selected patient subgroups. Carotid endarterectomy can be performed under regional anaesthesia or GA.

Cranial nerve damage

Many nerves, both cranial and peripheral, pass near the operative site and may be damaged. The prognosis depends on the degree of nerve damage (📖 p.418). Nerve function should be checked once the patient has recovered from the anaesthetic.

Hypoglossal nerve (cranial nerve XII) The nerve usually passes 3–5cm cranial to the common carotid artery bifurcation, but may occasionally be just above it. Damage to this nerve is the most common early complication after carotid endarterectomy. While it might be divided inadvertently, the commonest injury is a neurapraxia and is secondary to retraction during surgery. It manifests as deviation of the tongue to the affected side when protruded.

Greater auricular nerve The greater auricular nerve ascends on sternomastoid deep to platysma and may be divided in the upper part of the incision as it branches into anterior and posterior parts. The consequences are numbness over the parotid gland and ear lobe.

Superior laryngeal nerve The superior laryngeal nerve passes posterior to the internal and external carotid arteries, running adjacent to the uppermost curve of the superior thyroid artery, and may be damaged as this is mobilized. Injury results in a weak voice unable to make high-pitched notes, and one that tires easily.

Recurrent laryngeal nerve The recurrent laryngeal nerve supplies the intrinsic muscles of the larynx. Damage is rare, but may result from the pressure of a postoperative haematoma. It manifests as a weak voice that tires by the end of the day and that can't compete against a noisy background.

Stroke

A postoperative ispilateral hemisphere ischaemic event (stroke or TIA) occurs in up to 5% of patients. An immediate postoperative neurological deficit is an indication for emergency re-exploration. Most will be due to technical errors that can be addressed at re-operation. Intraoperative angiography can be performed, with thrombectomy or thrombolysis as appropriate.

The development of an ispilateral headache, with seizures and visual disturbance (flashing lights, blind spots), within hours/days of returning to the ward is due either to intracranial haemorrhage or cerebral hyperperfusion. Investigation is with emergency CT head. Treatment of hyperperfusion involves aggressive antihypertensive therapy with anticonvulsant therapy if seizures are present. If uncontrolled, intracranial haemorrhage will ensue.

Early postoperative complications: angiography/angioplasty/stenting

Complications following endovascular procedures are common. The main complications are bleeding, thrombosis, embolism, dissection, arteriovenous fistula, and false aneurysm.

Bleeding

Most haemorrhage occurs at the arterial puncture site and responds to direct pressure. Risk factors include anticoagulation, antiplatelet medication, multiple punctures, and large cannulae (e.g. those used when stenting). Diseased vessels predispose to bleeding since the calcified wall lacks the elasticity required to close the puncture site. Bleeding may also occur as a result of perforation by a guidewire. A high puncture in the external iliac artery instead of the common femoral artery cannot be satisfactorily compressed post-procedure and may be associated with a large haematoma in the retroperitoneal space. This is usually not evident on groin examination, but Hb is ↓. CT is required to make the diagnosis.

Thrombosis

Fibrin and platelet aggregates form along the side of the catheter, and when the catheter is removed these adhere to the side of the vessel. Clot propagates and thrombosis of the vessel follows. Presentation is as an acutely ischaemic limb (□ p.332). Treatment usually involves anticoagulation and surgical exploration of the vessel.

Embolization/trash foot

Emboli may arise from the catheter itself, or the catheter or guidewire may dislodge debris from the wall of a blood vessel. Occasionally, part of the catheter, guidewire, stent, or angioplasty balloon may break off and embolize. Microemboli or cholesterol emboli lodge in the small vessels of the feet if a femoral puncture was performed and result in trash foot.

Large emboli may be removed at exploration. Microemboli require anticoagulation to prevent clot propagation and supportive treatment is appropriate.

Dissection

The catheter guidewire may deliberately, or accidentally, enter a false lumen outside the intima and within the media. Blood tracks through this false passage as an arterial dissection. If the blood does not re-enter the true lumen distally the dissection will result in acute ischaemia.

Deliberate dissection is employed as a method of bypassing an occluded superficial femoral artery. There is an inherent risk that the false lumen will perforate through the adventitia, rather than re-enter the true lumen beyond the obstruction. If this occurs an expanding haematoma forms, visible at angiography. It can usually be managed angiographically, but may result in worsening of the distal ischaemia and necessitate urgent surgical exploration.

False aneurysm

A false aneurysm (pseudoaneurysm) occurs where the puncture site continues to communicate with a cavity within the haematoma outside the vessel. The aneurysm continues to enlarge and may rupture outside the haematoma. In most instances the false aneurysm thromboses spontaneously, and this can be hastened by the application of pressure over the neck of the aneurysm using a duplex ultrasound probe. Thrombosis may be hastened by injection of thrombin into the sac or with the administration of platelets or FFP to patients on antiplatelet or anticoagulant therapy, respectively.

Contrast nephropathy

Deterioration in renal function occurs in up to 10% of patients, and starts within a couple of days of the angiogram and usually lasts 10–14 days. Contrast nephropathy is uncommon in patients who are adequately hydrated, have normal baseline renal function, and do not have diabetes. Where patients are at risk, and contrast angiography is essential, a low osmolality non-ionic contrast agent should be used, IV fluids given the night before, and NSAIDs and aminoglycoside antibiotics avoided (e.g. gentamicin). Watch urine output closely and monitor U&Es. The treatment of renal impairment is supportive (📖 p.342).

Early postoperative complications: thrombolysis

Thrombolysis is commonly used in an attempt to revascularize acutely ischaemic thrombosed limbs. Thrombolytic agents include streptokinase, alteplase, reteplase, and urokinase.

Haemorrhage

Haemorrhage is the most feared complication of thrombolysis. Bleeding commonly occurs at failed venous cannulation/phlebotomy sites and the intravascular cannulation site for delivery of the fibrinolytic. Place pressure over the bleeding area and resuscitate with IV fluids. Ongoing bleeding requires the thrombolysis to be reduced or stopped. More severe bleeding may occur elsewhere, including the upper (📖 p.190) or lower (📖 p.280) GI tract, intracerebrally, or into the retroperitoneum.

Distal embolization

As the occluded vessel reopens, fragments of undissolved clot embolize into distal vessels, necessitating continuation of thrombolysis for some time after patency of the main vessel is restored. In some circumstances, such as in the presence of a popliteal aneurysm, so many clots can be dislodged into the distal circulation that the lytic ability of the thrombolysis is exceeded, and the foot becomes irreversibly ischaemic. Trash foot is common.

Reperfusion syndrome (📖 p.346)

Anaphylaxis

Most common with streptokinase. Avoid repeated use.

Early postoperative complications: amputation

Phantom limb pain

This is a painful sensation perceived to be in the amputated limb. This is more common where ischaemic pain was present preoperatively, and can be minimized by pre- and perioperative epidural anaesthesia. Once present, it can be moderated by amitriptyline, carbamazepine, or gabapentin.

Wound infection

Usually due to skin organisms such as *Staphylococcus aureus*, it is more common when ischaemia is still present in the stump tissues. It is difficult to treat, but may be improved by IV antibiotics and negative pressure occlusive dressings. Wound infections delay mobilization and often result in revision to a higher level amputation.

❶ Necrotizing soft tissue infections (e.g. gas gangrene) may also occur (📖 p.478). Sepsis and confusion are often present. Check for crepitus on palpation of the stump. Always consider this in a confused patient post-amputation.

Early postoperative complications: open varicose vein surgery

Open surgery for long saphenous vein (LSV) territory varicose veins usually consists of ligation of the LSV at the sapheno-femoral junction, stripping to the level of the knee, and multiple avulsions of calf varicosities. USS-guided foam injection and thermal ablation techniques are increasing in popularity.

Femoral vein damage

Groin dissection to expose the LSV may result in damage to the femoral vein or artery. Failure to correctly identify the saphenous vein can result in ligation of the superficial femoral vein. This causes a painful, cyanotic swollen leg. Urgent duplex USS followed by re-exploration is the management of choice, but may not be possible if the superficial femoral vein has already occluded with thrombus.

Haematoma

A groin haematoma results from ligatures slipping off tributaries of the LSV, or from the sapheno-femoral junction itself. Thigh haematomas occur from the tunnel from which the LSV has been stripped, and into which its tributaries still flow. These should have been controlled by leg bandaging at the time of surgery. For both types of haematoma, the treatment is to lie the patient head-down, reducing venous pressure, and to place pressure over the haematoma. In most cases no further treatment is necessary.

An early extensive groin haematoma might need re-exploration, a procedure that should be undertaken by an experienced surgeon.

Deep venous thrombosis (📕 p.322)

Nerve damage

The most common nerve to be damaged is the saphenous nerve as it passes below the knee, intimately related to the LSV to supply cutaneous sensation over the medial calf down to the hallux. It is damaged by stripping below the knee, and presents with numbness in its area of distribution. Damage is avoided if veins are stripped to the knee, and not below. There is no treatment. The femoral nerve is sufficiently lateral to avoid damage by all but the most hapless surgeon.

Paediatric surgery

Introduction

The management of sick children demands specialist skills. Many of the conditions seen in children are distinct from those seen in adults. Conditions that occur in both often present differently in children (e.g. appendicitis).

You may have limited paediatric experience and dealing with anxious parents makes this especially stressful. However, the on-call paediatric team will be more than happy to advise and assist you, and basic surgical principles in children are identical to those in adults.

Managing paediatric patients requires an understanding of the physiological differences between children and adults.

- Age determines normal physiological parameters (Box 14.1).
- Maintenance fluid volumes and resuscitation bolus fluid volumes are based on weight (Box 14.2).
- Children compensate for hypovolaemia more effectively than adults. Circulatory collapse can therefore occur with little warning.
- Children have a high energy requirement and should not be kept NBM for periods beyond those that are absolutely necessary (p.14).

Interdisciplinary co-operation

In larger teaching hospitals, on-call specialist paediatric surgeons review children under a certain age, usually 4 years. However, in the majority of hospitals, the on-call general surgical team may be called to see children of all ages. The surgical team may require paediatric input for:

- fluid and electrolyte management of dehydrated children;
- assistance with gaining IV access;
- advice on analgesia;
- excluding non-surgical causes for acute abdominal pain.

❶ Have a low threshold for discussing management with your seniors and the paediatric team. Children with sepsis, severe dehydration, or significant medical problems require joint care.

Assessment of children with acute abdominal pain

Most children seen by the surgical on-call team have acute abdominal pain. The following should be kept in mind.

- White coats are intimidating—take them off before seeing children.

History

- This is usually taken through the parents, and is often incomplete.
- Family history may be especially important, e.g. hypertrophic pyloric stenosis.
- If gastroenteritis is possible, enquire after recent contacts and siblings.

❶ Listen carefully to a parent's concerns. They know their children best.

Examination

- Co-operation may be difficult, especially in infants. If necessary, examine the child while they lie in their mother's arms. Distracting them with a toy can be useful.
- With older children, establishing rapport is essential. Get down to their level, smile, and make your examination as gentle as possible.

Box 14.1 Physiological parameters and age

Heart rate and respiratory rate
- < 1 year old: HR 110–160/min, RR 30–40/min
- 1–2 years old: HR 100–150/min, RR 25–35/min
- 2–5 years old: HR 95–140/min, RR 25–30/min
- 5–12 years old: HR 80–120/min, RR 20–25/min
- > 12 years old: HR 60–100/min, RR 15–20/min

Blood pressure
- Systolic BP = 80 + (2 × age in years)
- Diastolic BP = 2/3rd systolic

Urine output
- 0–3 years old: 2mL/kg/h
- 3–5 years old: 1mL/kg/h
- 6–12 years old: 0.5–1mL/kg/h

Box 14.2 Paediatric fluid requirements

Daily maintenance fluid requirements
- For the first 10kg: 100mL/kg
- For 10–20kg: 50mL/kg
- For 20–50kg: 20mL/kg

For example, for a child weighing 38kg, daily maintenance fluid requirement is (10 × 100) + (10 × 50) + (18 × 20) = 1000 + 500 + 360 = 1860mL. This is usually given as 0.45% saline + 5% dextrose.

Resuscitation bolus Give 20mL/kg crystalloid (normal saline or Hartmann's).

- Assess the level of hydration by examining the mucous membranes, skin turgor, and the fontanelles in neonates.
- Examination of the ears and throat is mandatory in children < 10 years old to exclude an URTI.
- Do not check for rebound tenderness in children when trying to elicit early signs of peritonitis. It causes unnecessary pain. Check for pain on coughing or percussion instead. In young school-age children, use the hop test. Ask the child to hop on one leg—localized abdominal pain on hopping is a significant finding.
- DREs should not be performed routinely. Discuss with your seniors if you think it necessary.

Investigations
- FBC and U&Es are routine, while serum amylase and LFTs are often not required. PT/INR and APTT are rarely necessary. Use anaesthetic creams before venepuncture.
- Request a CXR in febrile children with vague abdominal signs to exclude pneumonia.
- All children with abdominal symptoms or signs should have a urine dipstick to exclude a UTI.

- Radiological investigations using high doses of ionizing radiation (e.g. CT) should be avoided but may require sedation if essential. USS is often more useful.

❶ Don't forget—you must involve your seniors **early** when asked to assess a child. Sick children are quiet and lethargic and don't want to get up to play. Consultants should be informed as soon as possible if an acutely unwell child is admitted under their care.

Other emergencies

Surgical emergencies in the neonate are not covered in the following sections, as these children invariably present to paediatricians first. Many are detected on antenatal USS and are usually managed by specialist regional paediatric surgery units. This includes necrotizing enterocolitis, oesophageal atresia/tracheo-oesophageal fistula, duodenal atresia, anorectal abnormalities, meconium ileus, diaphragmatic hernias, gastroschisis, and exomphalos. Acute scrotal pain (📖 p.372) and appendicitis (📖 p.262) are discussed elsewhere.

:Ö: **Hypertrophic pyloric stenosis**

Hypertrophy of the circular muscle of the pylorus occurs in 0.2–0.4% of neonates and infants. It nearly always presents between 3 and 8 weeks of birth and is more common in males, and firstborns. 10% of affected infants have a positive family history.

History
- Projectile, non-bile-stained vomiting beginning 2–4 weeks after birth.
- Vomiting usually occurs within 30min of a feed, and the child is hungry afterwards.

Examination
- Dehydration and weight loss are invariably present.
- Gastric peristalsis may be visible.
- A firm, olive-sized lump may be palpable in the RUQ.
- ❶ Abdominal examination is often completely normal.

Initial investigations
- FBC: usually ↔.
- U&Es: often show ↓ Na^+, ↓ K^+, and ↑ creatinine due to gastric fluid loss.
- Serum chloride is ↓ and ABG shows a metabolic alkalosis; both are due to loss of gastric HCl.

Initial management
Obtain IV access and re-hydrate with normal saline + K^+.

❶ IV access and fluid and electrolyte management require paediatric expertise. Involve the on-call paediatric team **immediately**.

Further investigations
- Test feeds can reveal gastric peristalsis and make palpation of the hypertrophied pylorus easier.
- USS: the investigation of choice if the hypertrophied pylorus is not palpable, it shows a hypertrophied pyloric sphincter.
  - If USS is inconclusive, contrast meal reveals complete pyloric obstruction.

Further management
Surgical correction is necessary but should only take place once fluid and electrolyte abnormalities are corrected.
- An NG tube is required to empty the stomach.
- Ramstedt's pyloromyotomy can be performed through a small trans-verse incision in the right upper abdomen or a periumbilical incision. A longitudinal incision is made through the thickened pylorus until the mucosa pouts through. The laparoscopic approach is increasingly popular.
- Feeds are re-introduced within a few hours postoperatively.

☼ Malrotation and midgut volvulus

Failure of the midgut to rotate 270° anti-clockwise during development leads to the caecum lying anterior to the duodenum (malrotation). The base of the small bowel mesentery is therefore very narrow, predisposing to volvulus, and occlusion of the superior mesenteric vessels, causing midgut ischaemia. Midgut volvulus commonly occurs in the first few days of life. The majority of cases present within the first year of life but can also present later in childhood or in adults. The volvulus may be partial and intermittent, confusing the clinical picture and delaying diagnosis.

History

- Bile-stained vomiting.
  - ❶ Bile-stained vomiting in a baby is malrotation volvulus until proved otherwise.
- Sudden onset of abdominal pain, manifested by screaming.
- Ischaemic bowel leads to bloody diarrhoea.

Examination

- Inconsolable, dehydrated infant.
- Abdominal distension is mild, due to the high obstruction.
- Abdominal tenderness is diffuse.
- Later, generalized peritonitis and shock develop.

Initial investigations

- FBC: ↑ WCC.
- U&Es: ↑ creatinine due to dehydration, ↑/↓ Na^+ and K^+ also.
- Supine AXR: the first part of the duodenum and the stomach are distended with flecks of gas in the bowel distally, although radiographic signs are variable.

Initial management

- Obtain IV access, and give a 20mL/kg crystalloid bolus. Further boluses may be required.
- Parenteral analgesia (e.g. IV morphine) may be required. Discuss with the on-call paediatric team.
- Insert an NG tube.
- Start broad spectrum IV antibiotics.

❶ If midgut volvulus is suspected, discuss with your senior and inform the on-call paediatric team **immediately**.

Further investigations and management

These depend on the clinical state of the child.

▶▶ If peritonitis is present, urgent laparotomy is required after fluid resuscitation. The bowel is untwisted and gangrenous bowel is resected. The base of the mesentery is 'widened' by a Ladd's procedure.

If peritonitis is not present and the diagnosis is in doubt, an emergency contrast meal and follow-through indicate an abnormally positioned duodenal–jejunal flexure with a cut-off. Urgent laparotomy is required, as in the previous paragraph.

☼ Inguinal hernias

Inguinal hernias occur in children when the processus vaginalis fails to close. They are common in the first 2 years of life, especially in boys (4:1), on the right, and in those born prematurely. Reducible inguinal hernias can be repaired electively. However, irreducible (incarcerated) inguinal hernias often present as an emergency. Strangulation (📖 p.174) is rare. In females the ovary is often within the hernial sac and may be mistaken for an enlarged lymph node.

Clinical features

- The parents notice a lump in the groin or scrotum, usually when the child cries.
- On examination, the lump in the groin may extend into the scrotum and is usually obvious. Bilateral hernias may be present.
- The lump enlarges and becomes firmer when the child cries.
- The spermatic cord cannot be identified above the swelling. This differentiates a hernia from a hydrocele. Check for transillumination.
- Gentle, sustained pressure may reduce an initially irreducible hernia.
  - ❶ Significant tenderness and/or colour changes indicate strangulation. Reduction should **not** be attempted.
- Abdominal distension implies obstruction, and is usually a late feature.

Investigations are usually not necessary. If the child is systemically unwell or if there is evidence of obstruction, take blood for FBC and U&Es.

Management

Children with inguinal hernias that do not reduce with gentle pressure require admission. These hernias can then nearly all be reduced after analgesia and sedation. Discuss with the local general paediatric surgeon and on-call paediatric team.

▶▶ If there is evidence of strangulation, emergency herniotomy is required. If local expertise is not available, **immediate** referral to the regional specialist paediatric surgical team is required. If significant dehydration is present, give a 20mL/kg crystalloid bolus IV, and discuss with the on-call paediatric team.

:Ö: **Intussusception**

This occurs when the proximal bowel (the intussusceptum) telescopes inside the distal portion (the intussuscipiens). The peak age for presentation is 6 months, but intussusception can occur at any age. It is usually located at the ileocolic junction, and is thought to be due to peristaltic action on enlarged Peyer's patches within the ileal wall. Any mucosal abnormality (e.g. polyp, tumour, Meckel's diverticulum) predisposes to intussusception and should be suspected in cases of recurrent intussusception, or if this condition presents in the older age group.

History
- Intermittent, severe abdominal pain (manifested as screaming in infants). The child may be well between episodes.
- The child may appear pale during attacks.
- Passage of 'redcurrant jelly' mucus or stool.
- Vomiting is a late feature.

Examination
- The child may be inconsolable during episodes with the legs drawn up.
- A sausage-like mass may be palpable, usually in the upper abdomen.
- Distension appears late.
- Peritonitis indicates bowel ischaemia or perforation.
- DRE may reveal blood-stained mucus. The intussusception may be palpable.

❶ Intussusception can rapidly lead to severe dehydration and sepsis.

Initial investigations
- FBC: ↑ WCC.
- U&Es: ↑ creatinine.
- Supine AXR. Distended loops of bowel can be visible, with a paucity of gas in the RIF. A soft-tissue shadow is often present.

Initial management
- Obtain IV access and, if dehydrated, give a 20mL/kg crystalloid bolus. Further boluses may be required.
- Parenteral analgesia (e.g. IV morphine) may be required. Discuss with the on-call paediatric team.
- Insert an NG tube.

❶ If intussusception is suspected, discuss with your senior and inform the on-call paediatric team **immediately**.

Further investigations and management
These depend on the clinical state of the child.
- If intussusception is suspected, but a mass cannot be felt, arrange emergency USS. An intussusception in cross-section appears as a 'target' sign.
- If intussusception is suspected on USS, or is highly likely clinically, an emergency air enema can be both diagnostic and therapeutic.
- ❶ Radiological expertise is often unavailable out-of-hours. Transfer to a regional centre is usually necessary.

- In children with clinical evidence of peritonitis or after failed air enema reduction, emergency laparotomy is required. Reduction is performed by gently squeezing the distal bowel and pushing the intussusceptum proximally. Resection is required if the bowel is ischaemic or a mucosal abnormality is found.

① Swallowed foreign bodies

Preschool children often examine objects by placing them in their mouths, and can swallow foreign bodies. The narrowest part of the GI tract is the cricopharyngeal sphincter, superior to the oesophagus. If objects have passed into the stomach they are likely to pass all the way through the tract without incident. Occasionally objects may impact at the pylorus or terminal ileum.

- If the child is well and the object contains metal, confirm that it has passed into the stomach or beyond on AXR ± CXR. The object should pass within 7 days. Advise the parents to return if it has not done so, or if the child has abdominal symptoms.
- Children with abdominal symptoms require admission for assessment and observation. Objects in the stomach and duodenum may be retrieved by upper GI endoscopy. More distal obstruction or the presence of peritonitis requires laparotomy or laparoscopy.

▶▶ Ingested button batteries may contain mercury or other hazardous heavy metals (Box 14.3).

❶ Objects lodged in the oropharynx, laryngopharynx, trachea, or oesophagus are dealt with by ENT or paediatric surgeons.

Box 14.3 Management of ingested button batteries

The risk of damage with modern button batteries is low, as long as they have not lodged in the oesophagus.
- Obtain CXR + AXR, and refer to ENT **immediately** for emergency endoscopy if the battery has not passed into the stomach.
- Where the battery has passed into the stomach and the child is asymptomatic, further treatment is usually not needed.
- Discuss with the National Poisons Information Service.
- Advise the parents to return if it has not passed within 7 days, or if the child has abdominal symptoms.

:Ö: Rectal bleeding

Rectal bleeding may occur in children. As with adults, there are many causes (Box 14.4). Clinical features vary with the degree of blood loss and the underlying cause. If severe, symptoms and signs of shock may be present.

History

- Sudden onset of PR bleeding.
    - Bright red blood implies lesion in the distal colon, rectum, or anus.
    - Altered red blood usually originates from the distal small bowel or proximal colon.
- May be painless (e.g. polyps, arteriovenous malformations) or painful (e.g. anal fissure, intussusception).
- May be associated with either constipation (e.g. anal fissure) or diarrhoea/mucus (e.g. gastroenteritis, IBD).

Examination

- Check the lips and buccal mucosa for pigmentation suggesting Peutz–Jegher syndrome.
- Look for Henoch–Schönlein purpura on the buttocks and lower limbs.
- Abdominal tenderness may indicate intussusception, midgut volvulus, IBD, or gastroenteritis.
- DRE can be performed in older children.
    - Rectal prolapse may be seen as a lump at the anus (ΔΔ intussusception through the anus).
    - An anal fissure may be visible on exposure of the anal verge and significant tenderness is present on attempted insertion of a finger.

❶ Any suspicion of NAI/sexual abuse on history or examination should be discussed with the on-call paediatric team **immediately**.

►► If the child is shocked, involve the on-call paediatric team **immediately**.

Initial investigations

- FBC: ↓ Hb is present in significant bleeding.
- U&Es: Usually ↔, though creatinine can be ↑ if glomerulonephritis due to Henoch–Schönlein purpura is present.
- ESR: ↑ in IBD.
- PT/INR and APTT: exclude congenital bleeding tendencies (e.g. haemophilia).
- G&S: on all children with PR bleeding. Cross-match packed RBCs if bleeding is severe or shock is present.
- If diarrhoea is present, send stool for M,C, & S and virological culture.

Initial management

- Admission is required.
- The priority is to fluid resuscitate and replace lost blood. Give a 20mL/kg crystalloid fluid bolus. If more than 2 boluses are needed to maintain perfusion, give a 10mL/kg bolus of packed RBCs.
- If intussusception (🕮 p.364) or midgut volvulus (🕮 p.361) are possible, investigate and treat accordingly.

Box 14.4 Causes of rectal bleeding in children

- Gastroenteritis, bacterial (often *Campylobacter*), viral, protozoal
- Inflammatory bowel disease (IBD)
- Intussusception (📖 p.364)
- Midgut volvulus (📖 p.361)
- Trauma, consider NAI/sexual abuse
- Meckel's diverticulum (📖 p.265)
- Rectal prolapse
- Anal fissure (📖 p.311)
- Polyps, e.g. juvenile polyps, Peutz–Jegher syndrome, familial adenomatous polyposis (FAP)
- Arteriovenous malformations
- Henoch–Schönlein purpura

Further investigations

- In large volume, painless bleeding, Meckel's diverticulum is likely. The blood is usually dark red. Request a ^{99m}Tc radionuclide scan to visualize ectopic gastric mucosa. Sensitivity and specificity are each ~ 80%.
- ❶ Consider upper GI endoscopy in children with brisk bleeding to exclude a bleeding duodenal ulcer.
- As with adults, bleeding usually stops spontaneously. Lower GI endoscopy should be arranged as an outpatient. Sedation or general anaesthesia are required.
- ❶ Consider referral to a specialist paediatric gastroenterologist.

Further management

This depends on the underlying cause of the bleeding.

- Juvenile polyps are usually solitary and are often found in the rectum. These can be excised endoscopically.
- Peutz–Jegher syndrome requires endoscopic surveillance, and occasionally polypectomy.
- FAP requires screening of family members and, eventually, removal of the colon and rectum.
- Arteriovenous malformations can be ablated endoscopically. Large lesions causing recurrent bleeding may require surgical excision.
- Bacterial gastroenteritis can be treated with oral antibiotics (e.g. ciprofloxacin).
- IBD may require oral salicylates and steroids (oral or as enemas). Refer to the paediatricians.
- Rectal prolapse requires gentle reduction and reassurance. The condition is usually self-limiting, so recurrences require referral to a specialist surgeon.
- Anorectal trauma may require imaging (e.g. CT, MRI) to exclude perforation. A colostomy may be necessary if perforation is confirmed.

- A bleeding Meckel's diverticulum should be excised surgically. The bleeding may be from normal small bowel immediately downstream of the gastric acid-secreting diverticulum—this may need resecting also. Surgery may be necessary despite a negative radionuclide scan.
- Anal fissures should be treated with stool softeners. Vasodilator creams (e.g. GTN) may be required.
- Henoch–Schönlein purpura requires treatment with steroids. Refer to the paediatricians.

Urology

Acute scrotal pain: introduction

Acute scrotal pain can affect males of all ages, although some conditions are more common in certain age groups. **Two key emergency diagnoses not to miss are testicular torsion and Fournier's gangrene**.

❶ If the diagnosis is unclear, ask a senior colleague to review urgently, and always have a low threshold for surgical exploration.

☠ **Torsion of the testes**

Testicular torsion is a surgical emergency. It is most common in boys aged 10–15 years, and is rare in those > 30 years old. Irreversible ischaemic injury can occur within 4h from the onset of pain. The majority of testes can be saved if explored within 8h.

Clinical features

- There is a history of sudden onset unilateral testicular pain, often associated with nausea and vomiting.
- Young boys localize pain poorly and may complain only of abdominal pain; **always** examine the external genitalia as part of a routine abdominal examination.
- On examination, there is an exquisitely tender swollen testicular body, lying high in the scrotum often with overlying scrotal oedema and erythema.
- The contralateral testis may lie high and horizontally in the scrotum (bell-clapper deformity).
- The cord is shortened and thickened.
- ❶ Patients presenting late may have only moderate scrotal tenderness due to prolonged ischaemia.
- ❶ Torsion may be confused with minor scrotal trauma; beware of misdiagnosis.
- ❶ Torsion of an undescended testis presents as pain and/or swelling along the line of the inguinal canal. Check the scrotum for an absent testis.
- ❶ Young boys may not tolerate examination and, if the diagnosis remains uncertain, emergency scrotal exploration is required.

Investigations

❶ Investigations are rarely indicated, have high false positive and false negative rates, and should not delay surgical exploration.

- Scrotal/groin duplex USS is indicated in the case of inguinal pain and ipsilateral absent testis to diagnose and localize a torted inguinal testis.
- Do not delay for the results of blood tests/urine analysis.

Management

❶ Suspected torsion requires emergency scrotal exploration within an hour of the decision to operate.

- The patient should be consented for exploration, bilateral orchidopexy ± orchidectomy.
- Three-point fixation of a viable testis within a sub-dartos pouch should be performed with a non-absorbable material. The contralateral testis should always be fixed through the same incision.
- A non-viable testes should be excised to remove a potential focus of infection and prevent the development of anti-sperm antibodies.

☼ Torsion of the testicular and epididymal appendices

The testicular appendix (the hydatid cyst of Morgagni), and the epididymal appendix may both undergo torsion. This is most common in pre-teenage boys. Torsion of these structures is only important due to clinical mimicry of torsion of the testis.

Clinical features
- The onset of pain is usually rapid, but may be more insidious than testicular torsion.
- On examination, tenderness may be localized to the upper pole of the testis or epididymal head.
- A discrete tender lump may be felt separate from the testis, which may be visible through the illuminated scrotal skin as a 'blue dot'.
- Later presentations are difficult to distinguish from testicular torsion, with testicular swelling and tenderness, reactive hydrocele, and overlying skin oedema and erythema.

Investigations

As with testicular torsion, investigations are not usually indicated.

❶ Unless the diagnosis is clear clinically, the scrotum should be explored.

Management
- If the diagnosis is clear from clinical examination, the management is non-operative, with regular oral NSAIDs. The pain will usually settle within 3–4 days.
- If a torted appendix is found at exploration, simple excision is all that is required. Consensus regarding ipsilateral testicular fixation is lacking—follow the consultant's preference.

① Acute epididymo-orchitis

This is usually caused by pathogens ascending from the lower urinary tract, either spontaneously or following urethral instrumentation. In younger men the causative organism is usually *Chlamydia trachomatis*, and is sexually transmitted. In older men, coliform bacteria predominate. Epididymo-orchitis in young boys is rare, and may indicate an underlying genitourinary tract anomaly.

Clinical features
- The onset of pain and swelling is usually insidious, but may be acute, particularly in younger patients.
- The pain and swelling is usually unilateral, but may be bilateral in conditions such as mumps orchitis.
- Pain may be associated with local urinary symptoms of frequency and dysuria, or systemic complaints such as fevers and rigors.
- Orchitis may occur in children and the cause is frequently viral. The boy may have a concurrent URTI and lymphadenopathy.
- In early presentations, the epididymis may be tender and thickened on examination.
- Later, the entire hemiscrotum may be oedematous and erythematous, with difficulty assessing the underlying anatomy due to gross swelling of the epididymis and testis.
- In advanced cases, a fluctuant abscess may be detected.

Investigations
- MSU: dipstick urinalysis should be performed, although cultures may be sterile in 90% of cases.
- FBC: ↑ WCC.
- Scrotal duplex USS: may detect a hyperaemic, engorged epididymis.

Management
Patients presenting with mild epididymo-orchitis do not require admission.
- Prescribe oral ciprofloxacin 500mg bd (or doxycycline 100mg bd for 1 day then 100mg od). Oral ofloxacin 200–400mg bd covers chlamydia in younger patients. All antibiotics should be given for at least 2 weeks.
- Advise that symptoms may resolve slowly and that oral antibiotics may be required for 6 weeks or longer.
- Bed-rest, scrotal elevation, and NSAIDs help with pain.
- Advise younger patients (and their sexual partners) to attend the genitourinary medicine clinic for a sexually transmitted diseases screen.

Patients with advanced epididymo-orchitis, or those refractory to oral antibiotics should be admitted.
- Resuscitate with IV fluids and give IV gentamicin (usually 3–5mg/kg od).
- An abscess may be present. This requires incision and drainage. USS may be a useful diagnostic adjunct in equivocal cases.

☠ **Fournier's gangrene**

Fournier's gangrene is a life-threatening necrotizing fasciitis (📖 p.478) of the scrotum, perineal, and perianal region. It is usually associated with an infective source, either from the urinary tract, or from the anorectal area. Immediate wide surgical debridement is essential. Suprapubic catheterization is indicated if there is significant peno-scrotal involvement. Once all infected tissue has been cleared and the patient has recovered, delayed primary closure of the scrotal skin may be considered. Plastic surgical input may be required and a defunctioning colostomy may be necessary to facilitate wound healing.

Other causes of acute scrotal pain and swelling

Trauma
- Superficial scrotal lacerations can be explored and sutured under LA.
- If testicular disruption is suspected following blunt trauma, USS is diagnostic.
- If USS is inconclusive, or there is a history of penetrating trauma, surgical exploration should be performed.

Idiopathic scrotal oedema
- Usually in boys < 5 years old.
- Relatively painless and non-tender.
- Pathognomonic sign of a swollen hemiscrotum with scrotal erythema extending up to the inguinal region or the anterior abdominal wall.
- May be bilateral.
- Treatment is non-operative.

Others
- Inguinal hernia, either adult or paediatric.
- Varicocele.
- Communicating hydrocele due to a patent processus vaginalis.

❶ Consider the possibility of a testicular tumour or a bleed into a testicular tumour. If you have any concern that a mass is present, request an USS.

① **Renal tract colic**

Renal tract colic is caused by a stone in the kidney or ureter. In most cases the cause is a small stone passing spontaneously down the ureter, resulting in transient obstruction. Renal tract colic can also be caused by a blood clot, sloughed papilla, or, rarely, a ureteric tumour. Patients with uncomplicated renal tract colic can often be managed as outpatients.

❶ An obstructed, infected renal outflow tract is a urological emergency. Symptoms and signs of sepsis must be sought and, if present, management must be discussed with a urologist.

❶ Renal tract colic in a patient with a solitary kidney is an emergency and should always be discussed with a urologist.

History

- Sudden onset of severe colicky unilateral loin pain, often radiating into the groin, scrotum, or tip of the penis.
- Pain is not improved by lying still.
- Vomiting may occur.
- Rigors indicate sepsis.
- ❶ Anuria is an alarming sign suggesting obstruction of a solitary kidney.

Examination

- Patients may find lying still impossible.
- Unilateral loin or renal angle tenderness.
- Pyrexia or tachycardia may indicate sepsis, although the pain itself may cause a tachycardia.
- ❶ Feel for an AAA in patients > 50 years old (Box 15.1).

Box 15.1 Ruptured AAA and renal tract colic

Ruptured AAA (📖 p.326) with a unilateral retroperitoneal haematoma can mimic renal tract colic. It is rare for patients to present with a first episode of renal tract colic aged > 50, so ask yourself: could this be a ruptured AAA? Have a high index of suspicion, especially in patients with other risk factors for AAA. A ruptured common iliac artery aneurysm may also present like this. Aneurysms are often impalpable in the obese and dipstick haematuria is non-specific. Contact your senior early and consider emergency CT scanning.

Initial investigations

- FBC: ↑ WCC may indicate sepsis.
- U&Es: ↑ urea and creatinine may indicate dehydration, pre-existing renal impairment, or obstruction in a solitary kidney.
- LFTs and serum amylase: exclude biliary disease and acute pancreatitis.
- MSU and urine dipstick.
  - Microscopic haematuria in patients with appropriate symptoms and signs strongly supports a diagnosis of renal tract colic. Renal tract colic can occur without microscopic haematuria, however (e.g. sloughed papilla).
  - Leucocytes and nitrites indicate urinary infection and urine should be sent for M, C, & S.

- Macroscopic haematuria suggests clot colic.
- Take blood cultures if any signs of infection are present.
- KUB X-ray.
  - An adequate KUB (which must show the symphysis pubis) is useful. If the stone is visible, the patient may be followed-up with a single plain film rather than repeat IVU/CT.
  - 85% of renal and ureteric stones are said to be radio-opaque, though they are often difficult to see on KUB and difficult to distinguish from other opacities, especially in the pelvis
  - Look for stones along the line of the ureters (Figs 15.1 and 15.2).

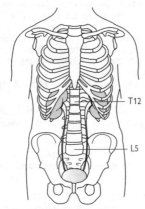

Fig. 15.1 On KUB X-ray, the ureters run along the tips of the lumbar transverse processes, over the sacroiliac joints, to the ischial spines, and (foreshortened) to the pubic tubercle. (Reproduced, with permission, from Hope, R.A. *et al.* (1998). *Oxford Handbook of Clinical Medicine*, 4th edn, Chapter 9, p. 373. Oxford University Press, Oxford.)

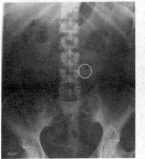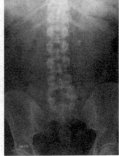

Fig. 15.2 (a) A small opacity is seen over the left L4 transverse process (circled). (b) A well-defined opacity is present adjacent to the left L2 transverse process.

Initial management

- Analgesia. Parenteral NSAIDs (e.g. diclofenac 75mg PR) are commonly given, but should not be administered to those with renal impairment. Parenteral morphine or pethidine may also be used.
  - ❶ Beware of opioid-seekers. A drop of blood from the fingertip makes very convincing dipstick haematuria! Warning signs include those with multiple admissions and no positive diagnosis, or those who cannot give a local address. If in doubt, consider alternatives, e.g. NSAIDs.
- Start thromboprophylaxis, if indicated (📖 p.26).
- Patients whose pain settles rapidly, and who have no evidence of renal impairment or infection can be discharged home with oral analgesia. Urgent outpatient imaging (either CT urogram (CTU) or IVU) and uro-logical follow-up should be arranged. Patients should be told to return if their pain is poorly controlled or if signs of sepsis develop.
- Patients with ongoing pain, renal impairment, or signs of urinary infec-tion require admission and urgent inpatient imaging.
  - Continue parenteral analgesia.
  - Adequate rehydration with IV fluids is essential, especially if IV con-trast is required for an IVU (Fig. 15.3).

❶ Patients with sepsis (📖 p.482) and those with significant renal impair-ment must be discussed urgently with the on-call urologist.

Further investigations

Non-contrast CTU (Fig. 15.4) is rapidly replacing IVU. It is fast, avoids the complications of IV contrast, and permits the diagnosis of other causes of abdominal pain.

Further management

- Patients with signs of mild infection can be given oral antibiotics (e.g. ciprofloxacin 500mg bd PO) and observed overnight for the develop-ment of sepsis.
- Those with overt signs of sepsis require IV fluid resuscitation, IV antibi-otics (e.g. gentamicin 3–5mg/kg od initially if the creatinine is normal, or ceftazidime 1g tds if abnormal) and emergency drainage of the infected urinary tract.
  - Drainage should be performed radiologically with a percutaneous nephrostomy tube, or surgically with a ureteric stent. Nephrostomy is preferred, as the rate of sepsis post-procedure is lower, but the choice depends on local availability. Adequate preoperative resusci-tation is essential before surgical stenting.
  - HDU/ITU expertise may be required in those with severe sepsis, the elderly, and those with significant co-morbidities.
- Stones < 5mm diameter usually pass spontaneously. Alpha-adrenergic blockers (e.g. tamsulosin 400mcg od PO for 2 weeks) may promote stone passage in the lower 1/3rd of the ureter.
- Stones > 5mm diameter may require intervention. The intervention used is dependent on the location and size of the stone, i.e. lithotripsy for smaller renal pelvis stones and upper 1/3rd ureteric stones, percu-taneous nephrolithotomy for large renal pelvis stones/staghorn calculi, and transurethral ureteroscopy for more distal ureteric stones.

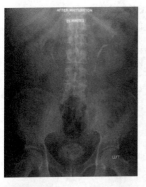

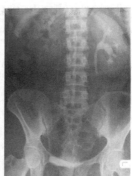

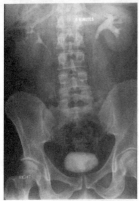

Fig. 15.3 (a) A normal IVU. The contrast has entered both ureters promptly and there is no dilatation of the ureters or renal calyces. (b) The opacity shown in Fig. 15.2(a) is shown to be an obstructing stone in the left ureter. (c) The opacity shown in Fig. 15.2(b) is shown to be a partially obstructing stone in the left renal pelvis with calyceal blunting.

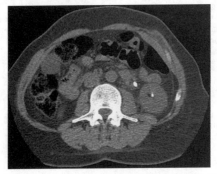

Fig. 15.4 Left lower renal pole and left ureteric stones are shown on CTU.

ⓘ **Acute urinary retention**

Urinary retention is defined as difficulty passing urine resulting in a distended bladder. It occurs predominantly in males and can either be acute or chronic (Box 15.2). Chronic retention may be painless, so acute retention is the more common emergency presentation and is discussed here. The initial management for both includes catheterization.

❶ Recent abdominal, pelvic, perineal, or genital trauma suggests bladder (📖 p.388) or urethral (📖 p.390) trauma and should be managed accordingly.

History
- Difficulty passing urine.
- Suprapubic discomfort or pain.
- Elderly patients may present with confusion/agitation.
- Precipitating factors may be present.

Examination
- Distended lower abdomen.
- Palpable or percussible bladder.
- Features of sepsis (📖 p.482) may be present if retention is due to UTI.
- DRE may reveal constipation, an enlarged prostate, or an irregular prostate (suggesting prostate cancer).

Investigations
- A portable bladder USS scan may be useful if the diagnosis is unclear.
- FBC: ↑ WCC in sepsis.
- U&Es: ↑ creatinine and urea indicate renal impairment.
- ❶ PSA can be falsely elevated in acute urinary retention. It is not required if the prostate feels benign and is only indicated if the prostate feels malignant.

Box 15.2 Acute versus chronic urinary retention

Features suggestive of acute urinary retention
- Short history (< 24h)
- Precipitating factors, e.g. constipation, recent surgery (especially pelvic, groin, or lower limb), UTI
- Painful retention
- Residual volume < 800mL
- No diuresis after catheterization
- Normal U&Es

Features suggestive of chronic urinary retention
- Longer history (> 24h)
- Previous history of urinary retention
- Painless retention
- Residual volume > 800mL
- Diuresis > 200mL/h after catheterization
- Abnormal U&Es

Management
- Urgent transurethral catheterization (📖 p.504); subsequent (dramatic) symptom relief confirms the diagnosis.
  - The residual volume **must** be measured and documented.
  - Send a CSU for M, C, & S.
- The patient can be sent home with a leg bag and α-blocker (e.g. tamsulosin 400mcg od PO) for a trial without catheter by the district nurse in 1 week if:
  - the residual volume is < 1000mL;
  - there is no evidence of sepsis or diuresis;
  - renal function is normal;
  - they have adequate care at home.
- Patients with sepsis require IV antibiotic cover for catheterization (e.g. gentamicin 120mg, or ceftazidime 1g if abnormal renal function) and admission for resuscitation and treatment.
- Patients with clinically obvious acute urinary retention where transurethral catheterization fails require a suprapubic catheter (📖 p.508). Observe overnight for potential complications.
- Start thromboprophylaxis, if indicated (📖 p.26).

Potential problems post-catheterization

Haematuria (📖 p.384) Check FBC, PT, APTT. Change to a 3-way catheter and put up irrigation if haematuria is heavy or if clot retention occurs. Resuscitate as required.

Diuresis > 200mL/h
- Alert patients who can take oral fluids with a normal plasma Na^+ should not need IV fluid replacement, as the diuresis is often physiological.
- In drowsy or less physically capable patients, aim to replace 90% of the hourly urine output initially (e.g. with Hartmann's solution), steadily reducing to maintenance fluids.
- Re-check U&Es regularly in all patients to guide fluid management and ask the nurses to maintain strict input/output charts.
- Daily weights are very useful.
- Watch for a 'salt-losing' diuresis.
- Elderly patients and those with cardiorespiratory co-morbidities may require HDU.

① **Frank haematuria**

Patients with frank haematuria may present as a urological emergency due to clot retention. Occasionally, bleeding may be severe enough to cause cardiovascular instability. Episodes of haematuria are usually self-limiting. Therefore, a patient presenting with a short history of frank haematuria who is voiding freely, haemodynamically stable, and with a normal Hb may be suitable for outpatient management.

Causes
- UTI.
- Post-urological procedures, e.g. transurethral removal of bladder tumours.
- Urinary tract tumours (bladder, ureter, kidneys, prostate).
- Renal trauma (📖 p.386).
- Bladder trauma (📖 p.388).
- Urethral trauma, e.g. inflation of a catheter balloon in the urethra.
- Post-catheterization in acute urinary retention.

History
- Recent urological procedures or trauma.
- Difficulty voiding and lower abdominal discomfort.
- Rarely, symptoms of shock.

Examination
- Usually unremarkable.
- DRE to check the prostate in males.
- Signs of shock (📖 p.52) or urinary retention may be present (📖 p.382).

Initial investigations
- FBC: ↓ Hb.
- U&Es: ↑ urea and creatinine if prolonged outflow tract obstruction.
- PT, APTT: both ↑ if severe bleeding.
- Send MSU for M, C, & S.
- ECG and/or CXR: if elderly or cardiovascular co-morbidities are present.
- G&S: in all patients. Cross-match 4–6 units of packed RBCs if shocked.
- PSA: only if the prostate feels grossly abnormal on DRE.

Initial management
- ❶ If symptoms and signs of shock are present, gain IV access with large-bore cannulae × 2, give high-flow O_2 and fluid resuscitate accordingly (📖 p.17).
- Give packed RBCs, if needed, and correct any coagulopathy (📖 p.22).
- Insert a 24F 3-way urinary catheter (📖 p.504).
- Perform a bladder washout using a bladder syringe and sterile saline until the most of the clots are evacuated. Connect up continuous irrigation with sterile saline.
- Titrate the irrigation so that the urine is light rosé or clearer.
- Further bladder washouts may be necessary if the catheter fails to drain well or is repeatedly blocking with clots. The patient **must** be

admitted to a urology ward with nurses who are familiar at performing washouts and handling irrigation.
- If severe bleeding persists, or if the patient is haemodynamically unstable, contact a urologist. Occasionally, a patient whose bladder is full of clot will require rigid cystoscopic evacuation or, rarely, an open cystotomy.

Further investigations

Flexible cystoscopy and upper tract imaging (usually an USS ± IVU) should be performed, either as an inpatient or urgently following discharge.

Further management

Once the urine is clear without irrigation, a trial without catheter may be performed.

:✪: Renal trauma

Most cases of renal trauma are minor blunt injuries, resulting in small sub-capsular haematomas. Severe injury can lead to life-threatening blood loss. Blunt trauma accounts for 90% of renal injuries and > 95% of these injuries can be managed non-operatively. The American Association for the Surgery of Trauma has developed a renal injury grading system (Box 15.3).

History
- Determine the mechanism of injury.
- ❶ Resuscitation and primary survey may take precedence over history-taking (🕮 p.42).

Box 15.3 AAST renal injury grading

Grade	Description
I	Renal contusion or subcapsular haematoma
II	Cortical laceration < 1cm parenchymal depth or non-expanding perirenal haematoma
III	Parenchymal laceration > 1cm depth without breach of the collecting system
IV	Parenchymal laceration involving collecting system or renal artery or vein damage with contained haematoma
V	Shattered kidney or avulsion of renal pedicle

Examination
- In blunt trauma, the only sign on abdominal examination may be loin or renal angle tenderness.
- Overlying bruising may be present.
- Signs of shock may be present.

Initial investigations
- FBC: ↓ Hb may be present in those with significant blood loss.
- U&Es: to assess baseline renal function.
- G&S: in all patients. Cross-match 2–6 units of packed RBCs as determined by the degree of shock and the presence of other injuries.
- MSU/CSU and dipstick: look for macro- and/or microscopic haematuria.
  - ❶ The degree of haematuria does not necessarily correlate with the severity of renal injury—a kidney avulsed from its vascular pedicle produces no urine.

Initial management
- Give O_2 to keep SaO_2 > 94%.
- Insert a peripheral cannula (2 large-bore cannulae if shock is present).
- Start IV fluids, initially crystalloid, although severe or ongoing hypotension requires transfusion of packed RBCs.
- If shock or heavy haematuria are present, insert a urinary catheter and maintain urine output > 0.5mL/kg/h.
- Correct any coagulopathy, e.g. with FFP.

Further investigations

The majority of haemodynamically normal patients (i.e. not requiring fluid resuscitation) with blunt trauma and microscopic haematuria can be discharged. Those with a significant mechanism of injury, major co-morbidities, shock, or significant pain or tenderness should be admitted.

- Renal tract USS: not usually helpful in cases of suspected minor renal trauma associated with microscopic haematuria.
- CT abdomen and pelvis (Fig. 15.5): This is the gold standard for imaging in renal trauma. This should only be performed in haemodynamically stable patients. Indications are:
  - blunt trauma with microscopic haematuria and evidence of significant blood loss, or a significant mechanism of injury;
  - blunt trauma with macroscopic haematuria;
  - haemodynamically stable patients with penetrating trauma, but no signs of peritonitis.
- Arteriography: permits identification and selective embolization of bleeding vessels in renovascular injury.

Further management

- Most patients with renal injuries diagnosed on CT require fluid resuscitation and observation only.
  - Watch for evidence of further bleeding, or signs of local or systemic infection that may indicate a collecting system leak not evident initially.
  - Repeat CT may be needed.
- Where the renal collecting system has been breached, a JJ stent should be placed, and any extrapelvic urinary collections drained percutaneously.
- Indications for laparotomy in renal trauma:
  - penetrating injuries with signs of shock or peritonitis. These patients often require laparotomy to exclude injuries to other viscera;
  - blunt injuries with haemodynamic compromise despite aggressive fluid resuscitation. These are usually grade V injuries.

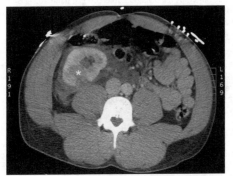

Fig. 15.5 CT showing a right grade III renal injury (*) with a surrounding retroperitoneal haematoma after high-energy blunt trauma to the right flank.

☼ Bladder trauma

Bladder trauma may result in contusions of the bladder wall, partial thickness tears, or complete ruptures. Injury may be caused by blunt or penetrating trauma, often in patients with a full bladder. Bladder trauma is usually associated with other injuries, especially pelvic fractures and urethral injury. Bladder ruptures can either be extraperitoneal or intraperitoneal.

❶ Most bladder ruptures are iatrogenic, e.g. during endoscopic bladder tumour resection, pelvic surgery, or cystoscopic biopsy.

History
- Determine the mechanism of injury.
- Symptoms are often non-specific, including diffuse lower abdominal pain and difficulty voiding.

❶ Resuscitation and primary survey may take precedence over history-taking (📖 p.42).

Examination
- Examination may reveal suprapubic bruising and tenderness, a distended abdomen, or absent bowel sounds.
- ❶ The non-specific clinical features of bladder rupture can lead to misdiagnosis. Features of late-presenting or missed bladder rupture include:
  - abdominal distension and vomiting due to prolonged ileus;
  - ↑ Na^+, K^+, urea, or creatinine;
  - hyperchloraemic metabolic acidosis.

Initial investigations
- FBC: Hb may be ↓.
- U&Es: usually ↔.
- G&S: in all patients. Cross-match 2–4 units of packed RBCs if shock is present.
- MSU/CSU and dipstick urinalysis: microscopic haematuria is universal; macroscopic haematuria is present in > 90% of patients with blunt trauma and 50% of those with penetrating trauma.

Initial management
- Give O_2 to keep SaO_2 > 94%.
- Insert a peripheral cannula (2 large-bore cannulae if shock is present).
- Start IV fluids, initially crystalloid, although severe or ongoing hypotension requires transfusion of packed RBCs.
- Insert a urinary catheter (📖 p.504), unless urethral injury is suspected (📖 p.390).

Further investigations
Unless other indications for laparotomy (📖 p.71) preclude it, imaging is essential when bladder trauma is suspected. Conventional or contrast-enhanced CT cystography are the modalities of choice. CT is increasingly

used as it is as accurate as conventional cystography, and allows the identification of other injuries. Indications for imaging include:
- blunt or penetrating abdominal trauma and gross haematuria;
- pelvic fractures and microscopic haematuria;
- penetrating pelvic injuries.

Further management

Management of blunt bladder trauma
- Bladder contusions, interstitial ruptures, and pelvic haematomas can be managed non-operatively, and may not require catheterization unless other injuries warrant it.
- Extraperitoneal ruptures and small (usually iatrogenic) intraperitoneal ruptures can be managed non-operatively using a urethral catheter. Prophylactic antibiotics (e.g. ciprofloxacin 500mg bd PO) should be prescribed. Cystography should be performed prior to catheter removal.
- Large intraperitoneal ruptures require surgical repair.
- If other injuries require laparotomy, extraperitoneal injuries should be explored and closed.

Bladder rupture due to penetrating trauma requires surgical repair.

☼ Urethral trauma

The urethra is divided into anterior and posterior portions. In males, the anterior urethra consists of the bulbar urethra, which runs from the uro-genital diaphragm to the penoscrotal junction, and the penile urethra. The posterior urethra runs from the bladder neck to the urogenital diaphragm. Most urethral injuries occur in the bulbar urethra.

History

- Determine the mechanism of injury. A fall astride an object is a common cause. Blunt or penetrating injury to the pelvis or external genitalia should arouse suspicion of a urethral injury, especially if pubic rami fractures are present.
- Inability to void or macroscopic haematuria suggests urethral injury.

❶ Resuscitation and primary survey may take precedence over history-taking (📖 p.42).

Examination

Urethral injury may be indicated by:
- blood at the meatus;
- bruising to the penile shaft, perineum, or scrotum;
- a 'high riding' or impalpable prostate on DRE. This is seen only in complete posterior urethral disruption.

Investigations

- Retrograde urethrogram. This can identify urethral contusion, incomplete or complete disruption, and localize the injury. Indications include:
  - overt signs of urethral trauma;
  - inability to pass a urinary catheter in a patient with pelvic trauma without signs of urethral trauma.

Management

Initial management involves providing urinary drainage without further damaging the urethra.

- In patients with pelvic trauma but no overt signs of urethral injury, an experienced surgeon may attempt gentle urethral catheterization (📖 p.504). If any resistance is encountered, the procedure should be abandoned, and a urologist called. Request a retrograde urethrogram.
- If imaging confirms only urethral contusion, gentle urethral catheterization may be attempted.
- In cases of significant urethral injury, or when a urethral catheter cannot be passed, a suprapubic catheter (SPC) should be inserted (📖 p.508), assuming that the patient is in retention. If the bladder is not palpable, a flexible cystoscopy and placement of a catheter over a guidewire may be needed.
- Definitive treatment is usually delayed, and is dependent on the location of the injury and the degree of disruption.

:O: Priapism

Priapism is a prolonged erection, usually painful and not associated with sexual desire. Two main types of priapism exist: low-flow (anoxic) and high-flow (arteriogenic). Low-flow priapism is most common. As their management is very different, it is important to accurately distinguish between them (Table 15.1). Advice from a urologist should be sought as soon as possible.

Low-flow priapism is believed to be due to obstruction of venous drainage, resulting in poorly oxygenated blood within the corpora cavernosa. Untreated low-flow priapism leads to smooth muscle necrosis after 24h and will ultimately result in corporal fibrosis and erectile dysfunction. Causes include:

- haematological disorders, e.g. sickle cell disease and polycythaemia;
- medication, e.g. antidepressants, anti-hypertensives;
- intracavernosal drugs for erectile dysfunction e.g. alprostadil;
- recreational drugs (e.g. sildenafil (e.g. Viagra®), marijuana, cocaine, Ecstasy);
- malignancy.

High-flow priapism is usually secondary to perineal trauma, sometimes perceived as fairly innocuous by the patient. Damage to the central penile arteries results in an arterio-sinusoidal shunt or aneurysm and impaired regulation of blood flow.

Clinical features

- A careful drug history, both therapeutic and recreational, is required.
- There may be a history of trauma, blood disorders, or malignancy.
- Systemic examination and examination of external genitalia is often unremarkable apart from the presence of the priapism itself.

Investigations

- Aspirate 10–20mL of blood from one of the corpora cavernosa via a green (21G) needle for blood gas analysis (Table 15.1). This may also relieve recent onset low-flow priapism.
- Duplex USS or arteriography is required if blood gas analysis fails to distinguish low-flow from high-flow priapism.

Management of low-flow priapism

- In early cases, detumescence may be achieved with exercise (e.g. climbing several flights of stairs) or ice packs.
- The β_2-adrenoreceptor agonist terbutaline (5–10mg PO) may reduce tumescence.
- If priapism persists, intracavernous α-adrenoagonists may be used.
  - Inject 100–200mcg of phenylephrine (0.5–1mL of a 200mcg/mL solution) into the corpora every 5–10min until detumescence occurs (maximum total dose 1mg).
  - ❶ This requires continuous BP and pulse monitoring. Take **extreme** caution in patients with IHD, hypertension, cerebral ischaemia or if they take antidepressants. This is best performed in an anaesthetic room with an anaesthetist standing by.
- Surgical treatment with caverno-spongeosal shunts is rarely indicated.

Management of high-flow priapism
- Arteriography is required to demonstrate the arterio-sinusoidal shunt and to embolize the internal pudendal artery.
- Surgical intervention is rarely required.

Table 15.1 Distinguishing between low- and high-flow priapism

Variable	Low-flow priapism	High-flow priapism
Onset	On wakening or following medication	Following trauma
Pain	Increasingly severe	Relatively painless
Corpora cavernosa appearance	Rigid	Turgid
Glans penis/corpus spongiosum appearance	Flaccid	Turgid
Cavernous blood appearance	Dark red	Bright red
Cavernous blood PO_2, PCO_2 (both kPa) and pH	$PO_2 < 4$; $PCO_2 > 10.5$; pH < 7.25	$PO_2 > 6.6$; $PCO_2 < 6.6$; pH > 7.5
Blood flow on duplex USS	Little or no flow	High arterial flow and/or shunt seen
Arteriography findings	Intact vessels	Arterio-sinusoidal shunt

☼ Paraphimosis

Paraphimosis develops when the foreskin becomes trapped behind the glans penis. The foreskin and glans become painful and oedematous. This often occurs following insertion of a urethral catheter when the foreskin has not been reduced at the end of the procedure. Paraphimosis requires immediate reduction.

❶ After urinary catheterization **always** replace the foreskin in uncircumcised men.

- Paraphimosis in the adult can usually be dealt with using LA. Reduction of paraphimoses in children often requires GA.
- If the oedema is severe, or the patient is in pain and unlikely to tolerate the procedure, a penile block should be performed.
- ❶ The LA must **not** contain epinephrine due to the risk of penile ischaemia.
- Alternatively, the foreskin and glans penis can be coated in 2% lidocaine gel, which acts both as a lubricant to ease reduction and as a topical anaesthetic.
- If the oedema is marked, gentle compression of the foreskin may lessen the swelling and facilitate reduction.
- Wrap a gauze swap around the penile shaft, just proximal to the constriction band, holding it in place with the index and third fingers of both hands.
- Using both thumbs, gently ease the glans back through the constriction ring.
- If reduction is not possible, the patient should be anaesthetized (local or general) and a dorsal slit performed. Call a urologist.
- Patients suffering recurrent episodes of paraphimosis should be offered circumcision.

☼ Penile fracture

Fracture of the erect penis involves disruption of the tunica albuginea, the tough fibrous membrane that surrounds the corpus spongiosum, and the two corpora cavernosa.

Clinical features

- There is a history of blunt trauma to the erect penis, almost exclusively during intercourse; the patient usually reports a loud snap, associated with the immediate onset of severe pain and subsequent bruising and swelling.
- On examination, there is marked bruising and swelling localized to the penile shaft if Buck's fascia remains intact; this bruising may spread to the scrotum and perineum if the fascia is disrupted.
- A defect in the tunica albuginea may be palpable at the site of the fracture.

❶ Blood at the meatus should raise suspicion of a urethral injury (📖 p.390); retrograde urethrography is indicated.

Investigations

- These are unnecessary if the clinical features are diagnostic.
- If the diagnosis is uncertain, a cavernosogram will distinguish a penile fracture from rupture of a vessel such as the superficial dorsal vein.
- ❶ If the patient is in urinary retention, suprapubic catheterization (📖 508) should be performed as well as a retrograde urethrogram to assess urethral integrity.

Management

Urgent surgery is needed—call a urologist. The penis is degloved, the clot evacuated, and the tunica albuginea repaired.

Early postoperative complications: nephrectomy

Nephrectomy can be performed open or laparoscopically. When performed laparoscopically the approach can be retroperitoneal or intraperitoneal.

Operative site bleeding (📖 p.154)

Bowel perforation

If the patient develops abdominal pain or sepsis, consider bowel injury, especially in laparoscopic procedures. Resuscitate, send bloods, arrange an emergency erect CXR, and call for senior help.

Pneumothorax

Pneumothorax can occur during open or laparoscopic nephrectomy.
- Give O_2 and arrange an emergency erect CXR.
- Insert a chest drain if confirmed (📖 p.522).
- If signs of a tension pneumothorax are present (📖 p.463), use needle decompression first (📖 p.516).

Haematuria

Some haematuria is to be expected post-nephrectomy. If heavy, the catheter can block off. Gentle manual washout can be performed with sterile normal saline via the Foley catheter. If this is unsuccessful, the Foley catheter can be changed for a 3-way catheter and irrigation connected. This should be discussed with the urologist on-call.

Early postoperative complications: radical cystectomy

This can be performed open or laparoscopically. In males the prostate is also removed and in females a hysterectomy may also be performed. The patient will be left with an ileal conduit or a reconstructed bladder, which is constructed from ileum, through which urine will drain.

❶ Read the operation note carefully.

Oliguria

This is commonly due to hypovolaemia.

- Check for signs of bleeding and send blood for FBC, U&Es.
- Give fluid challenges and transfuse as required.
- Urine output measurement may be complex—the patient may only have a urethral catheter to aid haemostasis.
  - Urine output is monitored via the ileal conduit.
  - In the case of a bladder reconstruction, the stents are frequently exteriorized so the urine output would be a product of the two abdominal bags.
  - The urethral catheter may be empty.
  - ❶ Do not flush the urethral catheter.

Sepsis (📖 p.482)

- Send bloods and blood cultures, fluid resuscitate, and give O_2.
- Check the chest, wound, and urine as sources by clinical examination, CXR, and urine dipstick.
- Consider anastomotic leak or bowel injury as a cause of peritonitis.
- Discuss with a senior **early**, as further imaging (e.g. CT) or return to theatre may be needed.

Prolonged ileus (📖 p.295)

Consider anastomotic leak of urine or GI contents as the underlying cause.

Early postoperative complications: radical prostatectomy

This can be performed open or laparoscopically.

Operative site bleeding (📖 p.154)

Oliguria/anuria

This may be due to a blocked catheter, ureteric damage, or hypovolaemia.

- Clinical features. Examine for signs of shock and check the drain output and wounds. Check for a distended bladder clinically, although this can be difficult postoperatively, so a bladder scan may be needed.
- Investigations. Check FBC, U&Es and cross-match 2–4 units of packed RBCs if bleeding is suspected.
- Management. If hypovolaemia is present, give a fluid challenge. The presence of a distended bladder implies catheter blockage. This needs to be managed promptly. A gentle washout can be performed, as commonly there will be a blood clot or mucus plug causing the blockage. If you cannot unblock the catheter then call for senior help. If the patient is anuric, but euvolaemic, and without a distended bladder, then ureteric injury may have occurred. Organize an urgent USS of the kidneys and ureters and call for senior help. The patient may require nephrostomies or possibly need to go back to theatre.

❶ Do not remove the urinary catheter.

Early postoperative complications: percutaneous nephrolithotomy (PCNL)

PCNL is the standard procedure for the removal of large renal stones. It involves puncturing the kidney and the collecting system, and dilating the track to allow passage of a nephroscope, through which the stone is evacuated. A nephrostomy catheter is left in situ to drain the renal pelvis.

Bleeding through the nephrostomy

- Perirenal haematomas are common; 5% of patients require transfusion.
- Transient clamping of the nephrostomy tube for 15min may tamponade venous bleeding.
- If bleeding fails to settle, or the patient is unstable, call a urologist.
- Urgent arteriography may be required to locate and embolize a bleeding vessel or arteriovenous fistula.

Sepsis (📖 p.482)

- Transient pyrexia following PCNL is common, especially in those with staghorn calculi.
- Persistent fever or sepsis requires fluid resuscitation and culture of blood, urine, and the nephrostomy drain output.
- Treat with IV antibiotics (e.g. benzylpenicillin 1.2g qds and gentamicin 3–5mg/kg od).
- Imaging may be required to rule out an infected urinoma or abscess.

Respiratory complications

Puncture of the upper pole calyx carries a risk of pleural damage, leading to pneumothorax or pleural effusion. Large or symptomatic pneumothoraces and effusions require drainage (📖 p.522).

Passage of retained stone fragment

As with lithotripsy, retained stone fragments may pass down the ureter, causing colic or even renal outflow obstruction when the percutaneous drainage is clamped off. If suspected, request a nephrostogram and unclamp the nephrostomy tube if obstruction is present.

Early postoperative complications: transurethral resection of the prostate (TURP)

TURP remains a commonly performed operation. Many centres are intro-ducing laser ablative, laser resection, and laser enucleation surgery, which have lower complication rates than traditional electrocautery TURP. TURP is often performed in elderly men with multiple co-morbidities.

Operative site bleeding (see also 📖 p.154)

Haematuria can be severe, usually in the first 12h postoperatively.
- Clinical features. Examine the patient for signs of shock and for clot retention. Patients in clot retention are in a lot of pain.
- Investigations. Check FBC, U&Es, and PT and APTT. Cross-match 2–6 units of packed RBCs if shock is present.
- Management. Shock must be treated with IV fluid resuscitation and packed RBCs. Correct any coagulopathy, e.g. with FFP. If the patient is not in clot retention, a bladder washout (Box 15.4) and continuous high-flow bladder irrigation may be all that is required. Gentle traction on the catheter (hang the catheter bag over the end of the bed) may tamponade prostatic bleeding. If clot retention is present, washout is mandatory (Box 15.4).

❶ Traction should not be prolonged beyond 15min as sphincteric ischaemia may occur.

TURP syndrome

This is due to absorption of water in glycine-based irrigation fluid, resulting in ↓ Na^+. Other more complex metabolic effects also occur. Patients become symptomatic (e.g. confusion, nausea, vomiting, hypertension, bradycardia, and fitting) when serum $Na^+ < 125$mmol/L. Mild dilutional hyponatraemia can usually be reversed with 40mg furosemide IV. Regular serum Na^+ measurement and monitoring is mandatory. Further IV furosemide may be necessary. In severe cases, discuss management with the on-call intensivist as HDU/ITU admission may be required.

Box 15.4 Bladder washout post-TURP

- Detach the catheter bag from the central lumen of the 3-way catheter. If the patient is in retention, try to aspirate from the bladder.
  - ❶ Flushing with 50mL of saline may exacerbate the situation or rupture the bladder.
- If you are unable to aspirate, inject 10 or 20mL of saline in an attempt to dislodge an obstructing clot.
- Try advancing the catheter to the hilt, and even deflating the balloon, both of which may permit aspiration and allow you to wash out the bladder with sterile saline.
- Once you are able to wash the bladder out, continue until you are getting very few clots out from the bladder and the washout is rosé-This may take > 30min—persevere!
- Once the washout is rosé, connect continuous high-flow irrigation and ensure the nursing staff do not allow the fluid to run out or the catheter to become blocked.
- If you are unable to drain the bladder, call for assistance. A change of catheter may be attempted after discussion with the urologist on-call.
  - ❶ On no account use an introducer to re-insert a catheter unless under the supervision of a urologist.
- Patients in whom bladder drainage cannot be established may require a return to theatre for washout. Cystotomy and open evacuation may be needed.

Early postoperative complications: transurethral resection of bladder tumour and cystoscopy

Bladder perforation (see also 🕮 p.388)

Don't dismiss the elderly patient with significant suprapubic pain and tenderness following a simple cystoscopy and biopsy, especially at the bladder dome, where the bladder wall is thinnest. Small defects following full thickness biopsies can open to result in significant intraperitoneal leaks.

Frank haematuria (🕮 p.384)

Early postoperative complications: scrotal surgery

Operative site bleeding (see also 🕮 p.154)

This can rapidly lead to a scrotal haematoma, which can subsequently become infected.

- Patients presenting with a stable scrotal haematoma, smaller than the size of a tennis ball, can be discharged on oral analgesia and antibiotics, e.g. ciprofloxacin 500mg bd PO for 2 weeks.
- If a large scrotal haematoma or signs of infection are present, a scrotal USS is needed to determine whether an abscess is present.
- Secondary haemorrhage, occurring 7–14 days post-procedure, is usually infective in origin.

Infection

- Simple scrotal wound infections can be treated with oral antibiotics e.g. co-amoxiclav 625mg tds for 1 week.
- Patients with more extensive wound infection should have a scrotal USS to exclude an underlying abscess, and may require IV antibiotics, e.g. gentamicin 3–5mg/kg od.
- Scrotal abscesses should be incised, drained, and packed.

Early postoperative complications: circumcision

Operative site bleeding (see also 📖 p.154)
Usually occurs on the day of the procedure. If direct pressure fails to stop the bleeding (which is often from the frenular vessels), the patient should return to theatre.

Infection
- Usually occurs after 3–7 days, and can be treated with oral antibiotics, e.g. co-amoxiclav 625mg tds for 1 week.
- Adjust the dose for children.
- Bleeding may cause an infected haematoma, requiring surgical drainage.

Early postoperative complications: lithotripsy

Lithotripsy is an outpatient procedure commonly used to treat upper ureteric and renal stones.

Passage of stone fragments
Patients present with renal tract colic (📖 p.378) and are managed accordingly.

Bleeding/haematoma formation
Many patients have transient macroscopic haematuria (📖 p.384) following lithotripsy, but clinically significant haematuria is rare. Renal subcapsular haematomas may occur and patients present with loin pain with tenderness on examination. A mass may be palpable if the haematoma is large. Frank haematuria may be present. A patient with a significant extracapsular bleed who is haemodynamically unstable should be resuscitated and transfused. CT is the imaging modality of choice to distinguish haematoma formation from renal tract colic. All patients presenting with pain and signs of bleeding should undergo urgent CT.

UTI
Infection may originate from the stone itself or from local tissue trauma allowing bacteria to enter the bloodstream. Patients with localized symptoms suggestive of post-lithotripsy infection may be treated with oral antibiotics (e.g. ciprofloxacin 500mg bd PO), but those with symptoms or signs of sepsis should be admitted for resuscitation, IV antibiotics (e.g. gentamicin 3–5mg/kg od) and observation.

Early postoperative complications: ureteroscopy

Biopsies and therapeutic interventions (e.g laser fragmentation of stones, ablation of small upper tract tumours) can be performed.

- Significant intraoperative complications, such as ureteric avulsion are rare, and require laparotomy and immediate repair or reconstruction.
- Clots or stone fragments can cause renal tract colic (□ p.378). Ureteric oedema can cause similar symptoms.
- Ureteric stents placed at the end of the procedure can cause severe bladder spasms. Treat with anti-cholinergics, e.g. oxybutynin 5mg tds PO.

Orthopaedic surgery

☢ Open fractures

Open fractures are an orthopaedic emergency due to the risk of deep infection. Consider every fracture with an overlying skin wound as being open, even if it is only an abrasion.

The Gustilo–Anderson open fracture classification is used to guide management, and is based on wound size, presence of neurovascular injury, degree of contamination, and degree of soft tissue injury (Box 16.1). The definitive grade should be assigned in theatre after debridement.

Box 16.1 Gustilo–Anderson open fracture grading

- Grade I. Wound < 1cm long with little soft tissue damage and no crushing.
- Grade II. Wound > 1cm long, with no extensive soft-tissue damage, flap, or avulsion. There may be slight or moderate crushing injury, moderate comminution of the fracture, or moderate contamination.
- Grade III. Extensive soft tissue damage and a high degree of contamination. There is often significant fracture comminution and instability.
  - Grade IIIA. Soft-tissue coverage of the fractured bone is adequate.
  - Grade IIIB. Extensive injury, or loss of soft tissue, with periosteal stripping and exposure of bone, massive contamination, or severe comminution.
  - Grade IIIC. Any open fracture associated with an arterial injury that must be repaired, regardless of the degree of soft-tissue injury.

Clinical features
- There is a history of recent trauma, with pain on movement or weight-bearing.
- On examination, signs of a fracture are present, with an overlying wound ± visible bone or bone fragments.

❶ Refer for senior orthopaedic review as soon as an open fracture is suspected.

Investigations
❶ The investigation and management of immediately life-threatening injuries take priority (📖 p.42).
- Photograph the wound: this documents the injury and ensures other clinicians don't have to remove sterile dressing once applied.
- Wound swab: although the organisms grown may not be those that later lead to deep infection.
- Request AP and lateral X-rays of the fracture **and** the joint above and below.
  - ❶ X-rays should only be performed **after** reduction (see 'Management').

Management
- Prophylactic IV antibiotics must be given **immediately**, according to the apparent grade of injury. Continue for 2–4 days.

- Grade I: first-generation cephalosporin, e.g. cefradine 1g qds.
- Grade II: first-generation cephalosporin ± aminoglycoside, depending on the level of contamination (e.g. gentamicin, given according to local protocol).
- Grade III: first-generation cephalosporin + aminoglycoside.
- ❶ Treat all farmyard injuries as grade III injuries and add IV benzylpenicillin 1.2g qds to cover clostridial organisms.
- ❶ Early administration of antibiotics is the most effective strategy for preventing deep infection.
- Give IV opiate analgesia with an anti-emetic.
- Remove gross contamination with sterile forceps and by gently irrigating with sterile normal saline. Apply a povidone iodine-soaked sterile dressing.
- Reduce any gross deformity and apply a splint. This reduces the pressure on neurovascular structures and limits further injury to soft tissues. Don't be too concerned about reducing a fragment of bone back into the body.
  - ❶ Check the distal neurovascular status before and after reduction.
- Give tetanus prophylaxis unless already covered (📖 p.94).
- Debridement, washout, and skeletal stabilization should be performed as soon as possible, once the patient is haemodynamically stable.

The principles of surgical management include the following.
- Wound extension and delivery of bone ends, followed by thorough debridement of non-viable tissue and contaminated tissue.
- Copious wound irrigation.
- Previously, internal fixation was thought to be contraindicated in open fractures; however, intramedullary nailing or plate fixation may be acceptable.
- Avoid primary wound closure. Consider a vacuum dressing for temporary closure.
- Book for re-look surgery after 48h. Repeat debridement may be necessary. Delayed primary closure of wounds may be possible.
- ❶ Plastic surgical consultation should be sought early in grade II and III wounds, preferably at the first debridement.

① Acute osteomyelitis and septic arthritis

Patients with acute osteomyelitis and septic arthritis often have a similar presentation. Both conditions may occur after haematogenous spread, trauma, or orthopaedic surgery. Likely causative organisms vary with age and patient co-morbidities (Box 16.2).

Box 16.2 Causative organisms and associations

- Neonates: *Staphylococcus aureus*, streptococci.
- Older children: *Staph. aureus* and occasionally *Haemophilus influenzae*.
- Adults: *Staph. aureus*. In sexually active individuals, *Neisseria gonorrhoeae*.
- The elderly: Gram-negative bacilli.
- Fungal osteomyelitis is a complication of intravascular catheter-related fungaemia, the use of illicit drugs contaminated by Candida species, and prolonged neutropenia.
- *Pseudomonas aeruginosa* infection is associated with IV drug abuse, long-term urinary catheterization, and plantar sole injection injuries.
- Salmonella osteomyelitis is associated with sickle cell anaemia.

Clinical features

- Patients present with local bony pain, sometimes with a history of trauma beforehand. Systemic symptoms and rigors may be present.
- On examination, pyrexia, swelling, and erythema over a bone or joint are seen.
- A joint effusion may be present. Any bone/joint may be affected, although haematogenous osteomyelitis in children tends to involve the metaphysis near the large joints.
- Joint movement is much reduced and causes severe pain in septic arthritis.
- ❶ Young children may present with a swollen joint and hemi-neglect, pseudoparalysis, or refusal to weight bear.

Investigations

- FBC: WCC is often ↑, but may be normal.
- CRP and ESR are both usually ↑↑ and are useful to monitor response to treatment.
- Blood cultures: may be positive, but in ~ 50% of cases no organism is identified, even following aspiration or surgery.
- Joint aspirate in septic arthritis: a synovial fluid WCC of > 50 000/mm³, with > 75% neutrophils suggests infection. The synovial fluid WCC may be ↓ in immunosuppressed individuals. Microscopy should be performed to look for crystals, e.g. in gout and pseudogout.
- Plain X-rays: useful to exclude other causes of joint pain, e.g. slipped upper femoral epiphysis in an adolescent with hip pain. Radiographic features of osteomyelitis usually take 10–14 days to appear. Look for periosteal elevation as the earliest radiographic sign.

- USS: may show joint effusion in septic arthritis, or a collection of subperiosteal pus in osteomyelitis.
- Nuclear medicine bone scan: may be cold, normal, or hot depending on the stage of the infection. Useful in detecting metastatic infection.
- MRI: the investigation of choice. Enables differentiation between osteomyelitis and septic arthritis.

Management

- Obtain all specimens (blood cultures, joint aspirate, intraosseous specimens) **before** starting best-guess IV antibiotics (e.g. flucloxacillin 2g qds + fusidic acid 500mg tds).
  - Begin IV cefotaxime in neonates or if Gram-negative or *N. gonorrhoeae* infection is suspected.
  - In MRSA colonized patients, or those with suspected MRSA infection, start IV vancomycin 1g bd.
- Septic arthritis should also be treated with washout of the affected joint in theatre.
- Acute osteomyelitis may require surgical debridement with decompression (drilling) of the affected bone depending on the extent and initial response to antibiotics. In adults, consider insertion of a tunnelled central venous line at the time of surgery to enable long-term IV antibiotic therapy.
- In children with haematogenous osteomyelitis and septic arthritis, IV antibiotics can be converted to orals once the organism has been identified and if clinical signs and symptoms improve rapidly.
- Monitor the response to treatment with serial inflammatory markers and regular clinical review.

Prosthetic joint infection

- Infection following elective prosthetic joint replacement is rare, e.g. 1% risk after total hip replacement.
- The most common organisms are: coagulase-negative staphylococci (30%) and *Staph. aureus* (20%).
- Prosthetic joint infection can be classified as early (< 3 months), delayed (3–24 months) or late (> 24 months after surgery). Early and delayed infections are usually acquired during implantation of the prosthesis; late infections are predominantly acquired by haematogenous seeding.

Clinical features

- Early infection: acute onset of a hot, swollen, painful joint. Cellulitis or a discharging sinus may develop.
- Delayed infection: subtle signs and symptoms, e.g. implant loosening, persistent joint pain, or both.
- Late infection: may present like early or delayed infections.

Investigations

- FBC: WCC is often ↔.
- CRP and ESR may be ↑ postoperatively.
- Blood cultures should be taken before starting antibiotics.
- Plain X-rays exclude mechanical problems and show the stability of the implant.

- Nuclear medicine bone scan: sensitive but not specific. Of limited value within a year of surgery due to false positives.
- Nuclear medicine white cell scan: may differentiate aseptic from septic loosening.
- Joint aspirate: do in theatre under sterile conditions. False negatives can still occur.
- Histology: when debriding the joint, tissue samples should be taken for histology and at least 3 deep tissue specimens are needed for culture.

❶ All blood cultures, joint aspirates, deep specimens should be taken **before** starting antibiotics unless the patient is unwell or septic.

Management
- Depends on the condition of the patient, the condition of the implant, the duration of infection, time since index procedure, causative organism, and antibiotic efficacy.
- Treatment options are multiple and include:
  - life-long antibiotics;
  - debridement, washout, retention of the original implant ± long-term antibiotic;
  - one- or two-stage revision joint replacement;
  - excision arthroplasty ± arthrodesis.

❶ Involve a microbiologist early, as antibiotic choice is complex.

:۞: **Compartment syndrome**

Compartment syndrome occurs when raised pressure within a closed osseofascial compartment compromises tissue perfusion at the capillary level, resulting in tissue ischaemia. Traumatized tissue is more susceptible to a rise in pressure since it has an increased metabolic rate. Compartment syndrome occurs most commonly in limbs, but can also occur in the abdomen (🕮 p.486).

Causes of limb compartment syndrome include:
- trauma, i.e. fractures, soft tissue contusions, crush injuries, electric shocks;
- post-ischaemic swelling due to reperfusion injury, e.g. after lower limb revascularization for acute limb ischaemia (🕮 p.332) or prolonged Lloyd–Davies position;
- tight casts or dressings;
- intracompartmental bleeding, often after anticoagulation;
- burns, especially if circumferential.

After 4h of tissue ischaemia, reversible muscle and nerve damage occurs. After 8h, muscle and nerve damage is irreversible.
- ❶ Maintain a high index of suspicion. Contact your senior **immediately** if you have **any** grounds to suspect a compartment syndrome.
- Errors in diagnosis and management are common (Box 16.3)—have a low threshold for surgical exploration.

Box 16.3 Pitfalls in compartment syndrome

- Distal pulses are often palpable in the presence of compartment syndrome.
- Compartment syndrome can occur in the thigh, upper arm, and hands, not just the forearm and the calf.
- Compartment syndrome can occur after open fractures.
- The pain associated with compartment syndrome eventually diminishes as nerve ischaemia develops.
- Clinical features of compartment syndrome can be difficult to detect in patients with impaired consciousness and in children. Consider prophylactic fasciotomy or continuous compartment pressure monitoring in those at risk.
- The use of pulse oximetry is misleading in the diagnosis of compartment syndrome.
- Regional or local anaesthesia may mask compartment syndrome.

History

Severe progressive limb pain, over and above that expected for a particular injury or operation.

Examination

- A tense, tender muscle compartment (this may not be palpable due to an overlying cast/dressing or if the compartment is deep).

- Pain on passive stretch of muscles within the compartment.
  - **❶** This is a **key** finding. As time progresses passive stretching is not possible.
- Paraesthesia and paralysis occur late.
- Pulselessness is a **very** late sign.

Investigations

❶ Investigations are usually not necessary—if you suspect it, treat it! Intracompartmental pressure can be measured, but the decision to investigate possible compartment syndrome should only be made by a senior surgeon.

- Pressure monitoring can be done with a commercially available set, or an ITU pressure transducer using a needle with a side port.
- Measure the pressure at multiple sites in **all** compartments of the affected limb.
- Compartment syndrome is suggested by either:
  - diastolic BP minus intracompartmental pressure ≤ 30mmHg;
  - intracompartmental pressure ≥ 30mmHg.
- ☛ The precise cut-off values are controversial. Some clinicians argue that diagnosis should be on clinical grounds alone.

Management

When signs are equivocal:

- correct reversible causes, e.g. split the cast and dressings (🕮 p.425), perform escharotomy, evacuate the deep haematoma;
- elevate the limb;
- if no improvement occurs in 30min, perform emergency fasciotomy.

Established compartment syndrome and compartment syndrome due to ischaemia re-perfusion injury require **emergency** fasciotomy in theatre.

- **All** of the osseofascial compartments of the involved portion of the limb must be opened via long skin incisions. This stops the skin acting as an unrecognized compartment envelope. There are 4 compartments in the leg (Fig. 16.1).
- Debride necrotic muscle (i.e. no bleeding, no twitch with diathermy). If further muscle necrosis is possible, check again in 24–48h.
- Delayed primary closure can occur 3–5 days later if the wound approximates without tension. Where delayed primary closure is not possible, split-thickness skin grafts are indicated.
- Postoperatively, check for reperfusion injury (🕮 p.346).

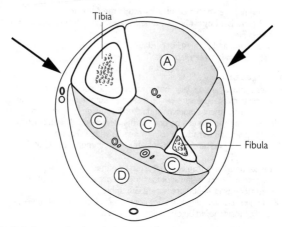

Fig. 16.1 Cross-section through the leg. There are four compartments. A, Anterior; B, lateral; C, deep posterior; D, superficial posterior. Fasciotomy incision sites are arrowed.

① Fat embolism

Fat embolism occurs when fat enters the systemic circulation. The aetiology is thought to be mechanical, with fat from traumatized pelvic or long bone medulla entering torn veins. Fat emboli can occur in those with extensive soft-tissue injury only, where circulating chylomicrons aggregate as a secondary metabolic effect of trauma.

Fat embolism syndrome (FES) encompasses a triad of respiratory, dermatological, and neurological features. Although systemic fat embolism can be detected in all patients during reamed nailing of fractures, only 1–5% develop FES. The likelihood of developing FES is determined by genetic factors, the absolute load of fat emboli, the presence of a patent foramen ovale, and pre-existing systemic inflammation Early stabilization of fractures reduces the incidence of FES.

❶ Mild FES is probably more common than appreciated, e.g. as a cause of first night postoperative pyrexia.

Clinical features
- There is a history of recent long bone/pelvic trauma or elective orthopaedic surgery. SOB and confusion are often present.
- On examination, a low-grade pyrexia, tachycardia, and tachypnoea are common. Other possible signs include:
  - acute confusional state or focal neurological deficit;
  - ↓ SaO_2;
  - petechial rash over the chest, axillae, or conjunctivae;
  - rarely, fat emboli can be seen in the retinal arteries on fundoscopy.

❶ Tachycardia, tachypnoea and pyrexia occur in SIRS, and the respiratory features of FES may be indistinguishable from ALI/ARDS (📖 p.151). The term FES should be used where definite evidence of systemic embolization exists, confirmed by the presence of two of the three major features (respiratory, cutaneous, or neurological).

Investigations
❶ It is important to exclude other causes of pyrexia, tachycardia, and tachypnoea in the postoperative patient (📖 p.131).
- FBC: Mild ↓ Hb, mild ↑ neutrophils, and ↓ platelets are common, but are non-specific.
- Blood cultures: take if a pyrexia is present.
- ECG: may show sinus tachycardia.
- CXR: Most useful in excluding other causes of respiratory distress, e.g. haemo/pneumothorax, pneumonia. Diffuse pulmonary infiltrates may develop later, as in ALI/ARDS.
- ABG: hypoxia is present.
- CT head: exclude intracranial pathology in those with a head injury and new confusion or focal deficits.
- Send urine and sputum for culture and microscopy to detect fat.

Management

Management is supportive.

- Give humidified O_2, titrated to keep $SaO_2 > 94\%$. Repeat ABGs to ensure that hypoxaemia is corrected.
- ❶ Increasing O_2 requirement, exhaustion, or rising $PaCO_2$ require **urgent** ITU/HDU referral for consideration of invasive monitoring, CPAP, or intubation and mechanical ventilation.
- Ensure adequate fluid resuscitation, but avoid overhydration, as this will worsen lung compliance and respiratory function.
- Arrange chest physiotherapy.
- Consider IV antibiotics in those with pyrexia and ↑ WCC to treat possible coexistent pneumonia.
- Nutritional support, e.g. NG feeding.

① **Peripheral nerve injuries: overview**

Peripheral nerve injuries are common following major limb trauma. Unlike the brain or spinal cord, axons within peripheral nerves have the potential for recovery.

Axonal disruption results in Wallerian degeneration to the distal axon. If the endoneurial tube surrounding the axon is intact, proximal axons can grow down it at 1–2mm/day. Destruction of both the axon and endoneurial tube leads to disorganized regeneration, even if continuity of the nerve is restored by surgical reconstruction.

Peripheral nerve injuries are classified according to the degree of injury of the surrounding endoneurial tube, which determines prognosis and management.

- Neurapraxia: local conduction block due to focal nerve demyelination without distal Wallerian degeneration. Examples include tourniquet compression or mild nerve stretching. Paralysis may be complete, but some sensory and autonomic function is preserved. Recovery is complete and spontaneous, although it may take many weeks.
- Axonotmesis: axonal damage with distal Wallerian degeneration, but an intact endoneurium. Examples include a severe blow or stretch injury. Spontaneous recovery proceeds at 1–2mm/day with a near-normal end result.
- Neurotmesis: complete division of the axon and endoneurium with distal Wallerian degeneration, e.g. stab injury or high-energy traction. Usually requires surgery to restore continuity and allow partial nerve recovery.

Both axonotmesis and neurotmesis present with complete loss of motor, sensory, and autonomic function.

Clinical features

- Determine the exact mechanism of injury (high-energy and open injuries are associated with more severe injuries).
- On examination, identify any open fractures or wounds. Determine the degree of motor, sensory, and autonomic dysfunction.
  - Grade motor and sensory abnormalities using the Medical Research Council (MRC) classifications (Boxes 16.4 and 16.5).
  - Absence of sweating indicates autonomic dysfunction.
  - Normal two-point discrimination is 4mm on the finger pulps.
- ❶ Reduce any fractures or dislocations immediately.
- ❶ Examination can be difficult in the acute trauma setting. Re-examine after 48h, if necessary.
- ❶ Nerves and arteries usually run together—always check for vascular injuries as well.

Investigations

❶ Thorough clinical examination is essential, and removes the need for complex investigations in the majority of cases. When necessary, the following may be of use.

- Neurophysiology (nerve conduction studies and electromyography): can identify distal Wallerian degeneration, but is unable to distinguish between axonotmesis and neurotmesis.

- MRI: allows accurate localization of the injury, especially in brachial plexus injuries. Complete lack of continuity confirms neurotmesis.

Box 16.4 MRC classification of motor nerve dysfunction

- M0   Complete paralysis
- M1   Muscle flicker
- M2   Power insufficient to overcome gravity
- M3   Movement against gravity
- M4   Movement against resistance
- M4+   Strong movement, but not normal
- M5   Normal motor function

Box 16.5 MRC classification of sensory nerve dysfunction

- S0   No sensation
- S1   Deep pain sensation
- S2   Touch, pain, and thermal sensation only
- S3   S2 with accurate localization. Unable to identify objects.
- S3+   S3 with object recognition. Poor two-point discrimination.
- S4   Normal sensation

Management

❶ The detection and management of life-threatening injuries take priority.

The mechanism of injury and examination findings determine early management.

In open fractures or penetrating injuries with loss of nerve function, neurotmesis should be assumed to have occurred. Early surgical exploration and repair are required once the patient is haemodynamically stable.

In closed injuries with loss of nerve function, management is more complex. If surgery is needed for fracture fixation, the nerve should also be explored. If surgery is not required for fracture fixation, nerve conduction studies 3–4 weeks after injury are helpful.

- Demonstration of a conduction delay but no Wallerian degeneration implies neuropraxia, and non-operative management is appropriate.
- The presence of Wallerian degeneration identifies axonotmesis and neurotmesis. Repeat neurophysiology at 6–8 weeks can identify re-innervation (implying axonotmesis). Surgical exploration and repair can be performed at 8 weeks if re-innervation is not found (i.e. neurotmesis).

Specific peripheral nerve injuries and their detection

Axillary nerve (C5, 6)

- Anatomy: winds around the neck of the humerus.
- Injury: shoulder dislocation, fracture of the proximal humerus, direct blow to the upper arm.
- Sensory: regimental badge area over the lateral shoulder.
- Motor: deltoid, teres minor.
- Motor test: unable to abduct shoulder (often difficult after dislocation).

Radial nerve (C5–T1)

- Anatomy: winds posteriorly and laterally around the humeral shaft near the spiral groove, coming anterior to the lateral epicondyle. As it crosses the elbow it divides into the posterior interosseus nerve (PIN; pure motor) and the superficial radial nerve (SRN; pure sensory).
- Injury: midshaft or distal 1/3rd humeral fracture midshaft (Holstein Lewis fracture).
- Motor: radial nerve supplies triceps, extensor carpi radialis longus (ECRL), brachioradialis. PIN supplies supinator, extensor carpi radialis brevis (ECRB), extensor digitorum (ED), extensor digiti minimi (EDM), extensor carpi ulnaris (ECU), abductor pollicis longus (APL), extensor pollicis longus (EPL), extensor pollicis brevis (EPB), extensor indicis (EI).
- Sensory: radial nerve supplies lower lateral arm skin; SRN supplies sensation to the dorsum of the 1st web space.
- Motor test: presents with wrist drop. Unable to strongly extend wrist, thumb, and fingers.

Ulnar nerve (C8, T1)

- Anatomy: runs posterior to the medial intermuscular septum in the upper arm, at the elbow it runs posterior to the medial epicondyle, then comes anterior through the two heads of flexor carpi ulnaris (FCU) to lie on the anterior surface of flexor digitorum profundus (FDP). At the wrist it passes through Guyon's canal into the hand.
- Injury: fractures around the elbow, elbow dislocation, penetrating forearm injuries.
- Motor: supplies FCU, and the ulnar half of FDP. In the hand it supplies abductor pollicis (AP), flexor pollicis brevis (FPB), the 2 medial lumbricals, the interossei, opponens digiti minimi (ODM), abductor digiti minimi (ADM), and flexor digiti minimi (FDM).
- Sensory: the medial aspect of the hand and the medial 1 and 1/2 digits, posteriorly and anteriorly.
- Motor test: presents with clawing of the ring and little fingers. Unable to abduct/adduct the fingers. Froment's sign: when asked to grip paper between the index finger and the thumb, the patient flexes the thumb interphalangeal joint (i.e. using flexor pollicis longus (FPL)—median nerve).

Median nerve (C6–T1)

- Anatomy: in the upper arm it runs deep to the short head of the biceps and lateral to the brachial artery. It crosses to the medial side of the brachial artery mid upper arm and descends to the elbow, where it lies deep to the bicipital aponeurosis and medial to the brachial artery. It then passes through the two heads of pronator teres descending to the wrist deep to flexor digitorum superficialis (FDS) and superficial to FDP. At the wrist it lies medial to flexor carpi radialis (FCR) and then enters the carpal tunnel.

- Injury: supracondylar elbow fractures in children (anterior interosseous motor branch), fractures/dislocations around the elbow, distal radial fractures with significant volar or dorsal displacement, penetrating wrist injuries.
- Motor: to all the long flexors in the forearm (except flexor carpi ulnaris (FCU) and the medial half of FDP) and pronator teres, palmaris longus, and pronator quadratus. In the hand, supplies abductor pollicis brevis (APB), FPB, opponens pollicis (OP), and the 1st and 2nd lumbricals.
- Sensory: the thenar skin of the palm and the radial 3 and 1/2 fingers.
- Motor test: poor grip strength, unable to make the 'OK' sign with the thumb and index finger, look for flexion of the interphalangeal (IP) joint of the thumb and distal interphalangeal (DIP) joint. For lesions at the level of wrist test abductor pollicis brevis (APB): patients are unable to lift their thumb up to the ceiling when their hand is flat on a desk palm up.

Femoral nerve (L2–4)

- Anatomy: a branch of the lumbar plexus, it descends between psoas and iliacus, and passes under the inguinal ligament lateral to the femoral artery.
- Injury: penetrating injuries in the groin.
- Motor: pectineus, sartorius, quadriceps femoris.
- Sensory: anterior thigh, medial knee, and down to the medial malleolus via the saphenous nerve.
- Motor test: knee extension.

Sciatic nerve (L4–S3)

- Anatomy: exits the pelvis through the greater sciatic notch below the piriformis muscle and descends down the back of the thigh. At a variable distance it divides into the tibial and common peroneal nerves.
- Injury: posterior dislocation of the hip, elective hip surgery using a posterior approach, penetrating injuries to the posterior thigh.
- Motor: superior and inferior gemelli, obturator internus, quadratus femoris, biceps femoris, semitendinosus, semimembranosus, adductor magnus. Via branches to all the muscles below the knee.
- Sensory: no cutaneous branches in the thigh. Via tibial nerve and common peroneal nerve supplies all sensation below the knee except for the medial aspect of the calf and ankle (saphenous nerve).
- Motor test: knee flexion, all movements of foot and ankle.

Tibial nerve (L4–S3)

- Anatomy: a branch of the sciatic nerve, the tibial nerve descends through the popliteal fossa down the back of the calf to terminate in the medial and lateral plantar nerves of the foot.
- Injury: penetrating injuries to the popliteal fossa, knee dislocation.

- Motor: gastrocnemius, popliteus, soleus, plantaris, tibialis posterior, flexor digitorum longus (FDL), flexor hallucis longus (FHL). The medial and lateral plantar nerves supply the intrinsic muscles of the foot.
- Sensory: posterior calf, lateral foot, sole of the foot.
- Motor test: ankle and toe plantar flexion.

Common peroneal nerve (CPN; L4–S3)

- Anatomy: a branch of the sciatic nerve, the CPN winds around the neck of the fibula and divides into the superficial and deep peroneal nerves (SPN, DPN)
- Injury: neck of fibula fracture or penetrating injury, knee dislocation, posterolateral knee ligament injury.
- Motor: DPN supplies the anterior leg compartment (tibialis anterior, extensor digitorum longus (EDL), peroneus tertius, extensor hallucis longus (EHL)) and the dorsal intrinsic muscles of the foot. SPN supplies the lateral compartment (peroneus longus and brevis).
- Sensory: DPN supplies sensation to the dorsal aspect of the 1st web space. SPN supplies the remaining dorsum of the foot except for that supplied by the lateral plantar nerve.
- Motor test: DPN—ankle, foot, and toe extension; SPN—foot eversion.

Early postoperative complications

The majority of problems in postoperative surgical patients are generic (📖 p.131). The points below apply to trauma and orthopaedic patients in particular.

Venous thromboembolism (see also 📖 p.149, p.322)

Patients undergoing many types of orthopaedic surgery are at high risk from postoperative venous thromboembolism (VTE), i.e. DVT/PE. The clinical features and management of orthopaedic patients with VTE can be different from those in other surgical specialties. After lower limb surgery, normal postoperative limb changes make the clinical diagnosis of DVT difficult. Anticoagulation after orthopaedic surgery may lead to a joint or wound haematoma, increasing the risk of prosthetic infection.

- ❶ Do **not** start anticoagulation without discussion with your senior.
- ❶ Have a high index of suspicion—VTE is common.

DVT management

Treatment depends on the extent of the DVT (calf versus thigh) and when it is picked up (< 48h versus > 48h postoperatively).

- Treatment of calf DVTs remains controversial: a large percentage will resolve with no long-term sequelae; only a small percentage will propagate proximally or give rise to a PE.
  - If detected < 48h postoperatively, operative site haematoma formation is a major concern. Consider re-scanning in 48h to detect progression, or anticoagulation once the risk of haematoma formation lessens.
  - If detected > 48h postoperatively, consider re-scanning in 1 week to detect progression, or anticoagulation. If the DVT has not spread to the thigh in 1 week, it is unlikely to and some would suggest that no anticoagulation is needed.
- Thigh DVTs have a much higher risk of PE. If identified < 48h following surgery, options include anticoagulation or using an IVC filter until it is safe to anticoagulate. Anticoagulate if identified > 48h following surgery.
- Anticoagulation can be achieved with a therapeutic dose of SC LMWH, according to local protocol. Load with warfarin, aiming for INR of 2.5. For calf DVTs, treat for 2–3 months; treat thigh DVTs for 3–6 months.

PE management If a PE is identified < 48h following surgery, options include anticoagulation as in DVT management, accepting the increased risk of bleeding, or using an IVC filter until it is safe to anticoagulate. Treat with warfarin for 6 months.

Postoperative pyrexia (📖 p.162)

As with other surgical patients, this is common, especially within 2 days of surgery. As well as considering other causes, look specifically for features of fat emboli (📖 p.416) and prosthesis infection (📖 p.408).

❶ Do not start antibiotics unless a clear focus is found or the patient is systemically unwell or septic.

Fat embolism syndrome (📖 p.416)

Compartment syndrome (📖 p.412)

Tight dressings, plaster casts, or backslabs

After any limb procedure, it is common for circumferential dressings to be applied. Immediately following a fracture, most patients are placed in plaster backslabs to allow for ongoing swelling, with a full plaster cast applied days later. Even with backslabs, the cotton wool and crepe bandages are circumferential. Any circumferential dressing or plaster cast may become restrictive, leading to increasing pain and a sense of tightness. Left untreated, this may progress to compartment syndrome (📖 p.412). If the dressing/cast/backslab is generally tight, but with **no evidence** of compartment syndrome, consider the following.

- Find the operation note as the surgeon may have left specific instructions.
- If no specific advice has been offered, ensure that simple measures to reduce swelling are used.
  - Gentle limb elevation (at or **just** above the level of the heart).
  - Cool the limb (e.g. Cryo/Cuff™).
  - Split the circumferential dressings or cast **down to skin** along its full length and gently prise open the plaster edges. Cutting through plaster requires a plaster saw (see 'Hints'). It is safer to do this and possibly lose fracture reduction, than to risk a compartment syndrome or local pressure sore.
  - Usually, once the cast or dressings have been split the patient immediately feels better. Don't remove the cast or backslab completely, but lightly wrap a crepe bandage around the limb.
  - If the patient experiences no benefit from the simple measures above or if the pain returns, consider the possibility of compartment syndrome.
- If a patient complains of a localized area of pressure or pain under a cast or backslab, cut out a window to check the skin. Replace the wool and bandage the plaster window back in place.
  - ❶ The edges of the window may create more pressure problems.

Hints

- When using a plaster saw, don't drag it along the skin, press down until you have cut the plaster. Lift it, and move further down and press down again. Be very careful cutting plaster in the presence of dried blood; it cakes the cotton wool dressings and makes it hard, which can then be cut by the oscillating saw.
- If a patient has a circumferential cast it can be difficult to split all the dressings including the cotton wool down to skin. If you are unable to prise the plaster open, instead remove a small channel of plaster by making two parallel cuts 2–5mm apart. The channel will enable you to cut the ortho wool with a pair of scissors and then prise open the cast a few mm. If needed, bivalve the cast (split down both sides).

Peripheral nerve injuries (📖 p.418)

These may be due to tourniquets, or poor positioning with inadequate padding. The majority of these injuries are neurapraxias and will recover spontaneously.

- ❶ Check that the patient has not had a peripheral nerve block for analgesia or local administration of a long-acting local anaesthetic. Read the operation note as nerve contusion and continuity may have been documented.
- ❶ Where the damaged nerve runs near an operative site, nerve transection may have occurred. Discuss the case with the surgeon and consider early wound exploration with nerve repair.

Neurosurgery

Introduction

Neurosurgery is concentrated in tertiary referral centres and many surgical trainees will not work with neurosurgeons directly. In spite of this, the ability to assess and manage patients with neurosurgical emergencies (especially head injuries) is important. Early and appropriate discussion with the regional neurosurgical service is essential as incorrectly managed patients can suffer potentially devastating long-term neurological sequelae.

Anatomy

The skull is made up of the cranial vault and the skull base. While the cranial vault is smooth, the skull base is irregular. The floor of the cranial cavity is divided into anterior, middle and posterior cranial fossae. The meninges cover the brain and consist of three layers (Fig. 17.1).

- Dura mater: a tough membrane tightly adherent to the inner surface of the skull.
  - The meningeal arteries lie between the dura and the skull.
  - The dura separates from the bone to form dural leaves (tentorium cerebelli and falx cerebri), dividing the brain into right and left and supratentorial and infratentorial compartments.
- Arachnoid mater: a thin membrane that lies deep to the dura, but is not adherent to it.
  - This creates a potential space (subdural space) into which haemorrhage can occur.
  - Cerebral arteries lie in the subarachnoid space.
- Pia mater: firmly adherent to the brain surface.

Cerebrospinal fluid (CSF) is produced by the choroid plexus in the cerebral ventricles. It flows from the lateral ventricles through the third and fourth ventricles to circulate in the subarachnoid space between the arachnoid and the pia. It is absorbed into the venous circulation by the arachnoid granulations projecting into the superior sagittal sinus.

Pathophysiology

The brain is encased within a bony box. The box also contains blood (arterial and venous) and CSF. The Monro–Kellie doctrine states that the total intracranial volume must remain constant due to its bony confines. If a mass (e.g. an intracranial haematoma) expands acutely within the cranial cavity, low pressure CSF and venous blood will be pushed out and the intracranial pressure (ICP) will initially remain constant. As the volume of the mass enlarges to > 100–150mL these compensatory mechanisms fail and ICP rises (Fig. 17.2).

Normal ICP is 5–10mmHg. ICP > 20mmHg is associated with a poor outcome after traumatic brain injury as it causes a reduction in the cerebral perfusion pressure (CPP) and cerebral blood flow. Further increases in ICP lead to brain herniation (📖 p.431). CPP is dependent upon ICP and mean arterial blood pressure (MABP): CPP = MABP − ICP. CPP must be maintained to ensure adequate perfusion of the brain.

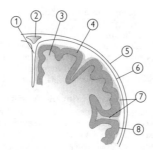

Fig. 17.1 Anatomy of the meninges ①, Falx cerebri—a folding of the inner layer of the dura mater; ②, venous sinuses are enclosed between the leaves of dura; ③, white matter; ④, grey matter; ⑤, outer layer of dura mater, fused with bony periosteum; ⑥, inner layer of dura mater; ⑦, arachnoid mater—dips into cortical sulci to form CSF cisterns; ⑧, pia mater—closely adherent to cortical surface at all points.

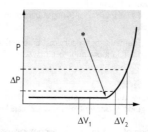

Fig. 17.2 Intracranial compliance curve. As the volume of a mass lesion in the skull increases, compensatory measures initially limit an increase in pressure (ΔV_1). Once this compensation has reached its limit (*), increases in volume (ΔV_2) cause exponential increases in pressure (ΔP).

Classification of intracranial neurosurgical emergencies

- Traumatic, e.g. intracranial haemorrhage (extradural, subdural, subarachnoid, intracerebral), skull fracture, scalp laceration.
- Spontaneous, e.g. subarachnoid haemorrhage
- Infective, e.g. intracerebral abscess, meningitis.
- Neoplastic.

Neurosurgical emergencies: principles of assessment

These can be summarized as follows.

- Accurate history-taking, in particular with respect to:
  - mechanism of injury;
  - changes to the level of consciousness;
  - symptoms of systemic sepsis.

- Using the GCS to document level of consciousness (📖 p.59).
- Identifying focal neurological signs.
- Identification of specific syndromes:
  - signs of basal skull fractures and CSF leak (📖 p.446);
  - raised ICP (morning headache, headache worse with coughing/straining, papilloedema, nausea and vomiting);
  - meningism (neck stiffness, photophobia, nausea and vomiting).

Neurosurgical emergencies: principles of management

As with surgical emergencies in other body systems, the management of neurosurgical emergencies starts before a diagnosis has been reached. Management principles include the following.

- Prevention of secondary brain injury:
  - good oxygenation and airway protection (📖 p.46);
  - maintenance of euvolaemia;
  - control of ↑ ICP;
  - seizure control;
  - prevention of infection.
- Frequent reassessment to detect complications:
  - further intracranial haemorrhage;
  - development of vasospasm (following subarachnoid haemorrhage) or hydrocephalus.

The diagnosis of traumatic neurosurgical emergencies rests on the appearances on head CT. Lumbar puncture may also be necessary in non-traumatic disease processes.

Control of raised ICP

In severe head injury, ICP monitoring using an intracranial transducer ('bolt') is used to guide treatment. Raised ICP can be reduced using a number of means:

- surgical (evacuation of mass lesions or decompressive craniectomy; see trauma craniotomy (Fig. 17.3));
- sedatives (reduce cerebral metabolism);
- induced hyperventilation (causes reflex vasoconstriction of cerebral vessels);
- hyperosmolar agents, e.g. mannitol (create an osmotic gradient that draws fluid across the blood–brain barrier);
- hypothermia (reduces cerebral metabolism).

❶ These treatments should only be given with ICP monitoring. Patients have an improved outcome if treated in the setting of a dedicated neuro-intensive care unit.

Seizure control

Patients with head injuries are susceptible to generalized seizures. This can be due to a localized lesion, e.g. a depressed skull fracture, or as consequence of diffuse axonal injury. Seizures increase ICP and raise the brain's requirements for oxygen and glucose at a time when these are in short supply. Prolonged seizures also impair ventilation and cause hypoxia. In the acute setting, phenytoin is the anti-epileptic of choice. The patient should be loaded with 15–18mg/kg IV over 30min with cardiac monitoring due to the risk of dysrhythmias. After loading, phenytoin should be continued at a dose of 300mg IV od until neurosurgical advice becomes available. Anti-epileptics should not be used prophylactically.

❶ A prolonged seizure lasting more than 30min (status epilepticus) is an emergency in itself and may require endotracheal intubation.

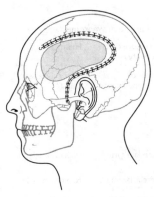

Fig. 17.3 The trauma craniotomy. In the trauma patient a wide fronto-temporo-parietal craniotomy allows access to mass lesions above the tentorium cerebelli. The crossed line shows a 'question mark' incision. The shaded area shows the area of bone removed.

Brain herniation and the unilateral fixed, dilated pupil

The inside of the skull is compartmentalized by the falx cerebri and the tentorium cerebelli. If the pressure in one of these compartments increases dramatically it can force portions of the brain from one compartment into another, compressing important structures (see Table 17.1).

In the context of head injury the finding of a unilateral fixed, dilated pupil ('blown pupil') most likely indicates the presence of an ipsilateral expanding intracranial haematoma causing transtentorial herniation (Fig. 17.4). Other causes of a blown pupil include direct trauma to the eye or a brainstem contusion in the region of the oculomotor nerve nucleus.

Brain herniation is a neurosurgical emergency because, if the pressure continues to rise, it will eventually force the cerebellar tonsils out of the foramen magnum ('coning'), fatally compressing the cardiorespiratory centres in the medulla oblongata. Cushing's response, consisting of hypertension and bradycardia, may immediately precede coning.

- ▶▶ The initial treatment for a blown pupil is to give 200mL of 20% mannitol IV **after discussion with a neurosurgeon**. As mannitol is a diuretic, any fluid lost in the urine must be made up in IV fluids to maintain the circulating blood volume. This might mean infusing a further 1–2L of normal saline.
  - Mannitol is an osmotic diuretic that is thought to reduce ICP by increasing serum osmolarity, drawing fluid across the blood–brain barrier, and reducing cerebral oedema. Ultimately, the cause of the

blown pupil must be dealt with surgically but mannitol can provide time for CT and transfer to a neurosurgical centre.
- ❶ The only indication for exploratory burr holes is a haemodynamically unstable patient in theatre for other surgery who blows a pupil on the table.

Table 17.1 Brain herniation syndromes

Type of herniation	Structure that herniates	Hiatus	Structures at risk
Transtentorial	Uncus of temporal lobe	Tentorial hiatus	Posterior cerebral artery
			IIIrd nerve nucleus
			Cerebral peduncles
			Periaqueductal grey matter
Subfalcine	Cingulate gyrus	Under falx cerebri	Anterior cerebral artery
Tonsillar	Cerebellar tonsils	Foramen magnum	Medulla oblongata

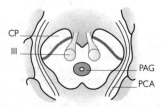

Fig. 17.4 A horizontal section of the midbrain at the level of the tentorial hiatus. Transtentorial herniation is shown. The structures that are compressed have the following clinical consequences: III, Oculomotor nerve nucleus (ipsilateral pupil dilatation); CP, cerebral peduncle (contralateral hemiparesis); PAG, periaqueductal grey matter (coma); PCA, posterior cerebral artery (ischaemia or infarction of the occipital lobes).

☼ Extradural haemorrhage

Extradural haemorrhage (EDH) is usually but not always, associated with a skull fracture, most commonly in the thin bone of the temple (the pterion). The fracture lacerates a branch of the middle meningeal artery which bleeds into the space between the cortical bone and the dura (hence extradural). As the blood is at arterial pressure, the haematoma enlarges rapidly and can lead to a dramatic deterioration in the patient's clinical state.

EDH may occur at other sites and can contain venous blood after laceration of a dural venous sinus.

Clinical features
- History of head injury (often trivial), e.g. a cricket ball to the temple.
- Recovery from transient loss of consciousness (lucid interval), then a rapid deterioration minutes-to-hours later.
- ❶ Patients with head injuries may initially appear normal but can have a significant underlying pathology. This is summed up by the phrase 'patients who talk and die'.
- On examination, there is tenderness over the injury site. Otherwise signs are variable, ranging from no signs to unilateral weakness, coma, or a unilateral fixed and dilated pupil (📖 p.431).

Investigation
Emergency head CT (Fig. 17.5). EDH appear as high density biconvex lesions outside the substance of the brain. They do not cross suture lines and most commonly occur over the pterion (the meeting point of the parietal, sphenoid, zygomatic, and temporal bones).

Management
- Prevention of secondary brain injury (📖 p.430).
- If the conscious state is impaired the patient requires rapid transfer to a neurosurgical centre for haematoma evacuation, ideally within 2h of deterioration.
- If a patient is awake and oriented and the EDH is small (volume < 30mL, thickness < 15mm, and midline shift < 5mm) on CT, the patient may not require surgery. Transfer to a neurosurgical centre is still required for observation. This allows rapid evacuation should the patient deteriorate.

❶ As there is often minimal underlying parenchymal injury the prognosis is usually good if the haematoma can be evacuated in time.

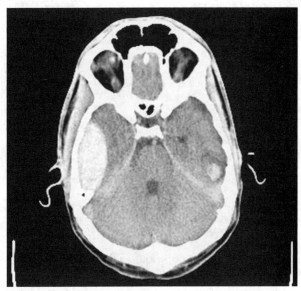

Fig. 17.5 A head CT showing an EDH. Note the contra-coup cerebral contusion in the left temporal lobe.

☼ Subdural haemorrhage

Acute subdural haemorrhage (SDH) must be distinguished from chronic SDH as their demographics, pathology, presentation, and management are very different.

Acute SDH

These are often the result of a **severe** impact and are associated with greater underlying brain injury than EDH. They are more common than EDH. Acute SDH usually arise as a result of a superficial contusion of the brain that ruptures into the subdural space and/or rupture of cortical veins. Rapid acceleration/deceleration forces can also shear the bridging veins that cross from the brain's surface to the venous sinuses on the inner table of the skull.

Clinical features As damage to the underlying brain is often severe, patients usually present with a decreased GCS post-head injury with no lucid interval.

Investigation Emergency head CT. Acute SDH appear as biconvex high density lesions that spread over the surface of the brain (Fig. 17.6). They can cross suture lines and compress the underlying brain.

Management
- Prevention of secondary brain injury (🕮 p.430).
- Patients with good pre-morbid function or large (thickness > 5mm) acute SDH require haematoma evacuation through a wide craniotomy with haemostasis of the underlying brain.
- Patients with multiple co-morbidities and small acute SDH do not require craniotomy. The haematoma can be left to resolve or evacuated once it becomes a chronic SDH.

❶ Acute SDH are associated with more underlying brain injury than EDH and have a worse prognosis.

Chronic SDH

Chronic SDH usually follows trivial trauma to the head that the patient may not remember. It is thought to occur in patients with brain atrophy where the bridging veins from the brain to the inner surface of the skull are fragile and susceptible to injury. It is most common in alcoholics, the elderly, and those on anticoagulants. An inflammatory membrane (neomembrane) forms around the initial bleed. As the blood within the haematoma is enzymatically digested there is an increase in the number of osmotically active molecules within the neomembrane. This progressively draws fluid into the collection, which gradually increases in size. The fluid within a chronic SDH is liquid.

Clinical features
- The patient may present many weeks after the initial injury.
- The most common symptoms are non-specific, such as drowsiness, forgetfulness, and clumsiness.
- Some present with focal signs such as hemiparesis.

Investigation Emergency head CT. Chronic SDH change their density when seen on CT. For the first 7 days they appear high density (whiter than brain), for the next couple of weeks they appear isodense (the same density as brain, hardest to spot; Fig. 17.7) before eventually becoming hypodense (darker than brain).

Management Two burr holes are placed at opposite ends of the collection and the fluid is drained by flushing copious warm normal saline from one hole to the other until the fluid runs clear.

This operation is much less invasive than a craniotomy. Neurological symptoms and signs are potentially completely reversible.

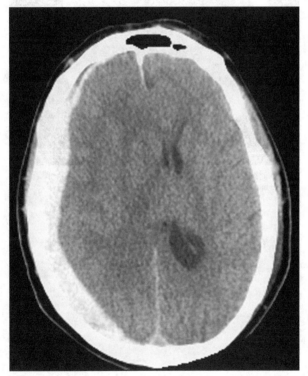

Fig. 17.6 CT appearance of an acute SDH. Significant midline shift, compression of the cerebral ventricles, and effacement of the ipsilateral cortical sulci are all demonstrated.

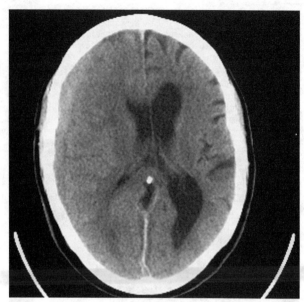

Fig. 17.7 CT appearances of a chronic SDH. In this scan, the chronic SDH is iso-dense to brain and difficult to spot. However, the midline shift gives it away.

☼ Subarachnoid haemorrhage

Subarachnoid haemorrhages (SAH) can be traumatic or spontaneous. Traumatic SAH is more common. Complications of both types include hydrocephalus and vasospasm. Subarachnoid blood can clot and directly obstruct the passage of CSF drainage through the ventricles (non-communicating hydrocephalus) or the blood breakdown products can obstruct CSF absorption in the arachnoid granulations (communicating hydrocephalus). These breakdown products also lead to vasospasm of the cerebral vasculature, and can result in brain infarction. Spontaneous SAH may also re-bleed.

Traumatic SAH is a common consequence of traumatic brain injury that does not require any special intervention over and above the standard treatment principles.

Spontaneous SAH

This is most commonly due to rupture of a 'berry aneurysm' at a branch point in the circle of Willis. These aneurysms are thought to be due to a congenital weakness of the arterial media. They have a higher incidence in women and rupture more commonly in hypertensives and smokers. SAH may also be due to arteriovenous malformations.

Clinical features

- Usually presents with a sudden-onset occipital headache described as the 'worst of my life'.
- On examination, signs of meningism are present, i.e. neck stiffness, photophobia, nausea and vomiting. Severe bleeds may produce coma.

Investigations

- Emergency head CT: shows blood within the subarachnoid space (Fig.17.8).
- Lumbar puncture: CT may not identify a small SAH (< 1% of cases) and lumbar puncture may show persistent blood staining of CSF and xanthochromia.
- Angiography: once stable, either conventional or CT angiography is required in order to look for an underlying aneurysm.

Management

- Flat bed rest and laxatives to avoid straining and spikes of BP until the aneurysm is secured.
- Adequate hydration with IV fluids.
- Oral nimodipine 60mg every 4h to reduce the incidence of vasospasm. If vasospasm occurs despite this, as evidenced by a focal neurological deficit or a drop in conscious state, 'HHH' therapy (Hypertension, Haemodilution, Hypervolaemia) is used to improve blood flow through the narrowed vessels.
- Close observation and repeat CT to detect hydrocephalus. This may require emergency external drainage of CSF from the cerebral ventricles. An internal ventriculoperitoneal shunt for long-term CSF drainage may be indicated if the hydrocephalus becomes chronic.
- Spontaneous SAH due to berry aneurysm:
  - surgical placement of a clip across the aneurysm neck;

- endovascular placement of metal coils within the aneurysm sac to occlude the lumen.

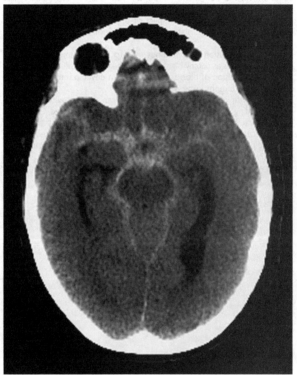

Fig. 17.8 CT appearance of a SAH. This demonstrates widespread blood (hyperin-tense on CT) filling the basal cisterns.

✪ Intracerebral haemorrhage

These are haematomas within the substance of the brain. They occur most commonly in the frontal and temporal lobes where head trauma causes the brain to move over the irregular inner surfaces of the skull. They can also occur at points of direct impact or opposite them, where the brain collides against the contralateral inner surface of the skull (contra-coup lesion, e.g. Fig. 17.5).

The term 'contusion' is sometimes used to describe an area of bruised brain that appears as patchy high density on head CT but doesn't represent a discrete collection of blood. Contusions can develop into haematomas and may require monitoring with repeat CT.

Patients with intracerebral haemorrhage can present with focal deficits, depending on the site of the lesion, or with decreased GCS. Most intracerebral haemorrhages are managed with non-surgical control of any associated rise in ICP. Eventually the haematoma is resorbed and any surrounding brain swelling settles. Surgical decompression should be considered if the haematoma causes significant mass effect (i.e. midline shift of > 5mm) or if the patient is comatose.

ⓘ **Concussion**

Concussion can be defined as a mild diffuse traumatic injury to the brain causing confusion or amnesia. Transient loss of consciousness may be a feature. There is no specific treatment, providing other pathologies are excluded. This may require head CT (📖 p.76). Patients can be discharged from the emergency department into the care of a responsible adult with appropriate head injury advice and an information sheet.

The 'post-concussive syndrome' describes a number of non-specific symptoms that can persist after concussion, including headache, irritability, visual disturbance, and loss of concentration. In most cases, symptoms resolve with time.

☼ Severe diffuse traumatic brain injury

Many patients with severe head injury have diffuse injury to the brain, particularly those sustaining high velocity injuries with a rotational element or rapid acceleration/deceleration. This injury is called 'diffuse axonal injury' histologically and is caused by shearing of axonal processes. It can occur together with an intracranial haematoma or independently. Treatment is targeted at reducing ICP (📖 p.430).

❶ These patients have severe and sustained brain swelling and often have a poor prognosis.

① Skull fractures

Skull fractures are a common consequence of head trauma. Before the widespread availability of CT, skull fractures found on plain skull X-rays were important risk factors for intracranial haematomas. As CT has now largely replaced skull X-rays, the significance of skull fractures has diminished, as the management of an associated intracranial haematoma takes precedence.

Classification
- Fracture configuration, e.g. linear, comminuted, depressed.
- Anatomical site, i.e. skull vault, base of skull (basilar).
- Communication with the environment, i.e. open or closed.

History
- History of trauma.
- Headache.
- Clear fluid dripping from the nose or ear.

Examination
- Tenderness over the injury site.
- 'Boggy' scalp swelling.
- Neurological signs from any underlying intracranial haematoma.
- Skull deformity.
- Signs of a skull base fracture:
  - anterior cranial fossa: raccoon eyes (periorbital ecchymoses), CSF rhinorrhoea, anosmia;
  - middle cranial fossa: Battle's sign (retroauricular ecchymosis), CSF otorrhoea (only seen in the presence of a perforated tympanic membrane), haemotympanum, damage to the facial or vestibulocochlear nerves.

Investigations
- Suspected skull fracture is an indication for emergency head CT (Fig. 17.9).
- ❶ Patients with skull base fractures and possible CSF rhinorrhoea or otorrhoea should have the leaking fluid tested for tau protein, a neurone-specific protein found only in the central nervous system.

Management
- ❶ Patients with skull fractures should be discussed with a neurosurgeon.
- Linear and comminuted skull vault fractures do not require intervention unless they are open or significantly depressed.
- Open skull fractures: as with any open fracture, this is a surgical emergency that should be considered for surgical debridement and thorough lavage, particularly as there may be communication between the fracture site and the underlying brain.
  - There is a risk of intracranial infection (intracerebral abscess or meningitis) and prophylactic IV antibiotics may be required initially, e.g. cefotaxime 1g bd with metronidazole 500mg tds.

- Depressed skull fractures: these fractures can result in underlying brain injury, breaching of the dura, and/or cosmetic deformity.
  - The rule of thumb is that fractures that are depressed more than the thickness of the skull require surgical elevation.
  - This allows correction of any cosmetic deformity as well as ensuring that there is no CSF leak or brain herniation at the fracture site.
- Base of skull fractures: the importance of recognizing these fractures is that there is a high likelihood of a CSF leak as the dura is tightly adherent to the skull base.
  - CSF leaks may be overt or occult, i.e. if CSF collects in the middle ear or paranasal sinuses.
  - Skull base fractures carry a risk of meningitis and the patient should be aware of the symptoms and signs to look out for before discharge. Prophylactic antibiotics are not indicated.
  - If a CSF leak is found, or suspected, the patient can usually be managed expectantly to see if it resolves spontaneously. Ongoing CSF leaks for > 5 days can be managed by reducing CSF pressure, e.g. with daily lumbar puncture, continuous drainage via percutaneous catheter, or surgical closure.

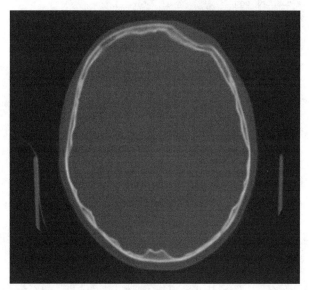

Fig. 17.9 CT of a depressed skull fracture. A depressed skull fracture is seen in the left frontal bone.

① Intracranial abscess

These result from either direct spread of infection or haematogenous spread. Direct spread can occur with:
- penetrating trauma;
- sinus or middle ear infection;
- surgery that breaches the dura;
- meningitis.

Haematogenous spread most commonly occurs from lung suppuration.

Clinical features

These are varied, but include:
- systemic signs of infection, swinging pyrexia;
- signs of raised ICP (morning headaches, headache worse with coughing/straining, papilloedema);
- seizures;
- focal neurological deficit.

Investigations

- FBC: ↑ WCC.
- ESR, CRP: both ↑.
- Urgent head CT with IV contrast: shows a mass lesion with ring enhancement.
- Lumbar puncture: often unhelpful and may be dangerous in the presence of raised ICP since it can precipitate tentorial herniation.

Management

- The mainstay of management is high dose IV antibiotics e.g. cefotaxime 1–4g tds and metronidazole 500mg tds for 2–4 weeks followed by a further 2–4 weeks of oral antibiotics.
- Surgery can be used to drain large collections, identify the causative organism, and exclude neoplasia.
- The exact treatment employed depends on the clinical state of the patient, likely causative organism, site of the abscess, and likelihood of neoplasia.
- These cases require careful liaison between neurosurgeons, neuroradiologists, and microbiologists.

☺ Meningitis

Meningitis is often a condition that is dealt with by physicians but it is relevant to surgeons as it may follow head trauma, ENT surgery, or neurosurgery. The patient presents with signs of systemic infection and meningism (neck stiffness, photophobia, nausea, and vomiting). CT is often used to exclude a significant space-occupying lesion before lumbar puncture is attempted. In bacterial meningitis, lumbar puncture shows ↑ neutrophils, ↑ protein, ↓ glucose, and bacteria on Gram stain.

❶ The importance of instituting rapid antibiotic therapy cannot be over-emphasized. Emergency microbiology advice is necessary to identify the likely organisms.

① Intracranial tumours

Intracranial tumours can be primary or secondary, benign or malignant. Primary (gliomas) and metastatic intracranial tumours have a similar incidence. Intracranial metastases arise most commonly from the lung, breast, kidney, GI tract, and malignant melanomas.

Clinical features

Brain tumours can present with:
- signs of raised ICP;
- seizures;
- a focal neurological deficit;
- endocrine disturbances (if the pituitary or hypothalamus is involved).

Investigation Urgent head CT with IV contrast. A ring-enhancing lesion (Fig. 17.10) is suspicious of a metastasis, particularly if there are multiple lesions or if the patient is known to have a malignancy elsewhere.

Management

- Patients presenting with seizures should be started on an anti-epileptic, e.g. phenytoin.
- In almost all tumours, significant brain oedema occurs and symptomatic relief can be gained by starting high dose corticosteroids e.g. dexamethasone 4mg qds PO.
- A brain biopsy may be required to reach a histological diagnosis when metastases are suspected with no known primary. Biopsy also allows exclusion of an intracerebral abscess, which can sometimes mimic neoplastic tumours.
- Primary brain tumours can be treated with a craniotomy and debulking, chemotherapy, or radiotherapy or a combination of these depending on the tumour histology and the patient's performance status.

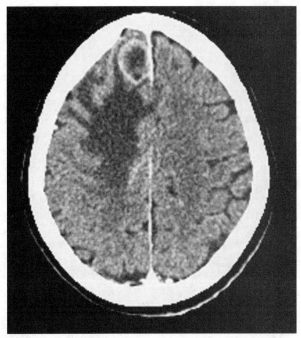

Fig. 17.10 Contrast-enhanced head CT. A ring-enhancing lesion is demonstrated in the right frontal lobe.

Cardiothoracic surgery

Rib fractures: introduction

Rib fractures are common and may be associated with underlying injuries to intrathoracic or intraabdominal structures. Multiple fractures can result in a flail chest.

❶ The associated pain prevents adequate ventilation and coughing, which can lead to pneumonia, particularly in smokers.

① **Single rib fractures** An isolated fracture of a single rib after trauma is uncommon. Following significant trauma, suspect multiple rib fractures and exclude injuries to underlying structures. Rib fracture following trivial injury may suggest a pathological fracture (see 'Multiple rib fractures').

⚙ **Multiple rib fractures**

The distribution of multiple rib fractures can indicate the severity of the injury and which underlying viscera might have been damaged. Younger patients have a more elastic chest wall than older patients so multiple rib fractures in young people imply a significant impact and a higher likelihood of associated intrathoracic and intraabdominal injuries.

- The upper 3 ribs are protected by the bony and muscular components of the upper limb girdle. Hence, fractures of the 1st or 2nd ribs suggest severe trauma. The potential for injury to great vessels, major airways, lungs, heart, and spinal cord exists. Investigate for aortic rupture (📖 p.472).
- The middle ribs (4–9) are most commonly fractured in blunt chest trauma (Fig. 18.1). Haemothorax, pneumothorax, and pulmonary contusion are common.
- The lower ribs (10–12) overlie the abdominal viscera. Fractures of these ribs should raise the suspicion of injury to the spleen (📖 p.252) or liver (📖 p.236).

Clinical features
- On examination, visible deformity, tenderness, and bony crepitus may be present.
- Look for features of injuries to underlying structures.
- ❶ Subcutaneous emphysema indicates an underlying pneumothorax.

Investigations
- CXR: may confirm fractures. More importantly, it will identify atelectasis, pneumothorax, haemothorax, or pre-existing bony or pulmonary pathology.
- ABG: if SaO_2 < 95%, or if pre-existing respiratory disease is present.
- CT chest and abdomen: if the mechanism of injury is significant and/or there is a possibility of underlying organ damage.
- ❶ If a pathological fracture is suspected, request FBC, U&Es, LFTs, Ca^{2+}, and serum protein electrophoresis.

Management
- Most patients with uncomplicated rib fractures can be discharged. Prescribe oral analgesia and advise return if pain worsens or if SOB or symptoms of pneumonia develop.

- Patients with $SaO_2 < 95\%$ or significant pain require admission. Have a low threshold for admission in the elderly and smokers.
  - Give O_2 to keep $SaO_2 > 94\%$.
  - Pain relief should be titrated to need without compromising respiratory drive. Use the 'analgesic ladder', i.e. simple analgesics, NSAIDs, parenteral opioids prn, opioids via a PCA, or regional anaesthetic techniques, e.g. intercostal nerve block, epidural analgesia.
  - Arrange physiotherapy to encourage coughing and prevent atelectasis and pneumonia.

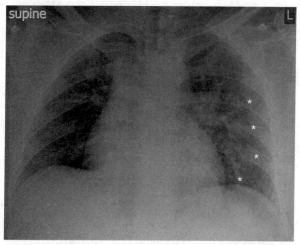

Fig. 18.1 Supine CXR of a young man after blunt left-sided chest trauma. Multiple rib fractures are seen (*), but there is no underlying haemo/pneumothorax present.

:O: **Rib fractures: flail chest**

Flail chest occurs when two or more ribs are fractured in two or more places (Fig. 18.2). This flail segment is paradoxically drawn in on inspiration and pushed out on expiration, causing inadequate ventilation. The severity of the trauma required will usually lead to an underlying pulmonary contusion and other injuries. The combination of pain, pulmonary contusion, and disrupted chest wall mechanics leads to hypoxia.

Clinical features
- Severe chest pain.
- On examination, paradoxical motion of the flail segment is often seen, with chest wall deformity, and bony crepitus.
- Features consistent with hypoxia or shock or damage to underlying viscera are commonly present.
- ❶ The flail segment may not be immediately obvious due to splinting of the chest wall.

❶ Resuscitation and primary survey usually take precedence over history-taking (📖 p.42).

Investigations
- As for 'Multiple rib fractures'. ABGs are mandatory.
- Other investigations are often necessary (📖 p.43).
- CT chest and abdomen: to exclude underlying injuries.

❶ One component of the flail segment may be due to costochondral separation and may not be revealed on a CXR.

Management
- Adequate oxygenation and analgesia are the priorities. A combination of high-flow O_2 and pain relief titrated to need may be sufficient.
- If shocked, fluid resuscitation should be guided by monitored CVP and physiological response. Excessive fluid replacement may exacerbate an underlying pulmonary contusion.
- Aggressive physiotherapy to minimize chest infection is vital once analgesia is adequate.
- The use of CPAP or intubation and mechanical ventilation may become necessary. Involve the on-call anaesthetic/ITU teams early. Hypoxia despite high-flow O_2 therapy, hypercapnia, increasing respiratory rate or work of breathing, or the tiring patient are all indications to consider more invasive ventilation strategies.
- Patients with large flail segments causing difficulty with ventilation should be referred to a cardiothoracic surgeon for consideration of operative fixation.

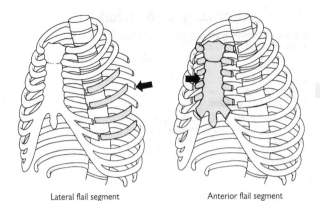

Lateral flail segment   Anterior flail segment

Fig. 18.2 Significant blunt trauma laterally or anteriorly can lead to a flail segment. (Reproduced, with permission, from Wyatt, J.P. et al. (2001). *Oxford Handbook of accident and emergency medicine*, 1st edn, Chapter 8, p. 351. Oxford University Press, Oxford.)

Pneumothorax: introduction

A pneumothorax may be spontaneous or acquired.
- Spontaneous:
  - primary (no underlying lung disease);
  - secondary (underlying lung disease, e.g. COPD).
- Acquired:
  - traumatic;
  - iatrogenic, e.g. central venous line insertion.

A traumatic pneumothorax may present as a simple, open, or tension pneumothorax and may be associated with a haemothorax.

☼ Simple pneumothorax

A simple pneumothorax is air within the pleural space without progressive increase in intrathoracic pressure. The lung partially or fully collapses, leading to a ventilation–perfusion mismatch and hypoxia.

Clinical features

Can be clinically occult (especially if small), or may include the following.
- Ipsilateral pleuritic chest pain.
- On examination, SOB, tachycardia, ipsilateral decreased chest expansion, and decreased air entry with hyperresonance of the ipsilateral side may be present.
- Subcutaneous emphysema may also be present.

Investigations

- CXR: reveals a thin pleural edge with loss of distal lung markings (Fig. 18.3(a)). This is best demonstrated on an erect CXR, especially in expiration.
  - ❶ A small pneumothorax may be difficult to detect on a trauma series supine CXR as the air lies anteriorly. Underlying bullous lung diseases can mimic a pneumothorax.
- CT chest: is more sensitive and specific than CXR and may be indicated if the diagnosis is unclear.
- ABG: perform if pulse oximetry shows $SaO_2 < 95\%$.

Management

- If hypoxia is present, give high-flow O_2.
- A small spontaneous simple pneumothorax may be managed expectantly or with pleural aspiration (📖 p.520).
- In contrast, a traumatic simple pneumothorax, **irrespective of size**, requires insertion of an intercostal chest drain (📖 p.522; Fig. 18.3(b)) as it can rapidly deteriorate into a tension pneumothorax.
- The requirement for positive pressure ventilation or aircraft transfer mandates intercostal drainage.
- Air leak (bubbling at the underwater seal) and failure of the lung to re-expand on CXR after insertion of a well-sited intercostal drain is an indication to apply low pressure suction (2.5–7.5kPa). Discuss further management with a thoracic surgeon.

(a)

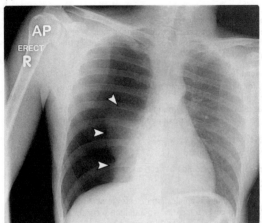

(b)

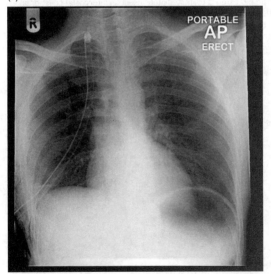

Fig. 18.3 (a) A large right-sided pneumothorax is seen on CXR. The lung edge is arrowed. (b) After chest drain insertion and underwater drainage, the lung has re-inflated on CXR. Note the subcutaneous emphysema.

☠ Open pneumothorax

Open thoracic wounds with a breach of the parietal pleura lead to air within the pleural space. If the defect remains open, air is sucked into the pleural space with each breath. If the defect is approximately 2/3rd of tracheal diameter or more, air preferentially enters the defect with consequent hypoxia and hypercarbia.

Clinical features
- As for a simple pneumothorax, plus presence of an open thoracic wound.
- Auscultation near the wound reveals air movement on respiration.
- A jet of air may be felt exiting the wound on coughing.

Investigations
CXR shows a pneumothorax.

❶ Investigations should not delay treatment.

Management
- Initial treatment is application of a sterile occlusive dressing large enough to cover the entire wound. Tape securely on three sides to provide a one-way flutter valve-type effect.
  - ❶ Taping all four sides may precipitate a tension pneumothorax.
- The next step is to immediately insert an intercostal chest drain (📖 p.522) into the ipsilateral hemithorax, remote from the wound.
- The patient should now be safe for further investigation and consideration of formal surgical closure of the wound. Discuss with a cardiothoracic surgeon.

☠ Tension pneumothorax

This is a life-threatening condition and must be treated **immediately** on diagnosis. A flap-like defect in the lung parenchyma leads to progressive passage of air into the pleural space with no means of escape. Rapidly increasing positive intrathoracic pressure causes ipsilateral lung collapse, mediastinal shift, and impairment of venous return with reduced cardiac output. Untreated tension pneumothorax results in cardiac arrest.

Clinical features
- Feeling of impending doom.
- On examination, there is tachycardia, severe tachypnoea, and hypotension. There is tracheal deviation towards the contralateral side with ipsilateral hyperresonance to percussion, and ipsilateral absence of breath sounds.
- ❶ Distended neck veins may be present, but this is an unreliable sign in trauma due to haemorrhage and hypovolaemia. In trauma patients the neck may be masked by a cervical semi-rigid collar.

Investigations
❶ This is a clinical diagnosis and no further investigations are warranted.

Management
- **Immediately** decompress by introducing a large bore (14G) cannula into the pleura via the 2nd intercostal space in the midclavicular line on the affected side (📖 p.516). A sudden release of air confirms the diagnosis.
- This should be followed by insertion of an intercostal chest drain (📖 p.522) and CXR.

☼ Haemothorax

The most common cause of blood in the pleural space is thoracic trauma. Haemothorax and pneumothorax often coexist (haemopneumothorax). After trauma, bleeding most commonly arises from intercostal or internal thoracic (mammary) vessels. Major bleeds are more likely to come from the pulmonary parenchyma, pulmonary vessels, heart, or great vessels. A large haemothorax will cause hypoxia and shock. Failure to evacuate blood within the pleural space may lead to an empyema or fibrothorax (clotted haemothorax). For this reason, a significant haemothorax requires drainage.

History
- A history of trauma or thoracic intervention is usually present.
- May present with SOB or pleuritic chest pain.
- Significant bleeding may cause symptoms of shock.

❶ Resuscitation and primary survey may take precedence over history-taking (📖 p.42).

Examination
- Tachycardia and tachypnoea.
- Signs of a pleural effusion, i.e. reduced chest expansion, dull to percussion at the base, decreased breath sounds.
- A large haemothorax may cause hypovolaemic shock (📖 p.52).

Investigations
- FBC: may show ↓ Hb.
- G&S: all patients. When shock is present, cross-match 4–6 units of packed RBCs and check PT and APTT.
- ABG: if SaO_2 < 95% on pulse oximetry or if shocked.
- CXR: appearances vary with patient position and size of haemothorax.
  - Erect CXR shows similar features to those of a pleural effusion.
  - Supine CXR shows relative haziness of the ipsilateral lung field.
  - ❶ Look for the underlying cause, e.g. rib fractures, mediastinal widening suggesting aortic rupture.
- CT chest: more sensitive and specific than CXR, but not usually required.

Management
- If SaO_2 < 95% or shock is present, give high-flow O_2 via a non-rebreathing mask.
- Treat shock (📖 p.54): get large-bore IV access × 2 and fluid resuscitate.
- Insert a 28–36F intercostal chest drain (📖 p.522) directed posteriorly and basally. Consider insertion through the 4th intercostal space rather than the 5th, as a diaphragmatic injury may have been obscured. In most patients the bleeding is self-limiting, and no further intervention is required.

- Emergency cardiothoracic referral for thoracotomy is indicated if:
  - initial chest drain output is 1500mL or more;
  - chest drain output > 300mL/h for 3 consecutive hours;
  - ongoing bleeding with hypotension or continued transfusion requirement.
- ❶ Massive ongoing bleeding after insertion of chest drain mandates preparation for immediate thoracotomy. This should be carried out by an experienced cardiothoracic surgeon in theatre, where at all possible.
- ❶ Massive haemorrhage may also result from inadvertent placement of the drain into the liver, spleen, great vessels, or heart.
- Haemodynamically stable patients may require chest CT to identify associated injuries, and the extent and location of retained/clotted blood. Thoracotomy may be necessary to repair associated injuries and/or evacuate a retained haematoma. Removal of haematoma may also be performed by video-assisted thoracoscopy.

:☼: **Tracheobronchial injuries**

Injuries to the trachea or main bronchi may result from penetrating or blunt trauma, inhalation injury, and iatrogenic endotracheal instrumentation. Traumatic tracheobronchial injuries are rare and have a high mortality. Most occur within 2–3cm of the carina. Major airway injury results in a large air leak into the surrounding tissues. Breach of the pleura results in a pneumothorax, either tension or simple. This may be precipitated by positive pressure ventilation.

Clinical features

- History of significant trauma or tracheobronchial instrumentation with haemoptysis and severe dyspnoea.
- On examination, marked subcutaneous emphysema is usually present with signs of a large simple or tension pneumothorax (📖 p.463).
- ❶ The diagnosis may only be suggested by the finding of a persistent large air leak on placement of an intercostal chest drain (📖 p.522), with failure of the lung to re-expand on CXR. Application of suction causes **increased** respiratory distress as air is preferentially sucked out of the bronchial tree.

❶ Involve a thoracic surgeon immediately if tracheobronchial injury is suspected.

Investigations

Awake flexible bronchoscopy confirms the diagnosis.

Management

- More than one intercostal chest drain may be necessary for lung expansion.
- Endotracheal intubation should be avoided where possible and should only be performed by a senior anaesthetist.
- Experienced cardiothoracic anaesthetists may be able to institute single lung ventilation with the use of a left or right bronchial tube placed under direct vision with a fibre-optic bronchoscope until definitive surgical repair occurs. This intervention is high risk and may worsen the initial injury.

☠ Aortic dissection

Aortic dissection occurs when blood passes through a tear in the intima into the media of the aortic wall. This creates a dissection plane that separates the intima and media from the adventitia. A false lumen arises with variable proximal and distal extension. The intimal tear commonly occurs in the proximal ascending aorta or the descending aorta just distal to the subclavian artery. There are two pathophysiological effects:

- separation of the components of the aortic wall causing weakness with the possibility of aortic rupture;
- the false lumen may compress the origins of branch arteries (e.g. coronary, carotid, mesenteric) causing ischaemia.

Proximal dissection into the aortic root can cause catastrophic aortic valve regurgitation. Rupture of the ascending aorta into the pericardium causes cardiac tamponade.

Risk factors for aortic dissection include hypertension, connective tissue diseases (e.g. Ehlers–Danlos syndrome, Marfan's syndrome) and cystic medial necrosis. Other associations include atherosclerosis, congenitally bicuspid aortic valve, aortic valve stenosis, coarctation of the aorta, and iatrogenic injury. The peak incidence is in the fifth decade, so suspect cocaine use when aortic dissection occurs in a young person.

History

- Sudden onset of severe tearing chest, interscapular, or neck pain. The site of pain moves as the dissection evolves.
- Stroke or syncope (cerebral ischaemia).
- Paraplegia (spinal ischaemia).
- Abdominal pain (mesenteric ischaemia).
- Leg pain (limb ischaemia (📖 p.332)).
- Severe dyspnoea (acute pulmonary oedema due to aortic valve regurgitation).

❶ The presentation of aortic dissection is highly variable, and a high index of suspicion is required.

Examination

Findings may include:
- shock;
- signs of cardiac tamponade;
- hypertension/hypotension;
- abdominal tenderness;
- differential systolic BP between upper or lower limbs (> 10mmHg difference) or absent pulses;
- aortic regurgitation;
- ischaemic limbs;
- hemiplegia or other neurological signs.

❶ Absent pulses may reappear as the blood flow switches from the false to the true lumen.

Initial investigations
- FBC: ↓ Hb with ↑ WCC can occur.
- U&E: ↑ urea and creatinine.
- G&S: all patients. Cross-match 2–6 units of packed RBCs if shock is present.
- ECG: sinus tachycardia, left ventricular hypertrophy, or acute myocardial ischaemia.
- CXR: widened mediastinum, left-sided pleural effusion (Fig. 18.4).

Initial management
- Give high-flow O_2 via a non-rebreathing face mask.
- Insert 2 × large-bore peripheral IV cannulae and begin IV fluids.
- ❶ Fluid resuscitation should aim for a systolic BP of 90–100mmHg. Higher BP requires rapid control (see 'Further management').
- Prescribe IV opioid analgesia.
- Keep NBM.
- Insert a urinary catheter (📖 p.504).

Further investigations

❶ Suspicion of aortic dissection mandates definitive imaging. Involve your seniors early.

Local availability and expertise determines which modality should be used.
- Contrast-enhanced CT has become the standard investigation due to its speed and accuracy (Fig. 18.5).
- MRI is also very accurate but availability may be limited.
- Transthoracic echocardiography can be performed at the bedside but is less accurate.
- Transoesophageal echocardiography has greater sensitivity than transthoracic echo, but is more invasive and requires an experienced operator.

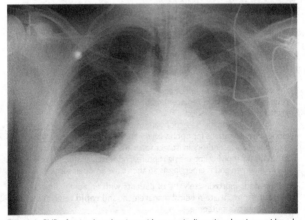

Fig. 18.4 CXR of an intubated patient with an aortic dissection showing a widened mediastinum and left pleural effusion.

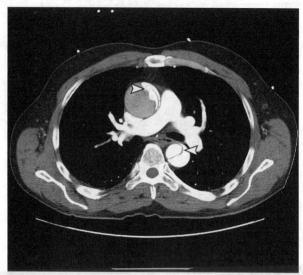

Fig. 18.5 Contrast-enhanced thoracic CT showing intimal flaps in the ascending and descending thoracic aorta (arrowed).

Further management

❶ Discuss with a cardiothoracic surgeon immediately.

Transfer the patient to ITU/CCU for invasive BP monitoring and BP control (systolic BP < 100mmHg) using IV antihypertensives, e.g. labetalol, sodium nitroprusside.

Definitive management is based on an anatomical classification (Box 18.1):
- Stanford type A aortic dissections require emergency open surgery (Fig. 18.6) to prevent life-threatening complications from rupture (e.g. cardiac tamponade) or extension of the dissection process across the coronary ostia (i.e. MI). Replacement of the ascending aorta is required. Aortic valve replacement and/or coronary artery bypass grafts may also be needed.
- Stanford type B aortic dissections are usually managed with BP control alone. The indications for open surgery are persistent pain, a rapidly expanding aorta, end-organ ischaemia, or the presence of a periaortic haematoma implying impending rupture. Endovascular stenting re-expands the true lumen and is emerging as an alternative to open surgery.

❶ Untreated, approximately 1% of patients with an aortic dissection die **per hour**. Appropriate medical management and **rapid** referral may dramatically improve outcome.

Box 18.1 The Stanford classification of aortic dissection

- Type A: involvement of the ascending aorta.
- Type B: no involvement of the ascending aorta.

❶ The proximal extent of the dissection process determines classification, not the origin of the intimal tear.

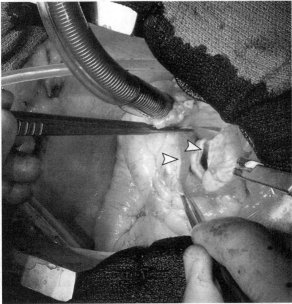

Fig. 18.6 Intraoperative photo of a dissection of the ascending thoracic aorta with the intimal flap and adventitia arrowed.

☠ Aortic rupture

Blunt aortic rupture (also known as aortic transection) is a sudden deceleration injury commonly caused by motor vehicle accidents or falls from heights of > 3m. Those who survive to hospital have a contained aortic rupture, where the aorta has ruptured and a haematoma forms in the periaortic tissues. **They are at risk of sudden exsanguination**.

The aorta is typically transected transversely involving all three aortic wall layers. Most ruptures occur at the level of the ligamentum arteriosum, just distal to the origin of the left subclavian artery.

History
- Significant mechanism of blunt injury.
- Symptoms may include SOB, back pain, and symptoms of shock.

❶ Resuscitation and primary survey take precedence over history-taking (📖 p.42).

Examination
- Multiple injuries are common.

❶ A high index of suspicion is required as there are no specific diagnostic features. Exclude aortic rupture in severe deceleration injuries.

Investigations
- FBC, U&Es, ECG, ABG, X-rays, etc. as adjuncts to the primary survey (📖 p.62).
- ❶ CXR may reveal signs of aortic rupture (Box 18.2), but a normal CXR does not exclude it.
- If the mechanism of injury or CXR suggests aortic rupture **and once the patient is haemodynamically stable**, CT chest should be performed.

Management
- ❶ Immediate senior cardiothoracic surgical involvement is mandatory.
- Patients should receive β-blockers/vasodilators to maintain systolic BP at 90–100mmHg as sudden surges may precipitate exsanguination. Death from haemorrhage occurs in **20%** of patients who survive to hospital.
- Emergency aortic repair can be performed open or endovascularly.

Box 18.2 Signs of possible aortic rupture on CXR

- Widened mediastinum (> 8cm)
- Mediastinum to chest width ratio > 0.25
- Tracheal shift to the right
- Blurred aortic contour
- Left haemothorax
- Irregularity or loss of the aortic knuckle
- Left apical cap (apical opacity due to collection of blood)
- Depression of the left main bronchus
- Opacification of the aortopulmonary window
- Nasogastric tube deviation to the right
- Wide paraspinal lines
- 1st or 2nd rib fracture, scapular fracture, or clavicular fracture
- Pulmonary contusion
- Thoracic spine fracture

☠ Cardiac tamponade

Cardiac tamponade is caused by an accumulation of fluid within the peri-cardial space. This may follow penetrating or blunt injury to the heart, great vessels, or pericardial vessels. Iatrogenic tamponade can occur after cardiac surgery or percutaneous catheter-based cardiac intervention (including central venous line insertion). Filling of the stiff pericardial sac leads to impaired venous return and reduced cardiac output.

History

- Blunt or penetrating thoracic trauma.
- Patients may complain of severe SOB.

❶ Resuscitation and primary survey take precedence over history-taking (📖 p.42).

Examination

- Shock (📖 p.52).
- Beck's triad:
  - hypotension;
  - distended neck veins;
  - muffled heart sounds.
- Pulsus paradoxus (↓ systolic BP > 10mmHg with inspiration).
- Kussmaul's sign (↑ JVP with inspiration).

❶ Diagnosis can be very difficult in a noisy resuscitation room. Most trauma patients are hypovolaemic and will not have distended neck veins.

❶ Note that the clinical findings are similar to those of tension pneumo-thorax. This should be promptly excluded by looking for tracheal devia-tion and unilateral absence of breath sounds (📖 p.463). If you are unable to exclude a tension pneumothorax, perform needle thoracic decompres-sion first (📖 516).

Investigations

- Bedside transthoracic echocardiography or FAST scan (📖 p.70) is highly sensitive and specific for pericardial fluid.
- CXR may show an enlarged, globular cardiac shadow.

❶ The treatment of suspected cardiac tamponade should **not** be delayed by investigations in haemodynamically compromised patients.

Management

- Prompt pericardiocentesis (📖 p.534) is **mandatory** once the diagnosis is suspected. The removal of just 15–20mL of blood can lead to clinical improvement.
- All patients with a history of trauma and positive pericardiocentesis for blood require formal exploration of the heart and great vessels and should be transferred to a cardiothoracic centre. Discuss with a cardio-thoracic surgeon immediately.

Miscellaneous conditions

① **Soft tissue abscess**

A soft tissue abscess may occur at any site, but is most common in the perianal area (📖 p.304), natal cleft, axilla, breast (📖 p.316), groin, scrotum, and neck. Recurrent axillary and groin abscesses are often due to hidradenitis suppurativa, a chronic inflammatory disease of apocrine sweat glands. The diagnosis and management of a soft tissue abscess is usually straightforward, but beware of pitfalls (Box 19.1). With the exception of perianal abscesses, most soft tissue abscesses are caused by staphylococci. Abscesses are more common in patients with diabetes.

History

Localized pain and swelling, with discharge of pus if spontaneous rupture occurs.

Examination

- Pyrexia may be present.
- Sepsis (📖 p.482) is uncommon.
- Abscesses result in erythema and swelling. They are painful on palpation and fluctuant. Pus may be pointing or discharging.
- ❶ The presence of crepitus or rapidly spreading cellulitis implies a necrotizing soft tissue infection (📖 p.478).
- ❶ Consider septic arthritis and osteomyelitis if the abscess is over a joint or bony prominence (📖 p.408).

Investigations

The diagnosis is usually clinical. Systemically well, young, fit people do not require preoperative investigation other than a CBG. If symptoms or signs of sepsis are present:

- FBC: ↑ WCC, with ↑ CRP;
- U&Es: ↑ urea and creatinine, reflecting dehydration;
- ABG: metabolic acidosis with ↑ serum lactate;
- blood cultures.

Management

Abscesses must be drained, as primary treatment with antibiotics is ineffective.

- Treatment is by incision and drainage under either GA or LA, depending on the site and size of the abscess, patient preference, and theatre availability.
- Occasionally, small fluctuant abscesses < 3cm diameter can successfully be aspirated using a syringe and green (21G) needle under ethyl chloride spray anaesthesia.
- Send pus for M, C, & S.
- Antibiotics are unnecessary in an otherwise healthy individual, except in the presence of widespread cellulitis or systemic sepsis. If necessary, start IV flucloxacillin 1g qds (+ metronidazole 500mg tds if the abscess is near the perineum).
- If sepsis is present, start aggressive IV fluid resuscitation, ensure adequate oxygenation, begin IV antibiotics after blood culture, and arrange for incision and drainage under GA as an emergency.
- Hidradenitis suppurativa requires outpatient referral to a dermatologist once drainage has been performed.

Box 19.1 Pitfalls in soft tissue abscesses

- ❶ Always be aware of underlying neurovascular structures when incising an abscess.
- ❶ An abscess in an area of previous surgery may be related to the original operation—consider an underlying fistula or an infected prosthesis.

Groin abscess

- ❶ **Never** incise and drain a groin abscess in an IV drug user without excluding an infected false femoral artery aneurysm. Overlying fibrosis may obliterate the pulsation. Order an urgent duplex scan first.
- An abscess pointing in the groin may originate from an intraabdominal or retroperitoneal focus, e.g. psoas abscess, sigmoid diverticular abscess.

Abdominal wall abscess

- Consider the possibility of an underlying bowel fistula, e.g. Crohn's disease, malignancy.
- Strangulated fat in a paraumbilical hernia may mimic an umbilical abscess.

Pilonidal abscess

- An abscess within 5cm of the anal verge may be anorectal (📖 p.304) rather than pilonidal. For this reason, and because of the high rate of recurrence, these patients need follow-up in a colorectal clinic.

☠ **Necrotizing soft tissue infections**

A wide variety of names have been used to describe severe infections within the soft tissue compartment (skin, subcutaneous tissue, superficial and deep fascia, muscle) associated with tissue necrosis. However, it is often impossible to distinguish between them clinically, and the principles of management are identical. They are therefore considered together under the term necrotizing soft tissue infections (NSTIs; Box 19.2).

Although commonly precipitated by such factors as burns, penetrating trauma, or operative wounds, most affected patients have chronic co-morbidities or immunosuppressive conditions e.g. diabetes, obesity, chronic renal failure, IV drug use. Most NSTIs are polymicrobial, with the majority of monomicrobial infections due to Gram-positive cocci. Although rare, NSTIs are rapidly fatal, and delayed diagnosis significantly increases mortality. Overall mortality is ~ 30%.

❶ Early features may be non-specific, and a high index of suspicion is essential. Distinguishing NSTI from severe cellulitis can be difficult. Severe cellulitis will respond to IV antibiotics; NSTIs require **immediate** surgical debridement.

Box 19.2 Types of NSTIs

- Necrotizing fasciitis. Infection of the deep fascia with secondary subcutaneous tissue necrosis. Often due to group A streptococci.
- Synergistic gangrene. A non-specific term covering polymicrobial NSTIs.
- Gas gangrene. Muscle necrosis due to gas-forming anaerobic clostridial species (commonly *Clostridium perfringens*), often after penetrating trauma or surgery. Non-clostridial gas-forming organisms can produce tissue crepitus, but this is not gas gangrene.
- Fournier's gangrene. Necrotizing fasciitis of the perineum, scrotum, or perianal areas (🕮 p.376). Usually polymicrobial.
- Meleney's synergistic gangrene. Postoperative polymicrobial NSTIs.
- 'Hospital gangrene'. An archaic term for all NSTIs.

History
- Progressive soft tissue swelling.
- Severe pain, often out of proportion to local clinical findings.
- Confusion.

Examination
- Pyrexia.
- Signs of systemic upset (confusion, tachycardia, hypotension).
- Tense soft tissue oedema with indistinct margins, followed by skin necrosis with surrounding cellulitis.
- Subcutaneous crepitus is a variable finding, but is indicative of NSTI.
  - ❶ **Always** palpate the area carefully in order to detect this important sign.

- Blisters and bullae (tissue fluid may initially be clear, but usually becomes haemorrhagic).

❶ The clinical presentation is variable and systemic features may be absent. The patient may look deceptively well.

Investigations

❶ Contact your senior **immediately** if an NSTI is suspected.

The diagnosis is primarily clinical; however, markedly deranged blood tests support a diagnosis of NSTI over severe cellulitis.
- FBC: ↓ Hb and ↑↑ WCC are common.
- U&Es: ↓ Na⁺ and ↑ creatinine and urea.
- CRP: ↑↑.
- PT, APTT: derangement may reflect DIC.
- Cross-match 2–4 units of packed RBCs, as surgery is often bloody. Clotting factors may also be needed.
- CBG: often ↑↑.
- Erect CXR: if history of cardiorespiratory disease.
- ECG: if history of cardiac disease or age > 40 years, to assess general fitness.
- ABG and serum lactate: metabolic acidosis supports a diagnosis of NSTI.
- Take blood cultures.
- Plain X-rays: the presence of soft tissue gas in the context of infection is highly suggestive of NSTI, but is rarely seen.
- CT and MRI may be useful if the signs are equivocal, or to determine the extent of the infection.
- Surgical exploration through a small incision can identify signs of NSTI e.g. necrotic tissue, thrombosed vessels, 'dishwater' fluid, and loss of resistance in tissue planes. Tissue biopsies may be useful.

❶ Unnecessary investigations delay diagnosis and increase mortality. Have a low threshold for surgery.

Management

Treatment principles include resuscitation, emergency aggressive surgical debridement, physiological support, and IV antibiotics.
- Give O₂ at 15L/min via a non-rebreathing mask.
- Start IV fluid resuscitation and correct deranged electrolytes.
- Correct any coagulopathy.
- Begin thromboprophylaxis (📖 p.26) if no contraindications are present.
- Consider an IV insulin sliding scale (📖 p.24) if CBG > 10mmol/L.
- Insert a urinary catheter and aim for output > 0.5mL/kg/h.
- Initial IV antibiotics should cover Gram-positive, Gram-negative, and anaerobic organisms, e.g. amoxicillin 1g qds + gentamicin (dosage according to local protocol) + metronidazole 500mg tds. Discuss antibiotic choice with a microbiologist as soon as the diagnosis is suspected.
- NSTIs are tetanus-prone wounds. Give tetanus prophylaxis (📖 p.94).
- Discuss with the on-call anaesthetist/intensivist as the patient may require a central venous line and/or arterial line. ITU admission is likely.

- Immediate, wide surgical debridement of all necrotic tissue is essential. Amputation may be necessary. Tissue and fluid must be sent for M, C, & S.
  - Repeat the surgical debridement every 24–48h until all infected material has been removed.
  - Delayed closure with skin grafts is often necessary once the infection has cleared.
- Consider using hyperbaric O_2 if available, although its value is uncertain.

☼ **Sepsis in the surgical patient**

Sepsis is a systemic inflammatory response to an infective process and is common in emergency surgical patients. Worsening sepsis leads to acute organ dysfunction (severe sepsis). One of the manifestations of cardiovascular dysfunction is hypotension despite fluid resuscitation (septic shock). A systemic inflammatory response syndrome (SIRS) may also occur in the absence of infection, e.g. acute pancreatitis, polytrauma, severe burns. Full definitions of SIRS and the sepsis syndromes are given in Box 19.3. In general surgical patients, sepsis commonly arises from:

- peritonitis, e.g. acute appendicitis, diverticulitis, perforated duodenal ulcer, penetrating trauma;
- intraabdominal collections, e.g. after an anastomotic leak;
- postoperative pneumonia;
- acute cholangitis;
- wound infection;
- soft tissue abscess, e.g. perianal;
- solid organ abscess, e.g. liver;
- urinary tract sepsis (e.g. infected obstructed kidney);
- infected lines, drains, and prostheses, e.g. mesh, vascular grafts.

❶ Severe sepsis has a mortality of ~ 25% and septic shock has a mortality of ~ 50%. Mortality can be reduced by early recognition and prompt resuscitation and treatment.

History

The general symptoms of sepsis include:
- sweats, rigors;
- malaise;
- vomiting.

Examination

- Confusion, especially in the elderly.
- Flushed initially, but may become clammy, with poorly perfused peripheries and mottled skin.
- Pyrexia **or** hypothermia.
- Signs of dehydration.
- Tachycardia with hypotension.
- Tachypnoea.
- ❶ Signs localizing to the source of the infection are usually present.

Investigations

Regardless of the underlying source, the following investigations are necessary to quantify the inflammatory response and assess organ dysfunction.
- FBC: ↑↑ WCC **or** ↓ WCC.
- U&Es: ↑ urea and creatinine.
- LFTs: ↑ bilirubin and mild ↑ ALT/AST/ALP with severe sepsis.
- PT, APTT: both ↑.
- CBG: usually ↑ but can be ↓.
- ABG: ↓ PaO_2 with ↓ pH, ↓ $PaCO_2$, and ↓ base excess is often seen.
- Serum lactate: ↑, reflecting poor tissue perfusion.

- ECG: often sinus tachycardia, but dysrhythmias or rate-related ischaemic changes are also common.

Box 19.3 Definitions of SIRS and sepsis syndromes

SIRS*

Present when more than one of the following are identified:
- T > 38°C or < 36°C;
- HR > 90/min;
- Respiratory rate > 20/min or $PaCO_2$ < 4.3kPa;
- WCC > 12 × 10^9/L or < 4 × 10^9/L.

Sepsis[†]

Documented or suspected infection and some of the following:
- T > 38.3°C or < 36°C;
- HR > 90/min;
- Respiratory rate > 30/min;
- Altered mental status;
- Significant oedema;
- Blood glucose > 7.7mmol/L in the absence of diabetes;
- WCC > 12 × 10^9/L or < 4 × 10^9/L or > 10% immature forms;
- Raised plasma CRP;
- Systolic BP < 90mmHg or MABP < 70mmHg;
- Hypoxia (PaO_2/FiO_2 < 40kPa);
- Acute oliguria (urine output < 0.5mL/kg/h for at least 2h);
- Serum creatinine rise ≥ 44μmol/L;
- INR > 1.5 or APTT > 60;
- Platelets < 100 × 10^9/L;
- Plasma total bilirubin > 70μmol/L;
- Serum lactate > 3mmol/L;
- Decreased capillary refill or mottling.

Severe sepsis[†] Sepsis + acute organ dysfunction, including hypotension.

Septic shock[†] Sepsis + persistent arterial hypotension despite adequate volume resuscitation, and in the absence of other causes of hypotension. Hypotension is defined as systolic BP < 90mmHg, or MAP < 60mmHg, or systolic BP ↓ more than 40mmHg from baseline.

* ACCP/SCCM Consensus Conference (1992). ACCP/SCCM Consensus Conference: definitions for sepsis and organ failure and guidelines for the use of innovative therapies in sepsis. *Crit. Care Med.* **20**, 864–74.

[†] Levy, M.M. *et al.* (2003). 2001 SCCM/ESICM/ACCP/ATS/SIS International Sepsis Definitions Conference. *Intensive Care Med.* **29**, 530–8.

Investigations to localize the source of the infection are also needed.
- Erect CXR: to detect pneumonia, lung abscess, and free intraabdominal gas.
- Samples for microbiology.
  - Blood cultures: one set from peripheral blood with one set through each intravascular cannula (unless < 48h old).

- MSU/CSU, wound swabs, sputum samples, drain fluid samples, line site swabs.
- Consider other cultures (e.g. CSF, ascites, pleural fluid), depending on the clinical situation.
- ❶ Obtain cultures before starting IV antibiotics.
- Where the source is not obvious, further imaging studies are necessary, e.g. CT abdomen, USS, nuclear medicine white cell scan, echocardiogram, MRI.

Management

The management of sepsis involves organ system support, antimicrobial therapy, and treatment of the underlying source of infection.

❶ In general surgical patients, treatment of the underlying source often requires emergency laparotomy once initial resuscitation has taken place.

- Give O_2 at 15L/min via a non-rebreathing mask to keep SaO_2 > 94%.
- Begin IV fluid resuscitation as soon as severe sepsis or septic shock is recognized.
  - Fluid challenge with 10–20mL/kg of crystalloid or 5–10mL/kg of colloid over 30–60min, and repeat as clinically indicated.
  - Aim to keep MABP ≥ 65mmHg and urine output ≥ 0.5mL/kg/h. Insert a central venous line and aim for a CVP of 8–12mmHg.
- Insert a urinary catheter if not already present.
- Aim to start empiric broad spectrum IV antibiotics appropriate to the suspected source of sepsis **within 1h** of recognizing severe sepsis or septic shock and **after** cultures have been taken.
  - Consider the effect of abnormal liver and renal function on dosage regimens.
  - Use local protocols to determine antibiotic choice.
  - ❶ Discussion with the on-call microbiologist is essential for those patients who are immunosuppressed, e.g. HIV infection, neutropenic sepsis, transplant recipients.
- Aim to maintain good blood glucose control (CBG < 9mmol/L).
- Give thromboprophylaxis, unless contraindicated (📖 p.26).
- Consider stress ulcer prophylaxis (e.g. H_2 receptor antagonists or PPIs).
- Once adequate resuscitation has occurred, treatment of the underlying source of infection is necessary. This may take the form of:[1]
  - drainage (surgical, radiological, endoscopic);
  - debridement, e.g. NSTI, infected pancreatic necrosis;
  - device removal, e.g. infected intravascular catheter or urinary catheter;
  - definitive control, e.g. amputation for NSTI, appendicectomy.
- Refer to ITU/HDU if:
  - failure to maintain MABP ≥ 65mmHg, systolic BP > 90, or tissue perfusion despite adequate fluid resuscitation (i.e. up to 60mL/kg);
  - other significant organ dysfunction.

☛ Recombinant human activated protein C (drotrecogin) can be given to patients with severe sepsis at high risk of death; however, this is an expensive drug that can cause life-threatening haemorrhage. Recent trials have not confirmed the initially promising results.

Reference

1 Dellinger, R.P. *et al.* (2004). Surviving Sepsis Campaign guidelines for management of severe sepsis and septic shock. *Intensive Care Med.* **30**, 536–55.

☼ Abdominal compartment syndrome

The abdominal and pelvic cavities make up a single compartment bounded by walls with varying degrees of distensibility. As with any other body compartment, raised pressures within it can lead to decreased organ perfusion and a compartment syndrome. Abdominal compartment syndrome (ACS) is increasingly recognized, most commonly in postoperative patients on ITU/HDU. Risk factors include:

- decreased abdominal wall compliance, e.g. tight abdominal wall closure, burns, obesity, mechanical ventilation;
- increased intraluminal contents, e.g. ileus, mechanical bowel obstruction;
- increased abdominal contents, e.g. haemoperitoneum, ascites, liver transplantation, retroperitoneal bleed (e.g. ruptured AAA);
- capillary leak, e.g. sepsis, massive transfusion, acute pancreatitis, abdominal trauma.

Normal intraabdominal pressure (IAP) is 0mmHg, but can be chronically raised to 10–15mmHg with no pathophysiological consequences, e.g. obesity, pregnancy. Acute rises in IAP lead to end-organ dysfunction, however, and intraabdominal hypertension (IAH) has been defined as a sustained pathological rise of IAP to ≥ 12mmHg.[1] As IAP rises, so does the risk of organ dysfunction. ACS can be defined as sustained IAP > 20mmHg associated with new organ dysfunction. Renal and respiratory dysfunction is common in patients with ACS.

❶ Patients undergoing laparotomy with multiple risk factors for developing ACS may benefit from having their abdomen left open and covered with a protective dressing (temporary abdominal closure).

History
- Risk factors for ACS.
- Abdominal pain.
- SOB.

Examination
- Dyspnoea, tachypnoea, poor SaO₂.
- Distended, tense abdomen.
- Decreased urine output.

❶ As examination findings are non-specific, a high index of suspicion is necessary

Investigations
- IAP measurement. This can be achieved in many ways, but is most commonly measured via a urinary catheter in the bladder.
  - The bladder must be empty and the patient must be supine.
  - Active abdominal muscle contractions should be absent, e.g. muscle relaxants or epidural anaesthesia.
  - Attach the urinary catheter to a manometer (water column or via a transducer).
  - Instil 25mL of normal saline into the bladder.
  - Zero the manometer at the mid-axillary line.

- Measure at end-expiration, 30–60s after installation to allow the detrusor muscle to relax.
- ❶ 1mmHg = 1.36cmH$_2$O.
- If IAH is present, imaging (e.g. CT abdomen and pelvis) is useful to detect mechanical bowel obstruction, intraabdominal bleeding, and ascites. CT may show a collapsed IVC.
- Other tests should be performed to exclude cardiorespiratory disorders (e.g. CXR, ABG, ECG). AXR cannot detect ACS.

Management

Patients with confirmed ACS should have their IAP reduced using non-surgical and surgical approaches. Organ dysfunction requires ITU admission and supportive treatment.

Non-surgical treatment

- Give analgesia to improve abdominal wall compliance.
- Avoid excessive fluid administration and use diuretics to treat over-hydration.
- Insert an NG tube, and empty the rectum using enemas.
- Percutaneously drain any intraabdominal fluid collections.

Surgical treatment Laparotomy with evacuation of blood and fluid. The abdomen should be left open and closed with a temporary abdominal closure (e.g. Bogota bag).

Reference

1 Malbrain, M.L.N.G. et al. (2006). *Intensive Care Med.* **32**, 1722–32.

Part 4

Procedures

Procedures

Introduction

These notes should not replace appropriate training or supervision. Instead, they should act as an aide memoir. Each procedure varies in complexity; the degree of difficulty and requirement for supervision has been graded * (straightforward, not requiring supervision) to ***** (complex, senior supervision required). In an emergency (e.g. needle thoracic decompression), there may not be enough time to wait for supervision. You should consider the following before each procedure.

Procedure

- Is this the **correct procedure** on the **correct patient** on the **correct side**?
- Do you know the **relevant anatomy**? Are you the appropriate person to be performing it? Do you require **supervision**?
- Are you aware of the contraindications and possible complications?
- Does the patient have abnormal coagulation and does it need to be corrected?
- If the procedure is close to a previous operation site, have you **read the operation note**, and does the surgeon need to be informed?

Equipment

- Is all the necessary equipment available?
- Is LA, IV analgesia, or IV sedation required, and does this require further patient monitoring?
- Do you need an assistant, chaperone, or someone present to reassure/monitor the patient?

Consent

- Is the patient fully aware of what you are planning to do and why? Discuss possible complications and alternative procedures. Have you explained what is required of him/her?
- Is written consent needed or is verbal consent adequate? Follow local policy.

Positioning and lighting

- Is the patient comfortable and suitably positioned, and is this adequate for you to perform the intended procedure?
- Is the lighting adequate? Consider the need for supplementary lighting.
- Has the patient's privacy and dignity been safeguarded?

Aftercare and documentation

- Discard your own sharps in a sharps bin.
- Do the nurses know what has been done, why it has been done, what complications to look for, and who to call if they occur?
- Are specific observations required?
- Do you need to check the patient again?
- Is further imaging required?
- Has the procedure been documented adequately, including the indication, consent obtained, level of supervision, technique used, drug usage, aftercare and management plan?

Superficial venous cannulation*

Indication Intravenous access.

Contraindications

- Overlying infection.
- In patients with renal failure, do not place cannulae in the cephalic vein at the wrist or in the antecubital fossae as this may compromise future sites for arteriovenous fistulae for haemodialysis.
- **Never** insert a cannula in the same arm as an existing haemodialysis arteriovenous fistula.
- Avoid placing cannulae in the arm on the same side as previous axillary surgery for breast cancer.

Equipment

- Use the smallest cannula needed to fulfil the task required:
  - orange (14G), grey (16G)—resuscitation of the shocked patient;
  - green (18G)—maintenance IV fluids;
  - pink (20G)—if IV antibiotics only;
  - blue (22G)—only when all else fails.
- Alcohol wipes.
- 5mL syringe and sterile normal saline for flush.
- Adhesive dressing.
- Tourniquet.
- Cotton wool and adhesive tape in case of failure.
- Non-sterile gloves.

Patient preparation

- An intradermal bleb of 1% lidocaine **without** adrenaline can be used if large cannulae are to be inserted or if the patient is anxious. In children, use topical anaesthetic cream placed 30min beforehand.
- In patients with difficult arm veins, try the following.
  - Wrap both arms in blankets for 30min beforehand.
  - Topical GTN spray.
  - Hang the patient's arm over the edge of the bed.
  - Leg veins can be used, but are fragile and often thrombose rapidly.

Procedure

- Place a tourniquet proximal to the elbow.
- Select the vein and clean the overlying skin with an alcohol wipe.
- Insert the cannula at 20–30° to the skin with the bevel of the needle facing upwards and enter the vein. Once a 'flashback' of blood occurs, lower the cannula to 10–15° and advance slightly.
- Remove the stylet partially and advance the plastic cannula up to the hilt. Occlude the vein proximally with your non-dominant hand, loosen the tourniquet, and then remove the stylet fully. Insert the screw cap into the end of the cannula or connect the IV fluids directly.
- Fix in place with an adhesive dressing and flush with normal saline. If significant resistance is met, the patient experiences pain on flushing, or a subcutaneous swelling appears, the cannula is outside the vein and should be removed once a successful cannula has been placed.

Complications
- Arterial puncture (remove the cannula immediately, apply firm pressure for 10min, and assess the distal circulation).
- Superficial thrombophlebitis or cellulitis (treat with cannula removal and consider oral flucloxacillin 500mg qds PO).

❶ Do not leave cannulae any longer than necessary, as they pose an infection risk. Generally, a cannula should not be in situ for more than 5 days.

Post-procedure care
- Patients with difficult veins require bandaging of the insertion site.
- Junior doctors are increasingly being encouraged to document IV cannulation in the notes.

Arterial blood gas sampling*

This is commonly achieved by percutaneous puncture of the radial artery. Samples can also be taken from the brachial, femoral, or even dorsal pedis arteries if necessary, although the difficulty and/or risk of complications are higher.

Indications

- Assessment of oxygenation, acid–base status, and/or CO_2 elimination.
- Rapid assessment of Hb, Na^+, K^+ (on some machines).

Contraindications

- Distal ischaemia.
- Distal arteriovenous fistula for haemodialysis.
- Overlying infection.
- Absent radial artery pulse.
- Abnormal coagulation is rarely a problem, but discuss with a senior.
- Positive Allen's test.
  - Ask the patient to make a tight fist, occlude both the ulnar and radial arteries, ask the patient to open their hand, release the ulnar compression only.
  - If poor perfusion of the hand is present more than 6s later, the test indicates inadequate ulnar flow, meaning that damage to the radial artery could result in hand ischaemia.

Equipment

- Pre-heparinized syringe and needle (if none are available aspirate a drop of 5000 units/mL unfractionated heparin into a 5mL syringe and use a blue (23G) needle).
- Alcohol wipes.
- Cotton wool and adhesive tape.
- Non-sterile gloves.

Patient preparation

- Place the patient's arm supine on a pillow, with the wrist extended.
- An intradermal bleb of 1% lidocaine **without** adrenaline can help in anxious patients.

Procedure

- Clean the skin with an alcohol wipe.
- Palpate the radial artery just proximal to the radial styloid with your non-dominant hand. Introduce the needle and syringe just distally, in line with the expected site of the radial artery, with the needle at 45° to the skin, bevel up.
- Advance slowly until arterial blood enters the syringe, or bone is encountered. Pre-heparinized syringes should fill with arterial pressure (5mL syringes require aspiration). Take 2–3mL of blood.
- Once the sample is obtained, withdraw the needle and press firmly over the puncture site for 5min. Ask the patient to maintain pressure over the area for another 5min.

- Expel all air bubbles from the syringe, cap the end, and ensure the heparin and blood mix fully. Take directly for analysis yourself, or pack in ice and send immediately to the lab.

Complications

- Haematoma (press firmly for another 10min).
- Arterial thrombosis, embolism, and arteriovenous fistulae are rare.
- Sampling the brachial or femoral arteries risks inadvertent needling of the median nerve or femoral nerve, respectively.

Post-procedure care

Document blood gas results and check the hand for complications.

Nasogastric tube insertion**

NG tube insertion is a procedure most commonly performed by nurses. You will be called when the experts have failed!

Relevant anatomy
The floor of the nasal cavity runs directly posteriorly.

Indications
- GI tract obstruction, either mechanical or paralytic.
- NG feeding.

Contraindications
- Significant head or facial injuries (risk of insertion into the cranial vault).
- Recent nasal or skull-base surgery.
- Relative contraindications include:
  - recent oesophago-gastric surgery;
  - oesophageal varices;
  - decreased level of consciousness and ability to protect the airway (risk of aspiration).

Equipment
- Non-sterile gloves and apron.
- Water-based lubricant jelly.
- Bladder syringe.
- Glass of water.
- Vomit bowl.
- Adhesive tape.
- pH indicator scale paper.
- NG tube.
  - For drainage, use a Ryle's tube (at least 14F) with drainage bag. Tubes kept in the fridge are stiffer and less likely to coil.
  - For NG feeding only, use a fine-bore tube (less than 10F).

Patient preparation
- Patient sitting upright in bed, glass of water nearby, and vomit bowl on lap.
- Look for nasal septal deviation and ask the patient to blow through each nostril in turn to confirm nasal airway patency.
- Suction should be available.

Procedure
- Uncoil the tube so that it is as straight as possible.
- Measure the distance from the tip of the nose to the earlobe and on to the xiphisternum. The tube will need to travel at least this far.
- Lubricate the tip and distal 10cm of the tube.
- Gently insert the tube into a nostril, aiming directly posteriorly.
- Advance slowly, and ask the patient to open their mouth.
- When the tip is visible in the oropharynx, stop advancing and ask the patient to hold a sip of water in their mouth.
- Ask the patient to swallow and advance the tube as they do so.

- If the tube advances freely, continue to advance. Give the patient more sips of water to swallow as you advance. **Never** advance if resistance is met.
- Once the tube has been inserted the predetermined distance check for correct positioning by aspirating gastric contents (check for pH < 5.5 with indicator paper if a fine-bore is inserted).
- If correct positioning is confirmed, tape in place on to the nose and cheek.
- In patients with GI tract obstruction, aspirate as much gas and gastric contents as you can; then attach the NG tube to a drainage bag.
- With fine-bore tubes, only remove the guidewire once correct positioning has been confirmed.

Complications and problematic insertions
- Aspiration of gastric contents with subsequent pneumonia.
- Insertion into the trachea or lungs may lead to coughing and laryngospasm.
  - **Remove the tube if the patient has difficulty breathing, coughs, or becomes cyanosed**.
  - Inserting NG feeds into an incorrectly placed tube leads to severe pneumonitis.
- Long-term placement may lead to oesophageal or gastric irritation or, rarely, perforation.
- Problematic insertions.
  - If there is difficulty in passing through the nasal cavity, remove the tube and try the other nostril.
  - Lidocaine jelly or spray can be used on the tube or oropharynx, but the patient should **not** then be asked to swallow water due to the risk of aspiration. The patient should remain NBM for 4–6h.
  - If gastric contents cannot be aspirated, advance the tube 10cm and try again. If this fails, lie the patient in the left lateral position and try again. Try also flushing 5mL of air down the tube to dislodge any blockages.

Post-procedure care
- For large-bore NG tubes, place on free drainage and inform the nursing staff how often it needs to be aspirated.
- For fine-bore NG tube insertion, request a CXR to confirm correct placement before beginning feeds (Fig. 20.1). The tip of the tube should clearly be within the abdomen. If the location is unclear, advance the tube further and repeat the CXR, or request a lateral view.
- Document consent, tube size, ease of insertion, and CXR findings.

(a)

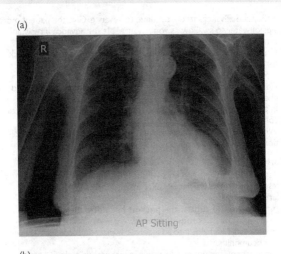

(b)

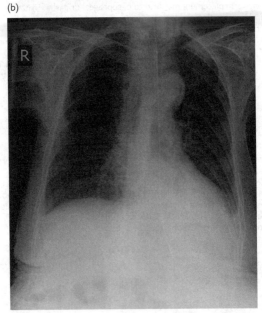

Fig. 20.1 (a) A fine-bore NG tube had mistakenly been placed into the left main bronchus. The patient was asymptomatic. (b) Correct placement.

Wound abscess drainage***

Relevant anatomy

- **You must be familiar with the technique used to close the wound/incision and the local anatomy. If not, read the operation note.**
- Laparotomy incisions are usually closed using a 'mass closure' technique with continuous sutures through both layers of the rectus sheath. The skin is commonly closed either with staples, or a continuous, absorbable, subcuticular suture.

Indications Superficial wound infection and wound abscess (📖 p.169).

Contraindications

- Wound dehiscence (📖 p.167).
- The presence of underlying prosthetic material (e.g. mesh). Thorough washout under GA ± mesh removal may be preferable. Check with your senior.
- ❶ Do not explore wounds overlying vascular grafts.

Equipment

- Absorbable pads.
- Dressing pack.
- Extra gauze swabs.
- Sterile suture cutters/staple removers.
- 2 × microbiology swabs.
- 30–40mL of sterile normal saline.
- 20mL syringe (for irrigation), 5mL syringe (for microbiology sample).
- Packing material (e.g. Sorbsan®, Kaltostat®) and dressings (e.g. gauze swabs/pads/adhesive tape).
- Sinus forceps are a useful aid, if available.

Patient preparation

- Patient lying supine, wound and surrounding area well-exposed.
- LA is not needed as the cutaneous nerves have already been divided.

Procedure

- Place absorbable pads under the patient. Prep with area with sterile normal saline and drape the area.
- Remove the staples or cut the subcuticular sutures in the area affected.
- Using one microbiology swab, **gently** open up the wound. More staples/sutures may need to be removed/cut. Healthy wounds are strong and will not open with gentle pressure. **Gently** deepen the cavity. Sinus forceps can be useful.
- **Any deep sutures you come across should not be cut!**
- Use the other microbiology swab and/or the 5mL syringe to take a sample of the pus/fluid for M, C, & S.
- Wash the cavity with copious normal saline.
- Gently pack the resulting clean cavity and cover with dressings.

Complications Rare, if performed correctly.

Post-procedure care
- Send the microbiology swab for culture and sensitivities.
- Document consent, sterile technique, findings, and dressing materials.
- Let the nurse looking after the patient know what has been done. The dressing will require changing once or twice daily, initially.

Transurethral bladder catheterization**

Female catheterizations are usually done by nursing staff; male catheterization is described here.

❶ If you are called to perform female catheterization, make sure you are familiar with the location of the female urethral meatus. If you are having problems visualizing the meatus, ask an assistant to retract the labia minora. In elderly women, the meatus is often more posterior than expected.

Relevant anatomy
- The male urethra is ~ 18cm in length with the prostatic urethra accounting for the proximal 3–4cm.
- The female urethra is only 3–4cm in length.

Indications
- Acute or chronic urinary retention.
- Monitoring of urine output.
- Inability to use a commode, bottle, or sheath.
- The bladder may form part of the contents of an incarcerated groin hernia and catheterization may facilitate reduction.

Contraindications (requires discussion with a urologist)
- Premature or traumatic removal of a catheter following recent radical prostatectomy (an absolute contraindication).
- Premature or traumatic removal of a catheter following recent trans-urethral surgery (a relative contraindication).
- Urethral trauma (📖 p.390).

Equipment
- Dressing/catheterization pack.
- Sterile gloves.
- Chlorhexidine or sterile normal saline.
- **Two** 2% lidocaine gel tubes (e.g. Instillagel®).
- Foley catheter: 14F routinely (most now have a 10mL syringe filled with **sterile water** to inflate the balloon as part of the pack). **Do not use normal saline to inflate the balloon as this may lead to inability to deflate it later**. Three-way catheters are much larger and require 30mL of water to inflate the balloon.
- Catheter bag (if an hourly urine output is needed use an appropriately calibrated bag).

Patient preparation
- Lying supine, with lower abdomen, external genitalia, and upper thighs exposed.
- Patients with mechanical heart valves, right-sided tissue heart valves, or recent orthopaedic prosthesis surgery should have one-off antibiotics (e.g. benzylpenicillin 1g IV and gentamicin 120mg IV).
- Patients who have had a traumatic catheterization should have a single shot of IV antibiotics (see above).

❶ Consider the need for prophylactic antibiotics in orthopaedic patients. Policies vary. However, as a rule of thumb, if the patient has had a joint replacement or large metallic implant (e.g. femoral intramedullary nail), insertion **and** removal of a urinary catheter should be covered with gentamicin 80mg. Give antibiotics 5min beforehand if administered IV; 30min if given IM.

Procedure

- Tear a small hole in the centre of the sterile drape and place around the penis. Use a gauze swab around the shaft of the penis to retract the foreskin and hold the penis while applying the antiseptic to the glans.
- Introduce all the gel into the urethra, keeping your dominant hand sterile.
- Straighten the penis, holding it vertically with the non-dominant hand, and introduce the catheter with the sterile hand. Introduce the catheter to the hilt. If it won't go up to the hilt, it's not in the bladder.
- **Only inflate the balloon after urine is seen**. Urine may take some time to flow through the catheter—it is usually blocked by the lidocaine gel. If this occurs, attach a bladder syringe to the catheter and flush with 20mL of sterile normal saline.
- Attach the catheter bag.
- **If the patient is not circumcised, replace the foreskin to prevent paraphimosis (📖 p.394)**.
- **Document the residual volume of urine**. This is important as urologists use it to predict whether the patient requires surgery.

Complications and problematic catheterization

Inability to pass the catheter beyond the prostatic urethra Ensure that the urethra is well-lubricated by using at least two tubes of lidocaine gel. **Gently** try a smaller 12F catheter. If this fails, **gently** try a larger catheter. If this fails and the patient is in acute urinary retention, a SPC is needed. In situations where the bladder is not distended, call a urologist.

Bleeding from the meatus Minor bleeding is occasionally seen, especially after difficult catheterizations. Ongoing bleeding, macroscopic haematuria, patient discomfort, or the appearance of bruising in the scrotum or perineum suggest significant trauma. Call a urologist.

Urethral stricture If you encounter firm resistance before 15cm or so of catheter has been passed, it is likely that the patient has a urethral stricture. Try a smaller 12F catheter. If this fails, SPC is required. In emergency situations where a SPC is not possible, an 8F or 10F catheter used for intermittent self-catheterization may be passed, but this cannot easily be secured within the bladder as there is no balloon.

Phimosis If the foreskin is too tight to allow catheterization then circumcision or dorsal slit of the foreskin is required. Call a urologist.

Penile oedema This often occurs in postoperative patients or those with fluid overload. Compression of the oedematous foreskin will force the fluid proximally, and allow gradual retraction to view the meatus. This may take some minutes, so be patient!

Meatal stenosis Requires dilatation under LA. Call a urologist.

Hypospadias The meatus is sited inferiorly, proximal to the tip of the penis, usually in the glans but sometimes subcoronal. Once located, introduce the catheter as normal.

Post-procedure bladder spasms These are due to either a blocked catheter (e.g. with blood clot) or too much fluid in the catheter balloon. Ensure that the urine is clear and running freely and consider deflating the balloon by 2–3mL.

Post-procedure care
- Document consent, sterile technique, catheter size and type inserted, volume of water used to inflate balloon, problems, complications, and residual volume.
- Inform the nurse how often urine output needs to be measured and recorded.

Suprapubic bladder catheterization****

This should only be performed when transurethral bladder catheterization is contraindicated or has been attempted and has failed.

Relevant anatomy In adults, the bladder is a pelvic organ until it contains > 300mL of urine, when it appears above the pelvic brim and enters the abdomen.

Indication Acute urinary retention when urethral catheterization fails.

Contraindications
- Presenting history of frank haematuria or past history of bladder cancer (causes tumour seeding).
- Laparotomy scars nearby (risk of bowel adhesions).
- Pregnancy.
- Abnormal coagulation is a relative contraindication.

❶ Beware the anuric/oliguric patient with an abdominal or pelvic mass (e.g. common iliac artery aneurysm). If there is clinical doubt, discuss with your senior or a urologist.

Equipment
- Dressing pack.
- Skin preparation fluid (e.g. povidone–iodine, chlorhexidine).
- Sterile gloves.
- 10mL of 1% lidocaine.
- 10mL syringe with orange (25G) and green (21G) needles.
- 12F (at least) SPC kit. **Do not** be tempted to use a Bonanno catheter—it will block rapidly and significantly complicate further management.
- Catheter bag.

Patient preparation
- Confirm that the patient is in urinary retention by palpating and percussing out the bladder. A bladder USS is advisable if the bladder is not readily palpable.
- Most patients find the procedure painful, not because of the incision, but because you are pressing down on an already distended bladder.
- A nurse should be present throughout to reassure the patient.
- The patient should be lying supine, with the lower abdomen, external genitalia, and upper thighs exposed.

Procedure
- Prepare and drape the abdomen from the umbilicus to the pubis.
- Palpate the pubis and infiltrate lidocaine into the skin two fingers' breadth above the pubic symphysis in the midline. Infiltrate with successive needles down to the bladder, staying in the midline.
- Using the same syringe, aspirate urine. In obese patients this may not be possible. If you cannot aspirate urine, do not proceed—call a urologist.
- Remove the syringe and make a transverse incision in the skin about 5mm in length, centred on where the needle was inserted.

- Advance the trocar and sheath through the skin, angling slightly towards the pelvis. Hold the trocar and sheath with the forefinger about 2 inches from the tip, allowing you to control the depth of penetration. There will be two 'gives': the first the linea alba; the second the bladder wall.
- Urine will run up the groove in the trocar once you enter the bladder. Advance slightly, then remove the trocar, keeping the sheath in place.
- Put a finger over the end of the sheath to maintain the distended bladder, insert the catheter through the sheath, and immediately inflate the balloon.
- Attach the catheter to the catheter bag. Gently withdraw the sheath and peel away the tearaway plastic strip. Discard the sheath.
- Place a dressing with a split cut in it across the incision and around the catheter. If the skin edges are bleeding, a suture may be needed.

Complications
- Frank haematuria.
- Bowel injury.
- Major vascular injury (IVC, abdominal aorta, iliac vessels).

Post-procedure care
- Document consent, sterile technique, local anaesthetic dose, catheter size and type inserted, volume of water used to inflate balloon, complications, and residual volume.
- Inform the nurse how often the urine output needs to be measured and recorded.
- Review later to exclude peritonitis.

Skin suturing***

Relevant anatomy

❶ You must be aware of the important neurovascular structures in the location that you are suturing.

Indications

- Wound closure.
- Securing drains/tubes/catheters.

Contraindications

Any wound that is grossly contaminated should be left open. Traumatic wounds that are tetanus-prone or more than 6h old should also be left open.

Equipment

- Sutures can be absorbable or non-absorbable, synthetic or natural, braided or monofilament. Outside of theatre, most sutures used are non-absorbable synthetic monofilaments (e.g. nylon, polypropylene). **Do not** use absorbable sutures to secure drains/tubes.
- Suture sizes: 2 > 1 > 0 > 1/0 > 2/0 etc. Chest drains require 1 or 0; facial wounds may need 5/0.
- Suture pack (must include forceps, needle holders, scissors).
- Gauze swabs.
- Skin preparation fluid (e.g. povidone–iodine, chlorhexidine).
- LA, usually 5–10mL of 1% lidocaine depending on wound size. Lidocaine with adrenaline 1:200 000 can be used, but **never on appendages** (penis, ear, nose, finger, toe) or tissue flaps. Maximum plain lidocaine dose is 3mg/kg.

Patient preparation

- Check tetanus status and manage accordingly (📖 p.94).
- The patient may still feel some pulling or pressure sensations, but they should not feel sharp pain. If they do, use more LA.

Procedure

- Make sure that the lighting is optimal.
- Give appropriate LA, usually as a field block. Give half before scrubbing, and keep the other half on your sterile tray. This gives you time to scrub and prepare your instruments.
- Prep and drape the area to be worked on.
- Test that the lidocaine has worked. Give extra if necessary.
- Deep sutures to fat may be needed to de-tension the skin edges. Use absorbable sutures. Senior advice is valuable.
- Do **not** place deep sutures to control bleeding without good access, light, assistance, and anatomical knowledge. Get help if any of these are lacking.
- Skin sutures are commonly interrupted, using non-absorbable monofilament sutures. Instrument-tied knots are easier than hand ties to perform (Fig. 20.2).

- Dressings are a personal preference. If you're not sure, ask the nurse what they recommend. Oozing wounds can be dressed with pressure dressings, but the latter should not be a substitute for proper haemostasis.

Complications
- Infection. Tell the patient to seek help if they notice increasing redness, pain, or discharge of pus from the wound. Wound infection requires removal of sutures and wound washout and packing (📖 p.502).
- Bleeding.
- Wounds across joints may lead to joint stiffness.

Post-procedure care
- Most non-absorbable sutures can be removed after ~ 7 days. Wounds in the back, buttocks, and legs should be left for 10–14 days. Facial sutures can be removed within 5–6 days.
- Document LA dose and technique, and number and type of sutures used. A diagram is useful.
- Oral antibiotics are necessary for human or animal bites, intraoral lacerations, or lacerations over exposed joints or tendons. In general, adequate debridement and washout is more important than antibiotic use.
- Arrange for the district nurse or GP practice nurse to change the dressings within a day or two.

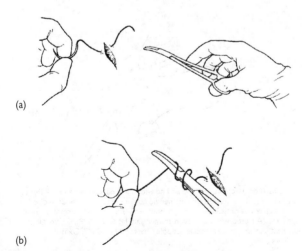

(a)

(b)

Fig. 20.2 An instrument tie. (a) After inserting the suture, pull through until just a short piece of suture is left. (b) Wrap the suture twice around the needle holder.

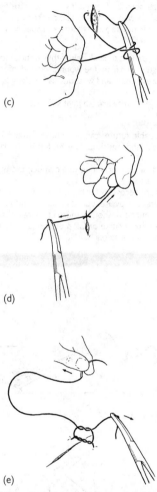

Fig. 20.2 (Cont.) (c) Grasp the loose end with the needle holder and pull through (d). (e) Wrap the suture around the needle holder once, in the opposite direction to the first throw, and again pull through. Another 2–3 throws are necessary to secure the knot. (Adapted, with permission, from Wyatt, J.P. et al. (1999). *Oxford handbook of accident and emergency medicine*, 1st edn, Chapter 9, pp. 426–7. Oxford University Press, Oxford.)

Rigid sigmoidoscopy ± flatus tube insertion***

Relevant anatomy

- The anus is 3–4cm long; the rectum is ~ 12cm long.
- The rectum follows the sacral curvature, turning posteriorly at the anorectal junction.
- Within the rectum there are sickle-shaped folds (the valves of Houston) that project into the lumen.

Indications

- Rigid sigmoidoscopy: investigation of PR bleeding, tenesmus, palpable mass, or to obtain rectal biopsies.
- Flatus tube insertion: decompression of a sigmoid volvulus.

Relative contraindications

- Recent anorectal surgery.
- Previous pouch procedures.

Equipment

- Disposable rigid sigmoidoscope tube and obturator.
- Rigid sigmoidoscope handle with light source, bellows, and tubing.
- Lubricant jelly, non-sterile gloves, absorbable pads, apron.
- Flatus tube (24–30 F), urinary catheter bag, connector, adhesive tape. **Check that the flatus tube fits completely through the lumen of the sigmoidoscope.**

Patient preparation

- The procedure can be uncomfortable for the patient, but should not be painful. Air insufflation will lead to a feeling a rectal fullness, and they may pass flatus during the examination.
- A nurse is necessary to chaperone and assist in positioning and reassuring the patient.
- Correct patient positioning is **vital**. (Fig. 20.3). Absorbable pads should be under their bottom and on the floor directly beneath.

Procedure

- Perform a DRE first.
- Assemble the rigid sigmoidoscope and check that the light is on.
- Lubricate the sigmoidoscope liberally.
- Holding the right buttock up with your left hand, and the sigmoidoscope in your right hand (with your right thumb pushing the obturator in), gently introduce the tip of the obturator and sigmoidoscope into the anus pointing slightly anteriorly (aiming towards the umbilicus).
- Once the sigmoidoscope tube is 2–3cm inside the anus, hold the handle in your left hand, and remove the obturator. Beware of flatus/faeces! Close the eye-piece and screw shut. Inflate the rectum using the bellows.
- Swing the sigmoidoscope posteriorly to follow the sacral curvature and locate the rectal lumen. Once the lumen is identified, advance the sigmoidoscope, inflating as needed. Getting 'around' the valves of Houston can be difficult. If the lumen is seen, keep on advancing as

much as patient comfort allows. **Never** advance blindly or if the patient complains of significant discomfort.

- Recto-sigmoid anatomy is variable: in some patients 20cm from the anal verge can be reached, in most 13–16cm is achievable. On withdrawal, ensure that all parts of the rectal wall are examined.
- If a flatus tube is to be inserted, insert the sigmoidoscope as far as possible, open the eye piece and insert the tube gently. Use the obturator to advance it while withdrawing the sigmoidoscope. Don't insert all the way into the anus, but grasp the flatus tube once the sigmoidoscope exits the anus. **Gently** advance the tube up to the hilt. **If significant resistance is met, stop. Stand back, as volvulus decompression can be 'explosive'.** Attach the catheter tubing and bag to collect flatus/faeces. Alternatively, place the end of the tube in a bucket underwater. Secure the tube to the buttocks with tape.

Complications

- Bowel perforation.
- ❶ Bleeding or post-procedure abdominal/pelvic pain is abnormal.
- Flatus tube blockage.

Post-procedure care

- Rigid sigmoidoscopy: document consent and findings.
- Flatus tube insertion: request an AXR to check decompression of the volvulus and flatus tube placement. Document consent, sigmoidoscopy findings, tube size, and AXR findings.

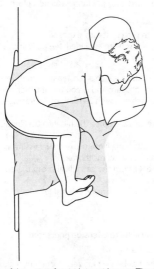

Fig. 20.3 Positioning of the patient for rigid sigmoidoscopy. The patient should be lying in the left lateral position, with their head on a pillow and their buttocks over the edge of the bed. The hips should be fully flexed with the knees partially flexed.

Needle thoracic decompression***

This is a temporizing measure for treatment of a tension pneumothorax, and is to be to be used in an emergency only. The tension pneumothorax will slowly recur unless an intercostal chest drain (ICD) is sited (📖 p.522).

Relevant anatomy
- The manubriosternal angle lies opposite the 2nd costal cartilage and rib; just below that is the 2nd intercostal space (ICS).
- The intercostal vessels and nerves run just inferior to each rib (Fig. 20.4).

Indications **Emergency** decompression of a suspected tension pneumothorax in a rapidly deteriorating patient.

Contraindications None.

Equipment
- Orange (14G) cannula.
- Adhesive dressing.

If time permits:
- Dressing pack.
- Sterile gloves.
- 10mL of 1% lidocaine.
- 10mL syringe with a green (21G) needle.
- Skin preparation fluid (e.g. povidone–iodine, chlorhexidine).

Patient preparation
- Lying supine, with the chest fully exposed.
- If a C-spine injury has been excluded, the patient can be sat upright.

Procedure
- ❶ Confirm the side in which a tension pneumothorax is suspected.
- **If time permits**, prepare and drape the anterior chest wall beneath the clavicle and infiltrate with 5–10mL of 1% lidocaine using a green needle.
- Insert an orange cannula up to the hilt into the 2nd ICS in the midclavicular line.
- Unscrew the plastic bung from the needle. Hissing air confirms the presence of a tension pneumothorax.
- Remove the needle from the cannula and cap the end off. Leave the cannula in place.
- Prepare to insert an ICD on the same side.

Complications
- Local bleeding.
- Lung laceration leading to a tension pneumothorax.

Post-procedure care
- Once the patient has been stabilized, document technique and findings.
- ❶ The procedure aims to temporarily relieve a tension pneumothorax. The tension pneumothorax can recur. An ICD with an underwater seal is

essential, therefore. If signs of a tension pneumothorax arise before an ICD is inserted, uncap the cannula or perform repeat needle thoracic decompression.

- ❶ If your presumptive diagnosis was incorrect, insertion of the needle and uncapping will cause a pneumothorax and an underlying lung laceration can cause a tension pneumothorax. Therefore, an ICD should be inserted even if a tension pneumothorax was not found!

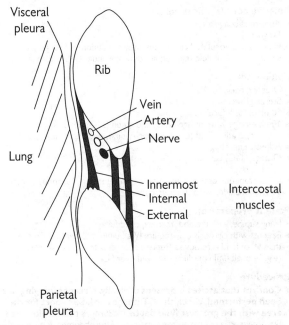

Fig. 20.4 Anatomy of the thoracic wall. (Adapted, with permission, from McLatchie, G.R. *et al.* (2007). *Oxford handbook of clinical surgery*, 3rd edn, Chapter 4, Fig. 4.4. Oxford University Press, Oxford.)

Peritoneal drainage (paracentesis)***

Relevant anatomy The inferior epigastric arteries arise from the external iliac arteries just medial to the deep inguinal ring and run supero-medially to enter the rectus sheath inferior to the umbilicus.

Indications

- Diagnostic aspiration of peritoneal fluid.
- Therapeutic drainage of symptomatic ascites.

Relative contraindications

- Abnormal coagulation.
- Pregnancy.
- Patients with loculated collections, previous abdominal surgery, or small volumes of fluid may require drainage under USS-guidance.

Equipment

- Dressing pack.
- Sterile gloves.
- 10mL of 1% lidocaine.
- 10mL syringe with orange (25G) and green (21G) needles.
- Skin preparation fluid (e.g. povidone–iodine, chlorhexidine).
- Adhesive dressing.
- Orange (14G) cannula.
- 20mL syringe.
- For therapeutic drainage, use a pigtail catheter (e.g. Bonanno), number 11 scalpel blade, and a drainage bag.

Patient preparation

- Lying supine, with the abdomen exposed fully.
- Patients with cirrhosis may require IV albumin replacement if more than 5L of fluid is removed. Replace according to local protocols (e.g. 5g of albumin per litre removed over 5L).

Procedure

- **Confirm that ascites is present clinically. If recent imaging has been performed, check the CT images or USS report for the area with the greatest fluid depth**. McBurney's point is often used. Do not insert a needle on the same side of the abdomen as a surgical scar as you risk perforation of underlying bowel adherent to the anterior abdominal wall.
- Prepare and drape the area.
- Infiltrate the skin and fat with 1–2mL of 1% lidocaine using an orange needle.
- Withdraw and change the orange for a green needle. Advance through the anterior abdominal wall injecting a further 2–3mL of lidocaine and aspirating as the needle is you go. A flash of ascitic fluid indicates entry into the peritoneal cavity.
- Withdraw the syringe, aspirating as you go until no further ascitic fluid is aspirated. Infiltrate the remainder of the lidocaine (~ 5mL) and remove the needle.

Diagnostic tap

- Insert an orange (14G) cannula attached to a 10mL syringe. Aspirate as you go and, once the flash of ascitic fluid is detected, advance the cannula and remove the stylet.
- Take 30–40mL of ascitic fluid for analysis (microscopy and culture, Gram stain, cytology, albumin, total protein, amylase).
- Remove the needle and cover the puncture with a small adhesive dressing.
- Take a blood sample for serum total protein and albumin.

Bonanno catheter insertion

- Assemble the catheter with the stylet inserted fully inside the catheter and a 5mL syringe on the end. Clamp the adaptor.
- Make a small stab incision with an number 11 scalpel blade.
- Insert slowly, aspirating with the syringe and supporting the catheter near the entry point with your non-dominant hand.
- Once ascites is aspirated, advance the catheter up to the hilt while simultaneously withdrawing the stylet. **Do not re-insert the stylet inside the catheter as this may damage the catheter**. Cover the end with your thumb and quickly connect the adaptor.
- Attach the adaptor to a drainage bag and unclamp. Ascites should flow freely.
- Inject lidocaine in the skin around the hilt and suture in place.

Complications

- Peritonitis due to perforated bowel.
- Bleeding.
- Hypotension due to fluid shifts.

Post-procedure care

- Document consent, local anaesthetic dose, technique, and findings. Send fluid to the laboratory for analysis if a diagnostic tap was performed.
- Alert the nurses to the possibility of peritonitis. Request that they call you immediately if the patient complains of abdominal pain. Monitor for hypotension and treat with colloids and/or albumin.
- There is no consensus on the maximum volume or rate of therapeutic ascitic drainage. Follow local protocols.

Pleural drainage/aspiration***

Relevant anatomy The intercostal vessels and nerves run just inferior to each rib (Fig. 20.4).

Indications

- Diagnostic aspiration of pleural fluid.
- Therapeutic drainage of a symptomatic pleural effusion.
- Aspiration of a small spontaneous pneumothorax—a large or traumatic pneumothorax requires insertion of an ICD (📖 p.522).

Relative contraindications

- Abnormal coagulation.
- Patients with loculated effusions, underlying bullous disease, or small effusions may require drainage under USS-guidance.

Equipment

- Dressing pack.
- 10mL of 1% lidocaine.
- 10mL syringe with orange (25G) and green (21G) needles.
- Skin preparation fluid (e.g. povidone–iodine, chlorhexidine).
- Adhesive dressing.
- Orange (14G) cannula.
- Three-way tap and 50mL syringe.
- Connector tubing and a sterile container to collect the pleural fluid.

Patient preparation The patient needs to be undressed to the waist, seated on the edge of a bed. Ask them to lean with arms forward on to a pillow placed on a bedside table at chest height.

Procedure

- **Confirm the correct side of the pathology by checking the CXR.**
- Examine the patient and percuss and mark the level of the effusion.
- For fluid aspiration, the point of entry should be over the posterior chest wall, lateral to the paraspinal muscles and inferior to the tip of the scapula. For pneumothorax aspiration, the needle should be inserted in the anterior chest in the 2nd ICS, midclavicular line.
- Prepare and drape the area.
- Infiltrate the skin and subcutaneous tissues with 1–2mL of 1% lidocaine at the point of entry low in the intercostal space.
- Advance the needle through the intercostal muscles into the pleural space, injecting a further 1–2mL of lidocaine and aspirating as the needle is advanced. A flash of pleural fluid (or air with a pneumothorax) with release of tension on the syringe indicates entry into the pleural space.
- Withdraw the syringe, aspirating as you go until no further pleural fluid or air is aspirated. Deliver the remainder of the lidocaine (~ 5mL) and remove the needle.
- Once the lidocaine has taken effect, ask the patient to inhale fully and then exhale slowly (say 'Eeeeeee') while an orange (14G) cannula attached to a 10mL syringe is introduced into the pleural space via the

same puncture site. Aspirate as you insert. Once the flash of pleural fluid or air is detected, advance the cannula, remove the needle and syringe. Remove a sample of fluid and send for cytology, microscopy, culture, protein, LDH, amylase, pH, and glucose.

- Attach a three-way tap. Connect the tubing leading to a container if necessary. It is important that the patient continues to exhale whilst the three-way tap is attached to minimize the risk of a pneumothorax.
- Attach a 50mL syringe to the three-way tap to aspirate the pleural fluid or air. Continue aspirating until resistance is met. Stop if the patient feels significant discomfort or coughing.
- Remove the cannula and place a small adhesive dressing.

Complications

- Pneumothorax, usually simple. Tension pneumothorax can occur but is rare.
- Bleeding from an intercostal vessel.
- Empyema (rare).

Post-procedure care

- Request a CXR, and look for:
  - amount of fluid remaining (an increase in the volume suggests an iatrogenic haemothorax);
  - presence/size of pneumothorax (may be manifest by loss of the pleural fluid meniscus);
  - lung re-expansion.
- Document consent, local anaesthetic dose, technique, and findings.
- Alert the nurses to the possibility of tension pneumothorax. Request that they call you immediately if the patient complains of SOB or chest pain.

Intercostal chest drain insertion****

The purpose of an intercostal chest drain (ICD) is to eliminate air or fluid from the pleural space. Small fluid or air collections can be drained with fine-bore catheters inserted using a Seldinger technique, but this is inappropriate in the trauma setting.

Relevant anatomy

- To ensure correct placement, count the ICSs. The manubriosternal angle lies opposite the 2nd costal cartilage and rib; just below that is the 2nd ICS.
- The intercostal vessels and nerves run just inferior to each rib (Fig. 20.4).
- ICDs should be inserted within the 'quadrangle of safety', bounded by the posterior axillary line, the anterior axillary line, and the 3rd to 5th ICSs. The usual site of insertion is the 5th ICS, just anterior to the midaxillary line.

Indications

- Traumatic pneumothorax.
- Moderate/large spontaneous pneumothorax.
- Tension pneumothorax after needle decompression.
- Symptomatic pleural effusions and other large pleural collections, e.g. empyema, gastric/oesophageal contents.
- Haemothorax (traumatic or spontaneous).

Relative contraindications

- Coagulation abnormalities.
- Suspected pleural adhesions.

Equipment

- Dressing pack and ICD instrument pack.
- 10–20mL of 1% lidocaine (maximum dose 3mg/kg). **The doses in this section are for a 70kg adult.**
- 10mL syringe, orange (25G) and green (21G) needles.
- Skin preparation fluid (e.g. povidone–iodine, chlorhexidine).
- Sterile gloves.
- Chest drain: standard sizes range from 28F to 32F, but in small patients a narrower tube may be needed.
- Underwater seal collection system with tubing, filled with sterile water.
  - ❶ The cap on the system must be open to room air.
- Heavy suture (1 or 0 gauge).
- Gauze swabs and adhesive dressings (e.g. Mefix®).

Patient preparation

- This procedure can be painful, although adequate LA infiltration will minimize this. Consider whether IV analgesia is necessary.
- The patient should be lying supine, undressed to the waist, with the shoulder abducted to 90°. The hand may be placed behind the head. The procedure may also be performed with the patient lying at 45°.
- A nurse should be present throughout to reassure the patient.
- Absorbent pads under the patient prevent soiling of the clothes or bed.

Procedure

- **In non-emergency settings, confirm the correct side of the pathology by checking the CXR again**.
- Prepare and drape the patient widely.
- Infiltrate the site of the planned incision with lidocaine (~ 5mL).
- Make a 1.5–2cm skin incision within the quadrangle of safety.
- Insert a single suture just posterior to the incision and tie down to the skin leaving both ends long. This will anchor the drain.
- Insert a mattress suture through the incision. This will act as a 'purse string' suture to close the incision when the drain is removed.
- Infiltrate further lidocaine (~ 10mL) into the targeted ICS and the ICS above and below to create a field block
- Blunt dissect with heavy artery forceps (e.g. Roberts) through the ICS. If significant pain is felt by the patient, use a further 5mL of lidocaine. Dissection should start at the lower margin of the ICS to avoid the neurovascular bundle.
- Continue blunt dissection through the parietal pleura when a gush of air or blood occurs.
- Open the Roberts fully to dilate the puncture site, and then insert the index finger to dilate the track. This is important as the track can be difficult to find again.
- Sweep your index finger inside the pleural cavity to detect any adherent lung tissue and exclude false passages and entry into the abdomen.
- Remove the trocar from the drain and **discard it**.
- Grasp the tip of the drain with a Roberts forceps and introduce it into the pleural space, aiming for the pleural apex (for drainage of air) or the base (for drainage of fluid). Ensure that all drainage holes are well inside the pleural space. The drain should be clamped.
- Once the drain is sited, attach it to the underwater seal via tubing **and unclamp it**. Entry into the pleural cavity is suggested by fogging of the tube, a respiratory swing, and bubbling of the fluid level on coughing. Cover the join between the two tubes with heavy tape.
- Fix the drain in position with the previously placed anchoring suture. Further sutures may be needed to close the incision.
- Dress with gauze swabs and cover with strong adhesive dressings.

Complications

- Major complications such as intraabdominal placement, diaphragmatic laceration, hepatic laceration, intracardiac penetration, lung and major vessel perforation are rare if the procedure is performed appropriately. Prolonged placement increases the risk of empyema.
- Minor haemorrhage can occur from bleeding intercostal vessels.

Post-procedure care

- Obtain a CXR to check that:
  - the drain is in the correct position and within the thoracic cavity;
  - the lung has re-expanded;
  - complications have not occurred.
- Check the patient to exclude complications and check that the drain is still swinging/bubbling. How much fluid has drained?
- Inform the nurse how often drain output should be measured.

- Document consent, LA dose, technique, drain size, fluid drained, and CXR findings.
- **❶ Tell the patient and remind the nurse that the underwater seal drain should NEVER be raised above the level of the chest**.
- Chest drain removal is usually performed by doctors.
  - Remove the dressings around the drain.
  - If a mattress suture is not already present for closing the wound, insert one now under LA, and leave it untied.
  - Cut the sutures anchoring the drain to the skin and ask an assistant to hold the drain securely until you are ready to remove it.
  - Ask the patient to take a deep breath in and then to breathe out **slowly** through pursed lips. Practise this a few times to make sure that the patient understands fully what is expected of them.
  - As the patient is breathing out, remove the drain fully and tie the mattress suture, closing the wound securely.
  - Place a dressing over the wound.
  - Request an urgent CXR to check that a pneumothorax has not occurred during ICD removal.

Venous cutdown****

Patients with severe shock may require surgical access to a peripheral vein if superficial venous cannulation has failed. This is most commonly achieved via the LSV at the ankle because of its constant anatomy and the absence of significant nearby neurovascular structures.

Relevant anatomy
- The LSV runs 1cm anterior to the anterior border of the medial malleolus.
- The saphenous nerve runs close to the LSV and may be adherent to it.

Indication
Emergency venous access.

Relative contraindications
- Proximal long bone or pelvic fractures.
- Proximal LSV injury.
- Ipsilateral varicose vein surgery or LSV harvesting (e.g. CABG, vascular surgery).

Equipment
- Venous cutdown instrument set.
- Scalpel with number 10 or 15 blade.
- Dressing pack.
- Skin preparation fluid (e.g. povidone–iodine, chlorhexidine).
- Sterile drapes and gloves.
- Large-bore venous cannula, e.g. orange (14G) or grey (16G).
- 5–10mL of 1% lidocaine and a 5mL syringe.
- Orange (25G) and blue (22G) needles.
- Absorbable and non-absorbable sutures (e.g. 3/0 polyglactin and 3/0 polypropylene, respectively).
- 10mL sterile normal saline for flush.
- Dressing.

Patient preparation
The patient should be supine, with the legs slightly abducted and externally rotated.

Procedure
- Put on sterile gloves.
- Widely prep and then drape the skin over the medial malleolus, proximal foot, and distal leg.
- If the patient is conscious, infiltrate 5mL of 1% lidocaine into the skin just anterior to the anterior border of the medial malleolus using an orange and then a blue needle.
- Make a 2–3cm long transverse incision through the skin with a scalpel, centred a finger's breadth anterior to the anterior border of the medial malleolus.
- Ask an assistant to retract the skin edges, and use scissors to dissect through the subcutaneous fat to find the LSV. This may be deeper than you expect.

- Dissect out a 3–4cm length of vein. You may need to lengthen your incision to ensure good access.
- Tie the vein distally with an absorbable suture. Using the same suture material, sling the proximal vein and retract on it, delivering it out of the wound.
- Make a small incision transversely in the vein between the two sutures, without dividing the vein completely.
- Insert the IV cannula through the venotomy into the LSV lumen. You may need to widen the venotomy or retract on its edges. Relax on the sling, allowing the cannula to pass proximally.
- Once the cannula is within the vein, tie it in place with the proximal sling.
- Close the skin wound around the cannula with non-absorbable sutures, connect to IV fluids, and place a dressing over the wound.
- Secure the cannula by inserting a non-absorbable suture through the skin and around the cannula.

Complications
- Cannula displacement.
- Skin infection.
- Thrombophlebitis.
- Saphenous nerve damage.

Post-procedure care
- Document indications, consent, LA dose used, sterile technique, type of cannula used, and any difficulties experienced in the notes.
- Once the patient's haemodynamic state is stabilized, more secure IV access should be inserted and the LSV cannula removed.

Central venous catheterization****

Large-bore catheters can be inserted into internal jugular vein (IJV), sub-clavian vein (SV), or femoral vein (FV). There are many different techniques for cannulation of these veins; only one is given for each below.

Relevant anatomy

- IJV: runs deep to the apex of the sternal and clavicular heads of the sternocleidomastoid muscle, with the common carotid artery medial and slightly posterior. The right IJV is cannulated most commonly in order to avoid the thoracic duct and the tortuous route to the heart followed by the left IJV.
- SV: lies anterior to the subclavian artery as they both arch over the thoracic inlet, posteriorly and then inferiorly to the clavicle. Either SV can be used.
- FV: lies just medial to the femoral artery, which itself lies medial to the femoral nerve. Either FV can be used, but the right is preferable.
  - The femoral artery emerges from under the inguinal ligament at the mid-inguinal point (halfway between the pubic symphysis and the anterior superior iliac spine).

Indications

- Central venous pressure monitoring or access for cardiac pacing (IJV and SV only).
- Administration of drugs not able to be given peripherally.
- Poor peripheral venous access.
- Administration of TPN.
- Large-bore single lumen catheters can be inserted into the femoral vein for fluid resuscitation.
- Haemodialysis or haemofiltration.

Contraindications

- Abnormal coagulation.
- Overlying skin infection.
- Arterial aneurysms nearby.
- Venous thrombosis.
- Avoid subclavian vein cannulation if apical bullae are present (risk of pneumothorax) or in patients with renal failure (subsequent stenoses can compromise future arteriovenous access).

Equipment

- Central venous catheter kit.
- Skin preparation fluid (e.g. povidone–iodine, chlorhexidine).
- Sterile drapes, gloves, and gown.
- 5–10mL of 1% lidocaine.
- Orange (25G) and green (21G) needles.
- Suture (e.g. 2/0 polypropylene).
- 10mL sterile normal saline for flush.
- Dressing.
- USS devices are increasingly being used to locate the IJV: its use is recommended in elective placements and in those with previous cannulations.

Patient preparation

- IJV and SV. Patients should be head down 15° to distend the veins and reduce the risk of air embolism.
  - The head should be turned away from the side of puncture.
  - Cardiac monitoring may be useful to detect ectopic beats.
- FV: supine, with hips slightly abducted and externally rotated.

Procedure

- Put on a sterile gown and gloves.
- Widely prep and then drape the appropriate area.
- **Check all equipment beforehand and ensure that the introducer needle, guidewire, dilator, and central venous line are not damaged and all run smoothly**.
- Flush all lumens of the central venous line with sterile normal saline and clamp and recap (**except for the port to the central lumen). If you forget to take off the cap over the central port you will push the guidewire inside the patient!**
- Infiltrate 1–2mL of 1% lidocaine in the skin and subcutaneous tissues around the target area using an orange needle.
- Insert a green 'seeker' needle on a 5mL syringe and advance, aspirating gently to locate the vein.
- IJV. Insert the needle at the apex of the two heads of sternocleidomastoid, with the needle at 45° to the skin, pointing towards the ipsilateral nipple (Fig. 20.5). The common carotid pulse will lie medially, but palpation of this during needle insertion may collapse the IJV and result in arterial puncture.

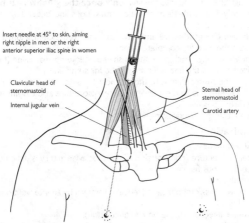

Internal jugular central line insertion

Insert needle at 45° to skin, aiming right nipple in men or the right anterior superior iliac spine in women

Clavicular head of sternomastoid

Internal jugular vein

Sternal head of sternomastoid

Carotid artery

Fig. 20.5 Anatomy of a right IJV cannulation. (Reproduced, with permission, from Myerson, S.G. et al. (2005). *Emergencies in cardiology*, Chapter 19, p. 291. Oxford University Press, Oxford.)

- SV. Insert the needle 1 cm inferior to the clavicle at the junction between the medial 1/3rd and lateral 2/3rd of the clavicle, aiming towards the suprasternal notch, with the needle 45° to the skin (Fig. 20.6)
- FV. Insert the needle a finger's breadth medial to the femoral artery pulsation, 2–3cm inferior to the inguinal ligament with the needle 45° to the skin and aiming towards the xiphisternum (Fig. 20.7). Feel the femoral artery pulse laterally.
- Once the vein is found (free aspiration of venous blood) remove the green needle, remembering where the vein was found.
- Using the larger introducer needle and syringe, insert and find the vein again. If you're unsure if the blood is venous or arterial, check for pulsations and pressure and send for blood gas analysis.
- Remove the syringe, cover the needle hub with your left thumb to stop bleeding, and insert the guidewire (J-tip first!). This should go in easily. Remove if resistance is met. Insert enough of the wire so that it is definitely beyond the introducer needle tip. Watch for cardiac dysrhythmias.
- **Holding the guidewire steady**, remove the introducer needle.
- Using the scalpel, make a 2–3mm incision in the skin around the guidewire. **Do not let go of the guidewire**.
- **Holding the guidewire**, slide the dilator down the guidewire, and insert just enough to dilate the subcutaneous structures and underlying vein. Dilate in the line of the wire; otherwise the wire can become kinked.
- **Holding the guidewire**, remove the dilator and have a gauze swab ready to place over the entry point to control bleeding.
- **Holding the guidewire**, slide the central venous line down, retrieving the guidewire as it emerges through the central port. Insert the line through the skin and into the vein **only once the guidewire is held securely**. Insert 10–15cm of the central venous line, depending on vein site and size of patient.
- **Remove the guidewire** and recap the port to the central lumen. Inspect the wire for complete removal.
- Aspirate through each port and flush with sterile normal saline (heparinized saline if the line will not be used for some time).
- Attach the suture clamps to the line near the skin entry point, infiltrate with 1% lidocaine, and suture into place. Also suture at the point where the three lines diverge.
- Place a transparent dressing.

Complications
For all techniques
- Arterial puncture (compression of the subclavian artery is difficult).
- Arteriovenous fistula.
- Air embolism.
- Guidewire loss/embolization (requires removal by an interventional radiologist).
- Catheter infection (higher in FV cannulation).
- Venous thrombosis.

Right subclavian vein central line insertion

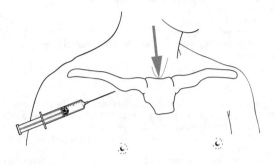

Fig. 20.6 Anatomy of a right SV cannulation. (Adapted, with permission, from Myerson, S.G. et al. (2005). *Emergencies in cardiology*, Chapter 19, p. 292. Oxford University Press, Oxford.)

Right femoral vein anatomy

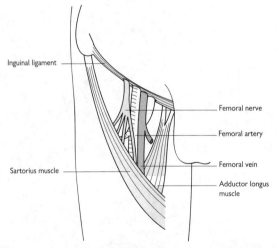

Fig. 20.7 Anatomy of a right FV cannulation. (Reproduced, with permission, from Myerson, S.G. et al. (2005). *Emergencies in cardiology*, Chapter 19, p. 293. Oxford University Press, Oxford.)

IJV and SV
- Pneumothorax (simple or tension); higher in SV.
- Haemothorax.
- Cardiac dysrhythmias.
- Cardiac tamponade.
- Nerve damage (e.g. vagus, sympathetic chain, brachial plexus).
- Chylothorax.

FV Retroperitoneal haemorrhage.

Post-procedure care

- Request a CXR (for SV and IJV catheters) and AXR (for FV catheters) to check placement and exclude complications. For IJV and SV lines the tip should be at the junction of the superior vena cava and right atrium. Withdraw the tip, re-suture, and re-X-ray if it is too far distal (risk of dysrhythmias).
- Document indications, consent, LA dose used, sterile technique, type of catheter used and site, any difficulties, and X-ray findings in the notes.
- Alert nurses to potential complications and when to call you.

Pericardiocentesis*****

This is a temporizing measure for the treatment of cardiac tamponade, to be used in a life-threatening emergency only. Although this is a potentially life-saving procedure it is associated with significant risks. Cardiac tamponade (□ p.474) can recur unless definitive surgical repair is carried out.

Relevant anatomy The pericardial sac sits on the apex of the dome of the diaphragm with the pericardial space separating the sac from the myocardium.

Indication Emergency decompression of a suspected cardiac tamponade in a rapidly deteriorating patient.

Contraindications None.

Equipment
- 14–18G IV catheter, 140mm length.
  - ❶ These cannulae are **much longer** than usual. They should be available on the resuscitation trolley, or from a central venous line pack.
- 20mL syringe.
- Adhesive dressing.

If time permits:
- dressing pack;
- sterile gloves;
- 5mL of 1% lidocaine;
- 10mL syringe with a green (21G) needle;
- skin preparation fluid (e.g. povidone–iodine, chlorhexidine);
- ultrasound guidance, if available, can be invaluable.

Patient preparation
Lying supine, with the chest fully exposed.

❶ The patient's continuous ECG trace must be visible to the person performing pericardiocentesis throughout the procedure.

Procedure
- **If time permits**, prepare and drape the epigastrium and lower sternum and infiltrate with 5mL of 1% lidocaine using a green needle.
- Insert the long IV catheter and syringe 1–2cm below and to the left of the junction between the xiphisternum and the costal margin at 45° to the skin. Aim for the tip of the left scapula (inferior angle) and advance the needle, while aspirating gently on the syringe (Fig. 20.8).
- When the needle enters the blood-filled pericardial sac, blood will be aspirated. Aspirate as much as possible. As little as 20mL of blood removed may improve the cardiac output.
- If the needle tip touches the myocardium, ECG changes will be observed (the 'current of injury'). These changes may include premature ventricular contractions, ST or T wave changes, or altered QRS complexes. Withdraw slightly if this occurs.
- Advance the catheter and withdraw the needle. Cap off the end of the catheter and secure it in place with a dressing.

Complications

- Entry into the peritoneum with subsequent hollow organ damage and peritonitis.
- Pneumothorax or haemothorax.
- Laceration of the myocardium, including damage to a coronary artery or vein (this may lead to subsequent cardiac tamponade or myocardial ischaemia).
- Dysrhythmias, including ventricular fibrillation.
- Entry into the ventricle or atria and aspiration of intracardiac blood.
- Damage to other thoracic structures, e.g. great vessels, oesophagus, thoracic duct.

Post-procedure care

- Once the patient has stabilized, document indications, technique, findings, and outcome.

❶ This procedure aims to temporarily relieve a cardiac tamponade. Ongoing bleeding into the pericardial cavity will again result in deterioration of the patient. **Aspirate further blood as required**. The patient requires definitive surgical repair of the underlying injuries and **immediate** discussion with the regional cardiothoracic service is essential.

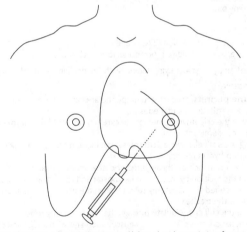

Fig. 20.8 Technique of pericardiocentesis. (Adapted, with permission, from McLatchie, G.R. et al. (2007). *Oxford handbook of clinical surgery*, 3rd edn, Chapter 4, Fig. 4.5. Oxford University Press, Oxford.)

Cricothyroidotomy*****

This should only be performed in an emergency when there is airway obstruction and less invasive techniques have failed to secure the airway. Although this is a potentially life-saving procedure it is associated with significant risks. Jet insufflation (🕮 p.48) may be used as a temporizing measure while the equipment is being set up.

Relevant anatomy The cricothyroid membrane lies between the cricoid and thyroid cartilages (Fig. 20.9).

Indication Failed orotracheal or nasotracheal intubation when a definitive airway is required.

Relative contraindication Avoid in children < 12 years old, as the cricoid is the only circumferential support to the upper trachea.

Equipment
- Scalpel with number 10 or 15 blade.
- Haemostat.
- Cuffed tracheostomy tube, usually size 5 or 6.
- 10mL syringe.
- Gauze tape.

If time permits:
- dressing pack;
- sterile gloves;
- 5mL of 1% lidocaine;
- 10mL syringe with a blue (22G) needle;
- skin preparation fluid (e.g. povidone–iodine, chlorhexidine).

Patient preparation Lying supine, with the neck in a neutral position.

Procedure
- **If time permits**, prepare and drape the area and infiltrate 2–3mL of local anaesthetic subcutaneously.
- Identify the cricothyroid membrane carefully, and hold the larynx with your non-dominant hand.
- Using the scalpel, make a 1cm transverse incision through the skin over the cricothyroid membrane.
- Make a 0.5cm incision through the cricothyroid membrane.
- Open the incision by inserting a haemostat and spreading the jaws.
- Insert a cuffed tracheostomy tube through the hole in the membrane and into the trachea.
- Inflate the cuff and ventilate through the tracheostomy tube.
- Check for correct placement by auscultation and with a CO_2 indicator.
- Secure the tube with tape or sutures.

Complications
- False passage subcutaneously or into the oesophagus.
- Laceration of the trachea.
- Intubation of the right main bronchus.
- Bleeding and aspiration.

Post-procedure care
- Ensure the tube is safely secured.
- Request a CXR to check the tube positioning.
- Document the procedure in the notes.

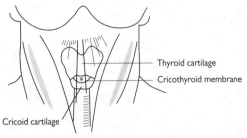

Fig. 20.9 Anatomy of the cricothyroid membrane (*).(Adapted, with permission, from Wyatt, J.P. et al. (1999). *Oxford handbook of accident and emergency medicine*, 1st edn, Chapter 8, p. 345. Oxford University Press, Oxford.)

Index